Dave, my dear friend and co

I am so grateful for all your tremendous support for these many years

A true friend, you're the best

Cheers

Daniel

A Humanistic Approach to Health Promotion

A Humanistic Approach to Health Promotion

By

David R. Buchanan

Cambridge Scholars Publishing

A Humanistic Approach to Health Promotion

By David R. Buchanan

This book first published 2020

Cambridge Scholars Publishing

Lady Stephenson Library, Newcastle upon Tyne, NE6 2PA, UK

British Library Cataloguing in Publication Data
A catalogue record for this book is available from the British Library

ISBN (10): 1-5275-5883-5
ISBN (13): 978-1-5275-5883-0

In loving memory,

Robert N. Bellah, 1927 – 2013,

an inspiration to all his students

Table of Contents

LIST OF CHARTS AND TABLES

ACKNOWLEDGEMENTS

One of the great pleasures of academic life is critical constructive dialogue with colleagues. I have benefited tremendously from the astute judicious feedback from many people who have challenged my thinking and pushed me to clarify the points that I am raising and their justification. This book is the product of a long and sustained conversation about the future of the field of health promotion.

I had the good fortune to spend three years at the National Cancer Institute mid-career on a fellowship focusing on public health ethics. There, I found the vocabulary for expressing my thinking in terms of ethical theories, where previously I had been operating within the social science framework and debates about qualitative versus quantitative research/ positivist versus interpretive or hermeneutic studies. I am deeply indebted to the many outstanding scholars that I had the opportunity to work with during my time there, collaborations that have continued to this day. At the NIH Department of Clinical Bioethics, I would particularly like to thank Franklin G. Miller, Dan Brock, Holly Taylor, Ezekiel Emanuel, Marion Danis and Christine Grady. At Georgetown's Kennedy Institute of Ethics, I benefited from the many stimulating dialogues with Tom Beauchamp, Robert Veatch, Maggie Little, Madison Powers, and Leroy Walters. At Johns Hopkins' Berman Institute of Bioethics, I am particularly grateful for the open door extended to me by Ruth Faden, Nancy Kass, Jeff Kahn and Jeremy Sugarman.

I have had a somewhat ambivalent relationship with the main professional organization representing the field of health promotion in the US, the Society for Public Health Education, as there was a strong push at the time I entered the field to put the profession on what was perceived to be more respectable, scientific grounds, rather than its earlier foundation in philosophies of education. Nonetheless, I want to thank John Allegrante, Ken McLeory, Bruce Simons-Morton and Patricia Goodson for the many provocative exchanges we have had over the years. Also in the field of health education but through more of a Berkeley connection, I have enjoyed the many collaborations with Meredith Minkler, Nina Wallerstein and Kathleen Roe. Also from Berkeley, I want to thank my mentor and inspiration, Dr. Robert Norton Bellah, for introducing me to another of his students, William Sullivan, who invited me to join a national task on the meaning of professionalism in America today.

At the University of Massachusetts, Amherst, I have benefited from working with George Cernada, Jane Zapka, and more recently, Louis Graham, Susan Shaw, Aline Gubrium, Donal Carbaugh, Michael Morgan and Dean Robinson. Over the last eight years, I have also been blessed by the friendship and camaraderie of the men involved with the Men of Color Health Awareness (MOCHA) movement, who have kept me grounded in the challenges of promoting social justice in America today. I would particularly like to thank Mr. Lamont Scott, Hank Douglas, Jr. and Al Hubert.

The author would like to thank the following publishers for permission to reuse material that originally appeared in their publications. From Oxford University Press, "Beyond Positivism: Humanistic Perspectives on Theory and Research in Health Education," *Health Education Research*, 13(3): 439-50, 1998; "Reflections on the Relationship between Theory and Practice," *Health Education Research*, 9(3): 273-283, 1994. "Social Marketing: A Critical Appraisal," *Health Promotion International*, 9(1): 49-57, 1994; and "Assuring adequate protections in international health research: A principled justification and practical recommendations for the role of community oversight," *Public Health Ethics* 1(3):246-257, 2008. From Sage Publications, "An Uneasy Alliance: Combining Qualitative and Quantitative Research Methods," *Health Education Quarterly*, 19(1): 117-135, 1992; "A New Ethic for Health Promotion: Reflections on a Philosophy of Health Education for a New Millennium," *Health Education & Behavior*, 33(3): 290-304, 2006; "The CEPA Project: A New Model for Community-Based Program Planning," *International Quarterly for Community Health Education*, 14(4):361-377, 1993-94, and "Promoting Dignity: The Ethical Dimension of Health. *International Quarterly of Community Health Education* 36(2): 99–104, 2016. From Elsevier, "Moral reasoning as a model for health promotion," *Social Science & Medicine*, 63(10): 2715-2726, 2006. From Johns Hopkins University Press, "Promoting justice and autonomy in public policies to reduce the health consequences of obesity," *Kennedy Institute of Ethics Journal* 25(4): 395-417, 2015; and, "Ethical Issues in Community Based Participatory Research: Balancing rigorous research with community participation. *Progress in Community Health Partnerships*, 2(1): 153-60, 2007. From the American Public Health Association, "Autonomy, Paternalism & Justice: Ethical priorities in public health," *American Journal of Public Health*, 98: 15-21, 2008. Finally, from Springer Publishing, "What types of Public Health Proposals Should Agencies Be Funding and What Types of Evidence Should Matter?

Scientific and Ethical Considerations," which originally appeared as Chapter 9 in Barbara Wallace (Ed.), *From Health Inequity to Equity in Health: A New Global Approach to Health Disparities*, 2007.

"God is real since he produces real effects."
—William James

PART I

1. WHY A HUMANISTIC APPROACH?

Many interesting and important questions about the human condition remain unresolved. Perhaps the most important is the question of free will, from which many other crucial questions derive. Can human beings make choices about how they want to live their lives? What is the basis for making choices about how one should live? Do human beings have the capacity to choose to act in accordance with moral principles and higher-order values? If so, where can we find these values?

For reasons explained in this book, because the rise of the empirical sciences has been so effective in enabling human control over the natural world, the prestige afforded modern science today has led most health researchers to assume that human nature is no different: human behavior can be analyzed and fully explained in terms of causal relationships. They assume that there is no such thing as free will; rather, behavior is the result of antecedent factors that cause the behavior in question (e.g., smoking, overeating, etc.). But, as we shall see, this is simply an unfounded assumption. We do not *know* this to be true.

In contrast, since ancient times, and now reflected in the worldwide division of the modern university into the sciences, social sciences and the humanities, a long tradition of scholars, intellectuals and philosophers has operated on the seemingly self-evident belief that people can and do make choices about what they want to do all the time. They believe that there is something palpably real about the experience of choice and that the ability to choose is the *sine-qua-non* of human morality. They believe that human conduct is motivated, at least in part, by the desire to do what is right and good. Perhaps not all the time but undeniably on occasion, people make choices on the basis of moral principles and values that matter. If this is the case, then the question becomes: how do we know–with reasonable assurance–what these values or principles are? Are love or justice, right and wrong, real? How do we know what they *truly* are? Where can they be found? Are they mere figments of our imagination, as empirical scientists who deny free will are wont to suggest? Although the scientific method has provided unprecedented knowledge about empirical cause-and-effect relationships found in the natural world, it cannot answer questions about the meaning and significance of human values, for reasons this book delves into in depth. Yet, without taking the capacity for choice into account, the field of health promotion is missing something hugely important to understanding why human beings act the way they do.

If we want to know why people sometimes engage in behaviors that harm their health, then we need to develop a more comprehensive understanding of human decision-making. In many respects, health promotion found its unique calling based on the fact that people frequently appear to act irrationally and take up self-destructive activities (such as smoking), and that making them aware of the dangers is insufficient to lead them to stop; hence, the field's *raison d'etre* has been seen to lie in the search for currently unknown mysterious underlying causes. This book shows that we cannot simply assume that behavior is caused by independent variables that inexorably drive human acts. We need to come to terms with the idea that people might choose to act against a superficially obvious interest in self-preservation, and decide to smoke, or eat too much, or get drunk, smoke pot, fail to wear condoms, avoid strenuous exertion, and on and on, for reasons that evidently take precedence over a putative desire to live longer (e.g., the desire for immediate pleasure) (Sullum, 1998; Metzl and Kirkland, 2010; Tavernise, 2014). Is there anything more important than individual gratification, anything that might provide a basis for making a different choice? We need the humanities to make sense of human conduct. We need the humanities to clarify moral principles and values that matter and so appreciate how they guide us in making choices that enable us to become the kind of person we long to become. It is only by incorporating this knowledge into the work of health promotion that the field can begin to move towards the goal of helping people to be healthy and flourish as human beings, with all of the distinctive capabilities unique to the human condition.

This chapter sets the stage for the essays that follow and presents a preliminary framework for health promotion that takes the possibility of free will fully into account. I cannot maintain that this assumption is any more certain than its rejection, but I am convinced that operating on the alternative humanistic assumption will make work in the field more perceptive and sympathetic, more consistent with lived experience and observation, and more in line with the professed goal of taking action to expand the sphere of justice in the world. It will also help to explain why efforts to control behavior have thus far failed to pan out. *A Humanistic Approach to Health Promotion* explains how a humanistic approach offers more worthwhile goals for the field and a more ethically robust means for achieving them.

The text starts with a brief history of health promotion and the evolution of the types of health problems driving the leading causes of morbidity and mortality. It then tracks these developments to the parallel rise of modern science. This background lays the foundation for understanding the current challenges facing the field posed by the central role of behaviors in contributing to premature sickness, disease and death today. To the extent that the reader accepts the argument that human behavior is categorically distinct from the cause-and-effect relationships that govern events in the natural world, then we will be in a better position to grapple with the complex questions of epistemology, ontology and ethics that must be addressed to bring health promotion in line with a more plausible and comprehensive account of human behavior. To anticipate, it will require us to examine the role of subjective consciousness in perceiving values and the role of language in bringing those values into human experience.

A Brief History of Health Promotion

The key point of this section is that the methods of research and practice in public health today have not kept pace with the changing nature of disease etiology. Due to a phenomenon referred to as the epidemiological transition, the leading causes of morbidity and mortality today are no longer led by infectious diseases but by chronic diseases, which are associated with behaviors such as smoking, obesity and physical inactivity. Thus, to achieve the goal of improving population health, the field needs to address the role of human behaviors in contributing to disease and death. But changing human behaviors poses categorically distinct challenges compared to efforts aimed at controlling the pathogens that cause infectious diseases. The field has yet to come to terms with this new challenge.

The respective proportions of infectious and chronic diseases present in the world today are summarized in the table below produced by the World Health Organization (WHO, 2008; see Table 1.1). For definitional purposes, **infectious diseases** are caused by pathogenic microorganisms, such as bacteria, viruses, parasites or fungi; the diseases can be spread, directly or indirectly, from one person to another. In contrast, **non-communicable diseases** (NCDs), also known as **chronic diseases**, are not transmitted from person to person. They are of long duration and generally slow progression. The four main types of non-communicable diseases are cardiovascular diseases (like heart attacks and stroke), cancers, chronic respiratory diseases (such as chronic obstructed pulmonary disease and asthma) and diabetes.

Table 1.1: Leading Causes of Mortality Source: WHO, 2008				
		World (%)	**High income (%)**	**LMIC* (%)**
Communicable Diseases		32.3	7.0	36.4
	Infectious & parasitic	19.3	1.9	22.1
	Respiratory	6.8	4.4	7.2
	Perinatal	4.5	0.4	5.1
Non-Communicable		58.5	86.5	53.8
	Cardiovascular	29.1	38.3	27.6
	Cancer	12.5	26.0	10.2
Injuries		9.2	5.9	9.8
	Unintentional	6.3	4.0	6.6
	Intentional	2.9	1.9	3.1
* - LMIC = Low & Middle Income Countries				

Currently, chronic, non-communicable diseases account for an overwhelming proportion of disease burden in high income countries, 86.5%, and these days even a greater burden (53.8%) than infectious diseases in low- and middle-income countries too. The role of human behaviors in disease etiology today is actually even higher, to the extent that certain prevalent infectious diseases, in particular, HIV/AIDS and STIs, are also associated with behaviors such as unprotected sex, and many injury deaths are also due to behaviors such as car crashes (drunk driving), homicide and suicide. The significance of this shift has yet to be fully appreciated by researchers seeking to develop more effective prevention and control measures to reduce chronic disease burden. Instead, researchers continue to use the same research methods to analyze and explain chronic diseases that they use to explain the mechanisms of infectious disease pathology. Because the scientific method has been so effective in providing the means to control infectious diseases, scientists seek to explain human behavior nowadays as if it was no different than the behavior of a bacterium, more complex to be sure but fundamentally governed by the same cause-and-effect laws found throughout the natural world. For better or worse, however, chronic diseases cannot be prevented by attempting to identify the causal analogs of immunizations or antibiotics.

One oft-cited indicator of the success of the scientific method is the doubling of the age of life expectancy over the last 100 years (see Graph 1). Most people view this as unmistakable evidence of progress in medical science. Fewer people are aware that the bulk of these gains in *average* life expectancy are attributable to sharp declines in the death rates for children under the age of five due to success in combatting childhood infectious illnesses. When people escaped or survived early childhood infections in 1900, they could expect to live to the age of seventy, not much different than today (Montagu, 1994; Olshansky, Carnes and Cassel, 1990). Making similar gains in controlling chronic diseases has proven much more difficult. Critics further argue that the slow progress in the war on cancer, for example, often measured in months not years, has come at the steep cost of severe deteriorations in quality of life and prolonged suffering (Callahan, 2002). Unlike the largely successful search for cures for infectious diseases, medical treatments of chronic diseases have been dubbed "halfway technologies"–they stabilize patients but generally do not restore complete normal healthy functioning (Chalmers, cited in Veatch, 2005).

Graph 1.1: Rising Life Expectancy Rates, 1850 - 1990

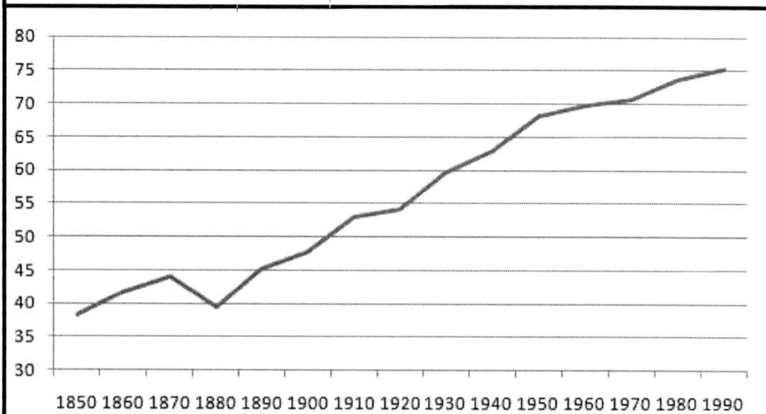

To appreciate how we have come to find ourselves in this situation, it is helpful to put these developments in historical context. There are many outstanding texts that offer detailed descriptions of advances in medicine (Porter, 1997) but a brief summary will suffice for our purposes here.

Hippocrates is generally considered the founding father of medicine, based on his text, *Airs, Waters, and Places*, written in 400 BC. His text had an enormous impact on the practice of medicine, held in esteem largely intact for the next twenty-plus centuries, a span of time that encompasses major milestones marking the beginnings of the field of public health. Public health professionals generally attribute the field's origins to the famous reports by Edwin Chadwick in his *Sanitary Conditions of the Labouring Population of Great Britain*, written in 1842, and its replication in the US, *Report of the Sanitary Commission of Massachusetts,* by Lemuel Shattuck in 1850. It is important to note that these reports were based on a pre-scientific understanding of disease etiology, where miasma theory attributed mortality rates to the "foul odours" exuded by corpses and other rotting matter. Set against a backdrop of the prevailing miasma theory, interest in cleaning up a polluted environment provided the backdrop for the legendary studies conducted by John Snow, the founding father of epidemiology, who tracked cases of a cholera outbreak in Soho, England, in 1854. Using a spot map to illustrate how occurrences of cholera were distributed around a central location, Snow traced the source of the outbreak to the Broad Street water pump. His investigation of the pattern of cases convinced the local council to disable the pump by removing its handle. Snow's work has since come to assume near-mythical status, including citation as the historical precedent for renewed interest in changing the environment advocated by proponents of the social determinants of health today. Yet it was not until 30 years later that the micro-organism, or agent of disease, present in the well's water was discovered.

It was not until the late 1800s that the methods of modern science became more widely accepted, codified and applied to explain the incidence and distribution of the most common diseases of the day. In 1884, Robert Koch advanced four postulates that laid the foundation for the germ theory of disease (see Table 1.2). Shortly thereafter, in a remarkable burst of scientific discovery, the microorganisms responsible for virtually all known infectious diseases were discovered and verified within short twenty-year time span between 1880-1900 (Rosen, 1993). Although effective immunizations and antibiotics were not discovered or developed for another 30-40 years, nonetheless, the germ theory of disease took root, putting medicine on firm scientific foundations.

Table 1.2: Koch's Postulates
• The microorganism must be found in abundance in all organisms suffering from the disease but should not be found in healthy animals. • The microorganism must be isolated from a diseased organism and grown in pure culture. • The cultured microorganism should cause disease when introduced into a healthy organism. • The microorganism must be re-isolated from the inoculated, diseased experimental host and identified as being identical to the original specific causative agent.

As new immunizations and antibiotics (such as penicillin) began to be discovered in the early decades of the 20th century, the germ theory of disease became the dominant paradigm for explaining disease causation. Its power to treat infectious diseases was wondrously impressive and its appeal became firmly entrenched in the minds of medical scientists. The growing use of vaccines early in the 20th century also raised new ethical and legal concerns, particularly relevant to the nascent field of public health. In the historic 1905 case of *Jacobsen v. Massachusetts*, the US Supreme Court upheld a Massachusetts law that authorized the state Board of Health to require all citizens to be immunized against smallpox, firmly establishing public health's authority to marshal the police powers of the state to protect citizens from the potential for widespread health threats. Citing the state's authority to legislate "for the common good, for the protection, safety, prosperity, and happiness of the people," the Court's ruling established the precedent of protecting the common good over individual liberty rights.

Buttressing the status of the germ theory of disease, another major milestone in medical science was the first-ever randomized controlled trial (RCT), a test of the effectiveness of streptomycin to treat tuberculosis, conducted in 1948 (Medical Research Council, 1948). Following these discoveries and other developments (e.g., refrigeration, improved sanitation), the diseases that were most prevalent in the US slowly began to shift, and sometime between 1930-1940, the prevalence of infectious diseases was eclipsed by chronic diseases for the first time. Appreciation of the categorical difference between infectious and chronic diseases, however, did not follow until decades later, in the '50s and '60s. As researchers grew frustrated with their inability to discover the germ that causes heart disease, a new longitudinal epidemiological case-control study was started in the early 1950s, the Framingham Heart Disease study.

The Framingham Heart Disease study is important for our purposes here on two counts. First, it introduced a new framework for thinking about disease etiology. Where the germ theory of disease found impressive success in identifying one-to-one, cause-and-effect relationships between the agent of disease (e.g., the Plasmodium parasite) and the onset of a particular disease (e.g., malaria), the Framingham Heart Disease Study re-defined causality in terms of statistical probabilities, associated with the new concept of "risk factors," which, in this pioneering investigation, were identified as smoking, high blood pressure and cholesterol. With the advent and increasing dissemination of the Framingham study results, the "cause" of chronic diseases was no longer explained in terms of a deterministic one-to-one relationship. Instead, researchers explained that risk factors were *neither necessary nor sufficient* to cause a heart attack. That is, a person could smoke and not die of a heart attack, while another person could have a heart attack without ever having smoked. As we shall see, the probabilistic risk factor framework makes hard-and-fast distinctions between scientific and humanistic approaches to health promotion more complicated, where choices might be more fruitfully understood in terms of probabilities, not absolutely determined but not completely free either.

The second major reason that this study is important is because it shifted the focus of attention in health research from identifying the *agent* of disease to the *behaviors* of the host, the human organism (Neubrauer and Pratt, 1981). Following on the heels of Framingham, the 1964 Report by the US Surgeon General on *Smoking and Health* stated that smoking "causes" heart attacks–a controversial assertion at the time, as the classic criteria for defining cause-and-effect relationships were not met (such that the assertion of a causal relationship between smoking and heart disease is still challenged by the tobacco companies [Michaels and Monforton, 2005]). Still, the significance of behavioral risk factors thereafter became the primary target of interest among health researchers and public health professionals.

Building on such findings, the 1979 *Healthy People* report, the first ten-year US national public health service planning document, announced that,

> A group of American experts developed a method for assessing the relative contributions of each of the elements to many health problems. Analysis in which the method was applied to the 10 leading causes of death in 1976 suggests that *perhaps as much as half of US mortality in 1976 was due to unhealthy behavior or lifestyle*; 20 percent to environmental factors; 20 percent to human biological factors; and only 10 percent to inadequacies in health care. [emphasis added]

To dispel any lingering confusions conveyed by reports on the "leading *causes* of morbidity and mortality," where heart disease, cancer and stroke regularly topped the lists, Dr. J. Michael McGinnis, MD, the Deputy Assistant Secretary for Health Promotion and Disease Prevention, and Dr. William H. Foege, MD, a former Director of the Centers for Disease Control and Prevention, published a report in 1993 in the *Journal of the American Medical Association*, cleverly titled, the "*Actual* Causes of Death in the United States." In their report, they confirmed that more than half of all deaths in the US were caused by behaviors, starting with smoking (400,000 deaths), poor diet and physical inactivity (300,000 deaths) and alcohol use (100,000 deaths). This report was replicated in a study by Mokdad, *et al*, in 2000, with virtually identical results. The central role of behaviors was re-affirmed in a 2014 report by Bauer and colleagues at the CDC, where they state, "The chronic disease burden in the USA largely results from a short list of risk factors—including tobacco use, poor diet and physical inactivity (both strongly associated with obesity), excessive alcohol consumption, uncontrolled high blood pressure, and hyperlipidaemia."

Finally, it would be remiss not to mention that considerable attention is being paid to the role of the social determinants of health (SDoH; see Table 1.3) to explain health outcomes these days (Marmot and Wilkinson, 1999; Wilkinson and Marmot, 2003). While the shift in attention from individual behaviors to the social determinants might initially seem welcome, I have two reservations. One, most SDoH proponents still rely on a physicalist definition of health. They advocate changes in the social structure, but those changes are recommended in order to reduce the number of heart attacks, not to strengthen autonomy or gain clarity about values that matter. This is shortsighted and self-defeating, as I hope readers will appreciate by the end of this book. Two, many advocates of the SDoH framework appear to have implicitly adopted a scientific behaviorist model, to the extent that they aim to modify positive/negative environmental reinforcement contingencies to effect the desired changes in behavior. For example, large numbers of proponents advocate raising taxes on soda pop to raise the costs (negative reinforcements) of choosing to drink sugary beverages (see Chapter 6 for a full discussion). In this case, proponents seem to have embraced behaviorist principles, perhaps unwittingly but nevertheless, in seeking to alter reinforcement contingencies, while discounting the significance of new restrictions on autonomy designed, in this case, to reduce obesity rates. Along these same lines, I am troubled by the term, "determinants," which seems too strong a word, essentially denying the potential for human agency. As I will show, Anthony Giddens's (1976) "agency-structure" framework better captures the tensions between the constraints imposed by the social structure and the capacity of agents to act to change the social structure.

Table 1.3: Social Determinants of Health
• poverty • racism • deficient education • unemployment • substandard housing • stressful neighborhoods with high crime rates and few public amenities • inequalities in wealth and status • stigmatization • lack of access to healthy foods, medical care and recreational areas • lack of transportation

The question addressed in this book is whether the evident role of behaviors in contributing to premature death, disease and disability today raises any distinct epistemological or ethical concerns in thinking about their prevention.

Why the Scientific Method Has Displaced Other Modes of Inquiry

The development of modern medical science closely tracks developments in the broader field of scientific research in general. In reviewing these parallel histories, I want to call attention to the slow pace of change in overturning the extant dominant paradigms of the day. Hippocrates's views on medicine prevailed for more than twenty centuries. The germ theory of disease emerges in the late 1880s and continues intact until the early 1960s. The central role of behaviors surfaces in the 1960s and it is only now, some 50-60 years later, that it is being challenged by growing interest in the social determinants of health. Similarly, this section reviews how the origins of the modern scientific method arise in the 16th century, yet secures philosophical warrant only in the 1930s, in the philosophical school of thought known as positivism. Allegations of the inappropriate and pernicious effects of applying the scientific method to study the human condition then surface in raging academic debates about the respective merits of quantitative versus qualitative research in the 1970s and '80s. These debates have quieted down to an extent in recent years, with an uneasy truce ostensibly signaled by more frequent calls for "mixed methods" among researchers with a positivist bent. Yet, at the same time, one sees signs of unremitting disenchantment in increasingly common reference to an ideology of "scientism" by philosophers and social scientists reflecting on the challenges of understanding the human condition. For my part, I think current controversies are indicative of a period of intellectual transition, which are typically slow-moving, as a review of historical challenges to the dominant paradigm of the day suggests.

The origins of the scientific method date back to the Age of the Enlightenment, notably in the works of Newton, Bacon, Galileo and Descartes. The scientific method is fundamentally empirical, and drawing on repeated observations, it seeks to discover causal laws to explain what has been observed. Such laws are often expressed as mathematical equations, such as $E=mc^2$, and from such equations, scientists make predictions about the effects of changes among the identified variables, predictions that are used to confirm or falsify the law itself. Laws are particularly prized for revealing the underlying dynamics that account for a diverse range of phenomena, like the identity of forces that explain apples falling and planets orbiting, and for their parsimony (their elegance in simplicity) and generalizability. Laws are considered universal and unchanging over time and space (see Table 1.4 below). Examples of such laws are Newton's universal law of gravitation and his three laws of motion, Kepler's three laws of planetary motion, Kelvin's laws of thermodynamics, Mendel's laws of genetic inheritance, Avagadro's law on the number of molecules in gases in closed containers, Dalton's Law of partial pressures, Ohm's Law, Coulomb's Law, and others (see Carroll, 2016, among many

Table 1.4: Key Characteristics of a Positivist Science
• **Empirical:** it relies on human powers of observation and sense-perception (sight, hearing, touch, smell and taste)
• **Verifiable:** where validity is equated with the power to predict and control; *If-then* hypotheses
• **Replicable:** where successful replication requires fidelity in reproducing the exact same methods used in confirming the original hypothesis
• **Generalizable:** where the results are not only applicable to the particular case at hand, but apply across the whole class or category of subjects, e.g., human beings as the class that includes both women and men, people of all races/ethnicities, people of all ages, etc.

sources). When laws are verified, they enable scientists to make highly accurate predictions about the effects of changes in any of the variables stated in the equation. The knowledge associated with such laws provides scientists with the power and ability to produce a desired result. Because laws are tested and verified by predicting the effects of a change in the "independent" variable(s) on the "dependent" variable in the equation, after verification, the application of these laws to effect desired changes by practitioners outside the laboratory is exactly the same as the researcher's, an identity of methods now known as fidelity in implementation. (See Chapter 2, for further discussion.) Down through the ages, applications of the scientific method were used by Robert Koch in the late 19th century, and later, provided the basic hypothesis-testing foundation for the first randomized controlled trial in medical research in 1948.

Pressure to accept the scientific method as *the* authoritative and exclusive source of all human knowledge is widely attributed to the rise of a philosophy of science known as positivism. One pivotal text propounding the tenets of positivism is A. J. Ayer's *Language, Truth and Logic*, published in 1936 (see also, Popper, 1959). Although the positivist school of thought has come under withering attack in philosophical circles for many years, in practice, this empirical, hypothesis-testing methodology now informs virtually all research supported by the US National Institutes of Health (see Table 1.3). To determine whether anti-retroviral (ARV) medications can control the course of HIV infection, medical scientists conduct double-blinded RCTs. In this line of thinking, the validity of evidence collected in different research designs can be rank-ordered to establish a lexical hierarchy of knowledge (see Table 7.1 in Chapter 7). In this hierarchy, the number of potential confounders or threats to the validity of the results are reduced at each step up the ladder, providing greater and greater confidence that results more accurately represent the true reality of the relationship between the hypothesized cause and the resulting effect. In medicine, this hierarchy was codified in the publication "Evidence-Based Medicine" issued in 1992. One key purpose of this publication was to put physicians on notice about the wide variations in practice observed in treating patients, intimating that they were clinging to an outmoded anachronistic belief in the "art" of medicine. They need(ed) to adopt a scientific evidence-based approach instead. These same standards have been adopted by the US Preventative Services Task Force in their authoritative reports on effective prevention measures. Following in medicine's footsteps, Brownson and colleagues advocated the need for public health to adopt the same evidence-based standards in 2009. These days, the need to implement only evidence-based interventions is almost invariably referenced in grant announcements supported by taxpayer dollars.

To summarize, current research and practice in health promotion are based on the assumption that there is no essential difference between the human condition and the natural world, where the laws of physics govern cause-and-effect relationships. Under the assumptions of the natural science paradigm, human behavior is caused by independent antecedent variables, which determine behavior and make people act in predictable ways. Behavioral health research is thus directed towards verifying cause-and-effect relationships. Researchers test hypotheses in experimental research designs, to confirm the hypothesized relationship between the independent variable(s) and the dependent variable of interest, a specified health behavior. Under this assumption, researchers use the exact same research designs and methods used to test the efficacy of new medications to treat HIV/AIDS, hypertension, or cancer as they use to determine the effectiveness of behavioral interventions aimed at reducing smoking or obesity.

To underscore the point, one of the most appealing features of the scientific method is that the process of verifying a hypothesis provides the very means for effecting a desired outcome. It provides the power to control events in the natural world. Based on Koch's postulates, we hypothesize that exposure to the tubercle bacillus will cause the person to contract tuberculosis (and not some other disease). If we introduce the microorganism into a healthy organism, we can then observe if it causes the specific disease in question or not. We hypothesize that streptomycin can kill the tubercle bacillus. We conduct an experiment by administering streptomycin and observing the result. If the course of the tuberculosis infection is stopped, our hypothesis is verified, thus providing the highest level of confidence known to humankind that we have discovered the truth about the nature and relationship of these events. In an amazing stroke of good fortune, we also come to learn that administering streptomycin is an extraordinarily effective way to treat tuberculosis; the patient can be cured, as long as one methodically follows the same procedures.

Lest I be misunderstood, I want to be clear: I fully accept, appreciate and am deeply grateful for the power of science to control events in the natural world, such as treating patients with HIV or tuberculosis. My quarrel is with the application of this same methodology to seek to control human behavior–to stop people from smoking, getting drunk or high, to effectively control people's weight, to make everyone get at least 45 minutes of aerobic exercise three times each week, to compel men to always wear condoms, and so on. There can be little doubt that the search for ever more effective behavioral interventions is precisely the direction that the field of health promotion is now headed. If this approach had demonstrated greater success over the last 50-60 years, then I would need reconsider my assumption that human beings have the capacity for free will. But I see little evidence that this approach is working; we still do not know how to make people lose weight, get more exercise, stop smoking, avoid opioid abuse, and so on (Michie, *et al*, 2018). Ironically, to the extent that decades of concerted, well-funded, sustained health behavior research have failed to demonstrate otherwise, this turn-of-events lends support to my contention that human beings can and do make choices that are not pre-determined by causal antecedents.

The Distinct Aims of the Humanities

One starting point for appreciating the need for a humanistic approach to health promotion is to ask what is missing from the empirical scientific view. The answer is everything that makes human beings distinctively human: free will, agency, autonomy, values, volition, creatures with the capacity for morality. What is missing is the contents of subjective consciousness. Why? Because we cannot see (or in any other way empirically observe) what people are thinking. But what then are we to make of this? Because there is no objective independent third-party position from which to observe thoughts and feelings, empirical scientists treat them as outside the scope of scientific inquiry, and thus lacking in trustworthiness or credibility. If one cannot measure something empirically and objectively, then scientifically, it is not something about which any claims regarding truth or validity can be verified. If the felt experience of making a decision is not part of objective reality, then positivists maintain that it is fruitless to discuss or debate its effect as there are no means to test and confirm the truth of any such assertions.

The quandaries posed by this doctrine have not passed unnoticed by health researchers. One relatively recent concern in medicine that captures the dilemmas here is the issue of symptoms, or “Patient Reported Outcomes” (PROs). (In medicine, symptoms stand in contrast to signs, which refer to objective, independent evidence of disease [e.g., temperature, blood pressure, tumor scans, etc.]) PROs refer to a broad category of patient experiences, such as pain, fatigue, depression, nausea, dyspnea (shortness of breath), perceived quality of life, anxiety, cachexia/anorexia, confusion, discomfort from constipation, intensity of hot flashes, hunger, thirst, etc. (The NIH database, Patient Reported Outcomes Measurement Information System [PROMIS] covers 70 different domains.) However common they may be, self-reports on such matters are viewed as decidedly, categorically unreliable (see, for example, Ferriera, Ferriera, Maher, Refsauge and Latimer, 2002, on the lack of agreement using different measures). Without the equivalent of a thermometer to measure a patient's temperature, how do we know whether the pain you claim to suffer is really as bad as you say it is, or whether it is more or less severe than the pain other patients say they feel? How do we square self-reports with the desiderata of unbiased, objective, empirical data? How much confidence do we have that they accurately represent reality? What is the basis for claiming confidence in their veracity?

We need the humanities to access the contents of subjective consciousness. The humanities are concerned with that which distinguishes the human condition. The tripartite division of the modern university is based on the recognition that the two pillars of human knowledge are the sciences and the humanities, reflecting human interest in both objective and subjective realities. (I come back to the purpose of the social sciences below.) Can you feel (see, or touch) someone else's pain? Can you measure justice? Are values, such as autonomy, equality, compassion, beneficence, generosity, or freedom, real? If science cannot measure and quantify values objectively, then how should we think about them? Does it mean they do not exist, are not real, and have no impact on human conduct?

Questions about the ontological status of values are critical for many reasons. For starters, the dismissive attitude of the sciences towards questions about the reality of human values erodes trust and confidence in their stature and place in human affairs. If they cannot be observed or otherwise measured directly, then empirical scientists are left only with what they consider problematic unreliable self-reports. From a scientific perspective, due to the lack of objective measures and consequent reliance on self-reports, values have come to be equated with individual desires. From this standpoint, there are no valid and reliable methods to calculate which desires are more important, have higher priority, or carry greater weight. Thus, short of the certainty and conviction that science provides, we have fallen into the trap of thinking that the only intelligible thing that can then be said about values is, different strokes for different folks. You have your opinion, I have mine, and that is all there is to say about the matter. I like drinking beer, you like fighting for social justice, but who is to say which is more worthwhile? How can one really know? As the press of science consigns values to an ambiguous netherworld presumed to be lacking substance and *ipso facto* causal consequence, the hegemony of the sciences in the modern world thus undermines the position that we can talk intelligibly about objective values. Another consequence of the high regard given the scientific outlook is the reversal of the classical relationship in ethics between the right and the good, where we now live in an era generally characterized as giving priority to the right over the good, a point to which we return below.

To grapple with questions about values, we need to recognize that the positivist/scientific method is capable of answering only certain types of questions, namely, questions about the direction and magnitude of empirical cause-and-effect relationships: If this [independent variable] happens, then that [dependent variable] will result. But testing hypotheses does not exhaust the kinds of questions that are relevant to understanding the human condition. As an indispensable complement to scientific knowledge, the humanities examine the inner workings of human consciousness, where human beings find meaning in events: how do I make sense of my attraction towards this person? the birth of a child? the death of a spouse? needless suffering and injustice in the world? Importantly, the humanities reveal the nuance of different words in describing subtle yet crucial differences in felt emotions, descriptions that are <u>not</u> available to direct empirical observation. We are not able to see or measure what goes on in someone's mind, but we recognize the differences captured by particular words, between, for example, feeling upset and feeling anger, jealousy and frustration, or feeling glad to see someone and feeling love or friendship. It is absurd to deny the impact of language in seeking to understand human behavior, or to deny the importance of articulating felt emotions more clearly.

Key characteristic differences between the respective domains of knowledge can be highlighted in a set of contrasts (see Table 1.5). Where the natural sciences focus on objective reality, the humanities focus on subjective reality. Where the natural sciences assume the sum total of "reality" exists independent of language, the humanities recognize that certain aspects of reality are revealed by language (e.g., the nature of justice). Where the natural sciences seek to identify causes, the humanities seek to articulate reasons. Where the central aim of research in the sciences is discovering truth, as in "Is this true?" the central aim of the humanities is discovering goodness, "Is this good?" Where the natural sciences conduct empirical analyses, the humanities conduct normative analyses. Where the natural sciences provide explanations about the truth of a proposition, the humanities provide justifications about the propriety of a course of action. Where the natural sciences aim to identify causes, which by definition occur in the past (i.e., they *must* precede outcomes), the humanities aim to imagine future possibilities (for example, the longing to create a just world). Raw data in the sciences consists of (empirical) observations; in the humanities, it is (normative) reasons. Finally, claims about the validity of conclusions are warranted by the results of hypothesis-testing experiments in the sciences, whereas the warrants of validity in the humanities are established by achieving coherence or wide reflective equilibrium. Such coherence often leads to agreement and consensus in a population, but consensus in itself does not guarantee the validity of an assertion (as, for example, the perceived social position of slaves historically demonstrates).

Table 1.5: Key Differences between Scientific and Humanistic Domains of Knowledge

Characteristic	Scientific Domain	Humanistic Domain
Focus of analysis	Objective reality	Subjective reality
Ontology	Language independent	Language dependent
Stimulus for human behavior	Causes	Reasons
Central research aim	Truth: Is this true?	Goodness: Is this good?
Type of analysis	Empirical	Normative
Goal of analysis	Explanation	Justification
Research objective	Identify causes of phenomena; establish facts	Determine best course of action; clarify values
Questions of interest	What are the causes of x? Does A cause X?	What is the best course of action? Should one do X?
Raw Data	Observations	Reasons
Warrants of validity	Experiments, hypothesis-testing, levels of evidence	Coherence, "wide reflective equilibrium," consensus

The Canadian philosopher, Charles Taylor (1985), highlights the distinct aims of the respective approaches:

> Technological payoff, or the greater ability to predict and manipulate things, is certainly a good criterion of scientific success on the post-Galilean paradigm of understanding. If understanding is knowing your way about, then modern technological success is a sure sign of progress in knowledge. But how is this meant to convince a pre-Galilean? For in fact he is operating with a different paradigm of understanding, *to which manipulative capacity is irrelevant, which instead proves itself through a*

> *different ability, that of discovering our proper place in the cosmos and finding attunement with it* . . . Each theory carries with it its own built-in criteria of success–*moral vision and attunement in one case, manipulative power in the other*–and is therefore invulnerable to the other's attack. In the end, we all seem to have gone for manipulative power, but this has to be for some extra-epistemic consideration, not because this mode of science has been shown to be superior as *knowledge*. [emphasis added]

Two noted ethicists offer additional distinctions to help clarify the differences. The first is by Tom Beauchamp (1980), the author of the Belmont Report, the work by the first US National Commission on Bioethics, which among other things prescribed standards for the ethical conduct of research with human beings:

> If science is inquiry into general causal laws and explanation, ethics is inquiry into non-causal justification and general action-guiding reasons. . . The foundations of normative ethics will be prescriptive (or at least non-descriptive), for ethics is an action-guiding discipline that provides reasons for human action and that attempts justifications of moral claims. Science, by contrast, deals with the causes of events and with causal explanations of phenomena. The statements in the two domains thus display an unbridgeable logical difference: one is based ultimately on non-descriptive sentences, and the other on descriptive sentences. Those familiar with modern ethical theory will recognize that this argument is merely a corollary of one use of the fact/value distinction.

The second by Anthony Kenny (1992), an Oxford-trained classicist, who explains Aristotle's distinction:

> Practical reasoning is reasoning which reasons out the good, as theoretical reasoning is reasoning which reasons out the truth. The conclusion of a piece of theoretical reasoning is a truth to be believed; the conclusion of a piece of practical reasoning is a good to be brought about. By setting out my theoretical reasoning I may explain why I believe a certain proposition; by setting out my practical reasoning I may explain why I am performing a certain action . . . The point of practical reasoning is the achievement of good, just as the point of theoretical reasoning is the acquisition of truth.

A humanistic framework is based on the assumption that human beings are endowed with free will, which enables people to choose between different courses of action. It is the ability to choose that provides the very foundation for ascribing moral responsibility. In this view, human action is guided by reasons, which provide the grounds for people to choose to act on felt desires–or to choose *not* to act on them–based on values that matter.

Research in the humanistic model is thus directed towards clarifying human values, good reasons for pursuing one course of action over another, and the moral considerations that support conclusions about the priority and propriety of certain actions over others.

It is our capacity for language that enables human beings to imagine alternative courses of action, and so see the need to make a decision. This is the essence of free will. Many intelligent people have wrestled with the question of free will since the dawn of recorded history; a final resolution of long-standing debates is not going to be ventured here. For our purposes, it is enough to note that empirical scientists start from the assumption that it does not exist. In contrast, one of the most prominent philosophers in America today, John Searle (2004), states unequivocally that this issue is absolutely unresolved and represents perhaps the most pressing and important question in philosophy at present (see Chapter 14 for further discussion). I must stress the point: behavioral health research is now founded on a contested questionable assumption. I do not wish to disparage the motives of behavioral health researchers, who I believe are motivated by the honorable goal of seeking to alleviate human suffering. But the blinkered search comes at a steep cost. To be successful, to develop *effective* interventions, scientists must demonstrate that they have the power to control human behavior–that is the gold standard for demonstrating the validity of their hypothesis. In pursing the scientific approach, they thus must ignore or deny the possibility of human agency and autonomy. B. F. Skinner's 1971 classic, *Beyond Freedom and Dignity*, makes the point explicit: in the modern scientific era of behavioral science, free will and dignity are illusions, archaic artifacts devoid of substantive meaning or relevance.

I am deeply concerned about the ethical implications of the current direction of the field. Seeking the capacity to effectively change behavior presumes that scientists know what subjects want better than they do themselves. This approach may seem reasonable if one accepts the scientific assumption that choice, morality, moral responsibility and accountability are all delusions, uncanny self-deceptions. In this perspective, questions about the ethical grounds for seeking the power to override whatever "misguided" choices people may make are moot; there is no need to uphold the principle of respect for autonomy if autonomy is not real but merely an illusion.

If, however, one feels reasonably confident that people can and do make choices, then the ethical implications of continuing on this course are deeply troublesome. (Personally, I suspect there would be much greater public uproar if scientists had in fact discovered how to make people lose ten pounds or stop smoking consistently, without fail, but, since the capacity for wielding such power does not appear imminent, most people now do not seem to be too bothered by the prospect.) But my ethical concerns derive from certain epistemological assumptions, such that my ethical concerns would be moot if the exercise of free will was known to be impossible. However, there are grounds–epistemological warrant, beyond wishful thinking–that support the plausibility of adopting the alternative assumption, the idea that people do indeed have free will.

There are two key warrants, one practical, one theoretical. In practical terms, the conspicuous lack of compelling evidence demonstrating the success of the natural sciences model in changing behaviors weighs in favor of reconsidering one's assumptions. Although defenders often suggest that the current dearth of compelling evidence is attributable to the relative youth of the social sciences (among others, see Glanz, *et al*, 1997), the historical record shows that scholars have persistently attempted to apply modern science methodology to explain human behavior at least since the publication of Hume's *A Treatise on Human Nature* in 1739. In theoretical terms, the most plausible account of how free will can possibly exist in a universe otherwise subject to universal natural laws may be found in the phenomenon of *emergence.*

In evolutionary terms, **emergence** is the rise of phenomena that cannot be predicted or explained by the properties and interactions of their constituent building blocks (Holland, 1998; Clayton, 2004; Macdonald and Macdonald, 2010). Emergence is the antithesis of reductivism, which holds that the properties of any higher order system are unconditionally, without qualification, reducible to the properties of lower level systems: physiology can ultimately be explained in terms of biology, biology in terms of chemistry, and chemistry in terms of physics. Against this view are many prominent examples of phenomena that could not have been predicted based on full knowledge of what each of the component parts has the potential to do. The emergence of life could not have been predicted as a result of combining the properties of inert inanimate objects. The emergence of motility could not have been predicted by examining the features of immobile objects. Given the number of other examples that could be cited, it seems plausible that free will emerged through the development of advanced language skills within human consciousness. In each of these cases, the emergent properties, although grounded in the physical, chemical and biological reactions of their elementary ingredients, are intelligible only in terms of a new previously nonexistent higher-order capability. Like life itself, free will is just such an emergent capacity.

Goals in a New Humanistic Approach to Health Promotion

Health promotion is widely referred to as the "social science wing of public health." The current application of social scientific theories in behavioral health research attempts to force the social sciences into the natural sciences mold, but the social sciences are better understood as the study of the interaction between objective and subjective realities (as the terms "social" and "sciences" suggest). In locating the social sciences at the intersection of the scientific and humanistic domains of knowledge, the purpose of the social sciences is to take up questions about how human beings understand and reconcile having feet in both worlds: our bodies exist in the natural world and are subject to those laws, while our minds are filled with language, desires, emotions, values, and moral principles that come into the realm of human experience in subjective consciousness, thereby creating the capacity for free will.

Acknowledging the essential humanistic dimension of the social sciences has major implications for the goals of health promotion. Instead of uncritically accepting that reducing heart disease (and hence, smoking and obesity) is the most important goal for health promotion, the purpose of health promotion in a humanistic framework is conceptualized in terms of fostering human autonomy: how can we collectively support each other in figuring out values that matter and the best ways of living in accordance with those values, as only human beings can do? What is a just world? How can we forge sufficient solidarity to move towards creating conditions in which more and more people are able to exercise autonomy in pursuing their life plans? We need the humanities to articulate goals befitting the human condition, in contrast to the measurable yet delimited objective of promoting regimens of physical fitness.

In laying the foundation for a new approach, three issues need to be addressed. The first is a defense of the idea that autonomy is essential to human well-being, more important than physical fitness. In defining autonomy, a second issue arises, namely, differentiating values from desires. Third, as testing empirical hypotheses is not possible or appropriate in a humanistic approach, I need to describe and explain the steps that can be taken to increase confidence in the validity of the decision, that is, that people are making the right decision in exercising their autonomy, and not making a foolish mistake.

Significance of autonomy

Philosophers have delineated three schools of thought regarding the meaning and scope of human wellbeing: hedonist, preference satisfaction and ideal or objective theories (Griffin, 1986). The first view is based on the idea that human wellbeing consists in pleasure, where the more pleasure one experiences, the higher one's level of wellbeing. The second school holds that people have preferences that are not reducible to hedonistic pleasures. People may decide to pursue interests that involve a great deal of hard work, often with many frustrations along the way, to gain the satisfaction of accomplishing something that they see important and worthwhile. The self-discipline required to become truly excellent at something is usually not described in terms of being "fun" or pleasurable, but in this school of thought, one experiences wellbeing by satisfying one's preferences even if such pursuits do not bring carnal pleasure. Finally, ideal or objective theories of wellbeing maintain that it is possible to define the good life for human beings as a whole, irrespective of individual pleasures or preferences. Wellbeing here is defined in terms of normative ideals. These ideals are considered an integral part of a good life for human beings, even if one is no happier as a result of, for example, being honest, or has no desire, for example, to be autonomous. This school holds that there are objective indicators of the good life for human beings, over and above what gives pleasure or satisfies preferences.

In objective accounts of wellbeing, many scholars cite autonomy as the most distinguishing characteristic of the human condition, of ultimate importance to defining what it means to thrive and flourish as a human being. Eminent proponents such as James Griffin rank autonomy among the top five objective characteristics of the good life for human beings (along with accomplishment, understanding, enjoyment and deep personal relationships). Similarly, Doyal and Gough (1991) cite physical survival and autonomy as the two most basic human needs. They are objective, independent of individual preferences, and universal; the loss of autonomy would cause anyone serious harm, it would cause people to be fundamentally disabled in the pursuit of their vision of the good. As they define it, "to be autonomous . . . is to have the ability to make informed choices about what should be done and how to go about doing it" (1991, p. 53). The founder of the capabilities approach to defining justice, Amartya Sen, states, "The 'good life' is partly *a life of genuine choice*, and not one in which the person is forced into a particular life– however rich it might be in other respects." Likewise, from the same capabilities approach, Nussbaum lists the "ability to form a conception of the good and to engage in critical reflection about the planning of our own lives" as one of ten essential capabilities that all human beings need. Elsewhere, in defending an essentialist account of human functioning, Nussbaum (1992, p. 219), writes, "All human beings participate (or try to) in the planning an managing of their own lives, asking and answering questions about what is good and how one should live." In linking autonomy directly to health, the epidemiologist Michael Marmot finds, "Autonomy, a sense of control over your life, and social connectedness–rather than actual financial resources or access to medical services–have the greatest impact on your health and life expectancy. The lower in hierarchy you are, the less likely it is that you will have full control over your life and opportunities for full social participation. Autonomy and social participation are so important for health that their lack leads to deteriorations in health."

I think these diverse thinkers are right for several reasons, most especially because it is difficult, if not impossible, for anyone to live a human life without this outlook: if one truly believes that people do not have the capacity for choice, then it would follow that there is no point considering what one should do as it is going to happen in any case. Such an outlook breeds fatalism, cynicism, nihilism. Why should I bother to consider different options, since I do not really have a choice in the end? Finally, although empirical scientists have focused on the goal of physical fitness, it is likely because it can be measured empirically, rather than an earnest belief that physical fitness represents the truest, most complete picture of human flourishing. Let us turn now to define autonomy, starting with a basic distinction between desires and values.

Defining autonomy

Because autonomy is a value without empirical referents, defining and understanding it is possible only by entering into an on-going historically-evolving discussion. In public discourse today, laypersons commonly conflate and use the terms "freedom" and "autonomy" interchangeably. Freedom is the absence of restrictions on one's ability to act on felt desires (typically, with the singular qualification that acting on one's desires must not harm others, *a la* John Stuart Mill). Autonomy, in contrast, is the exercise of reflective agency, where one might feel some desire or impulse but pause to reflect on whether one wants to act on it or not, based on reasons, which are expressed in terms of higher-order values. In this view, quenching one's desire for another fix of heroin does not make one free.

Here is the tricky part: values are grasped in subjective consciousness, but that does not make them the same as desires. Indeed, there is interesting and important scholarly debate about whether values should properly be considered objective or subjective (see, for example, Altieri, 2015; Antonoccia, 2000; Ellis, 2014), but a full discussion here would take us too far astray. Succinctly summarizing the issue, Griffin (1998) observes, "Values are puzzling; they are far from obviously part of the natural world, yet there is no other world obviously available to house them." Striding the line between objective and subjective realities, values are distinguished from desires by the intrinsic appeal to inter-personal validation for evaluating their relative worth. I may feel like having another drink on some night out, but I have the unique human ability to consider whether it is prudent or might interfere with my job or family responsibilities. I may feel like making a pass at a colleague but pause to reconsider in terms of the kind of husband and father I would then become–duplicitous, unfaithful, untrustworthy. Choices define who we are, and we become a good person by making good choices, based on values that matter. Drawing on a distinction originally made by Frankfurt (1971), Dworkin (1988) thus defines autonomy as follows:

> Autonomy is conceived of a second-order capacity of persons to reflect critically upon their first-order preferences, desires, and wishes, and the capacity to accept or to attempt to change these *in light of higher order preferences and values.* By exercising such a capacity, persons define their nature, give meaning and coherence to their lives, and take responsibility for the kind of person they are. [emphasis added]

Unlike the desire for chocolate or vanilla ice cream, values can be discussed and defended in terms of reasons. As Talcott Parsons notes, "A value is not just a preference but is a preference which is felt and/or considered to be justified." We can argue about the meaning of justice–affirming characterizations that deepen one's understanding while challenging assertions that appear shallow, incoherent or confused–in ways that we cannot debate your desire for vanilla and expect to be able to show you that you are mistaken. Confidence in the quality of our reasoning is strengthened through dialogue with others. "This course of action is better than that for the following reasons . . ." Emphatically, saying that one intends to do something "simply because I feel like it" does not qualify as a good reason. According to Taylor (1985), we make "qualitative distinctions of worth" between desires and values. As he states,

> Our desires are classified in such categories as higher and lower, virtuous and vicious, more or less fulfilling, more or less refined, profound and superficial, noble and base. They are judged as belonging to qualitatively different modes of life: fragmented or integrated, alienated or free, saintly or merely human, courageous or pusillanimous, and so on.

Values articulate the grounds for assessing the worth of felt desires from the point of view of people other than one's own self. As Dworkin puts it, "If we are to make reasonable choices, then we must be governed by canons of reasoning, norms of conduct, standards of excellence that are not themselves the product of our [personal] choices."

Qualifications: If autonomy is essential to human flourishing, then the goal of health promotion must not be to restrict it by seeking the power to effectively make people stop engaging in unhealthy behaviors, but rather to promote it. While highlighting the central role of autonomy in human flourishing, there are a couple of qualifications to keep in mind. First, our bodies are subject to the laws of the physical universe; even if we have free will, we are not absolutely free. We cannot, as a matter of sheer force of will, make Type I diabetes go away: bodies react to elevated sugar levels without regard for our feelings or intents about the matter. Thus, it is centrally important to gain a clearer picture of how we comprehend and negotiate having feet in both worlds, toward the goal of helping people strengthen their sense of autonomy while appreciating its limits, and not being driven blindly by poorly understood forces that elicit heated emotions and affect sound decision-making.

Second, just as health behaviors are associated with chronic diseases only probabilistically, so too it appears that structural, social and psychological risk factors "cause" unhealthy behaviors only in the weak, neither-necessary-nor-sufficient sense of increasing risk for adopting them. People make choices, but the press of social structural forces makes it more or less difficult for individuals raised and living in different environments to make autonomous choices that prioritize health over other needs. The full implications of these conditions are discussed in the final chapter

Gaining confidence in knowledge about values

A third challenge for a humanistic approach to health promotion is the process for justifying the assignment of different weights to different reasons. It is a matter of what scientists call "value judgements," and ethicists "normative analysis," which are based on non-quantitative assessments of the quality and soundness of the rationale and reasons presented (Daniels, 1996)

It is important to start off by acknowledging that the validity of normative claims does not (now?) match the certainty provided by the hypothesis-testing methodology of the natural sciences. Because of the subject matter intrinsic to the discipline, humanistic research may never achieve the same degree of certitude. But that does not make it irrational or unintelligible to discuss matters that cannot be tested empirically. Three steps to increase confidence in the validity of one's choices are: (1) reducing and eliminating potential sources of bias or error; (2) being open-minded, willing to consider the possibility that we may be mistaken and can see the error in our ways; and (3) putting forward a coherent case that achieves wide reflective equilibrium.

To increase confidence in the quality of one's decision, Brock (1995) calls for a public reasons process of deliberation. As a first step, one should eliminate as many potential sources of bias or error as possible:

> Considered judgments generally, not just considered moral judgments, are, first, judgments that are not made in conditions that we know from experience often lead to mistakes. Here are some examples of such conditions: (1) when we have insufficient time to consider the matter carefully; (2) when we lack significant, relevant information bearing on the question at hand; (3) when we have a relatively fixed commitment to a particular position on the question at hand that makes us inadequately open to a fair consideration of other positions; (4) when the question at hand requires technical knowledge or training that we lack; (5) when we must make a decision while distracted or emotionally overwrought; (6) when we lack sufficient relevant experience to appreciate fully some considerations and to integrate them adequately into our decision making; and so forth.

Second, it is important to listen carefully and humbly to the case being made by someone who disagrees with you, to see if they reveal flaws in your line of thinking or point out something that you forgot to take into account. Anderson (1993) captures the essence of reasoned argument,

> Like most of the elemental notions–justice, integrity–that guide our moral life, we do not have a sharply discriminating, operational definition ready at hand. Rather, we proceed by mutually intelligible intimations, affirming this, denying that, each claim suggesting an aspect of the whole that we vaguely discern but cannot readily grasp. . . This is what makes reasoned argument possible. We persist in trying to persuade our antagonists that there is some crucial element of the matter at hand that their case neglects, and we proceed in the good faith that, if we show them this perceptively, if we *illuminate* them, they may change their minds. And for our part, we presume that we may *learn* from the deliberation, which is to say, we keep

> open, and positively, the prospect that the case we are now earnestly making we will come to recognize as inadequate, because we will see a more significant, a larger truth in the matter.

We can change our minds, choose to go a different course, because we now see and understand the proposed alternative to be the better option.

Finally, in normative inquiry, one gains confidence in an analysis to the degree that it makes a coherent argument. A coherent argument involves more than avoiding logical inconsistencies, loose ends, and contradictions. Coherence (or "wide reflective equilibrium," in Rawls's phrase) is achieved when each of the pieces is sound in its own right and each supports, strengthens and/or reinforces other parts of the argument. Often, one works to achieve coherence by moving back and forth between the particulars of the case at hand and general moral values and principles, testing propositions in accordance with the normative maxim to treat like cases alike, and different cases differently. Is this choice like other ones that I have made in similar situations, or is there something crucially different, which leads me to think I should do otherwise? Like legal court cases, such deliberations typically build on precedents, but also always leave open the possibility that a key point may have been overlooked or not given due weight in previous judgments. In coherent arguments, one gains confidence in the analysis to the extent that it illuminates aspects of lived moral experience that we did not see or understand before, aspects that were previously unrecognized, opaque or only dimly appreciated. One gains confidence when others agree that the reasons put forward articulate sound compelling judgments.

Humanistic inquiry rejects the tenet that truth can only be determined *procedurally*, by following certain correct methods (e.g., empirical tests of hypotheses), and tackles such questions as the good life for human beings, which may yield only to *substantive* responses, the depiction and elucidation of the experience (Altieri, 2015). In humanistic studies, researchers reflect on the experience of self-consciousness, not just sense perceptions, but more significantly, encounters with the pain of losing a loved one, the satisfaction of a job well done, the fear of failing, the call of helping others in need, pangs of regret, and other values. They struggle to articulate those experiences as perceptively as possible. Confidence in the truth of statements about the meaning and significance of values grows through successive approximations, refinements made over time that enable human beings to see more clearly lives worth living. One gains confidence in the goodness of a decision as larger numbers of people come to see that it is the best thing to do (note: it is important to re-affirm that the validity of a judgment is based on the quality and coherence of the account, not because a majority of people say so). Despite doubts cast about the status of ethical principles, the Civil Rights and Women's movements are undeniable examples of moral progress (however far we may still have to go).

In a humanistic approach to health promotion, the task for public health professionals is to engage fellow citizens in discussing values that matter and how we can collectively live our lives attuned to these values. In the words of the eminent sociologist, Robert Bellah (1983),

> The purpose . . . is not to produce or control anything but to discover through mutual discussion and reflection between free citizens the most appropriate ways, under present conditions, of living the ethically good life. . . It is precisely the point about *praxis* that it has no extraneous product. It has an end, namely, the good of human beings, but that end is attained through itself, that is, through action or practice that is ethical and political. . . For 'helping professionals', this would involve toleration of high levels of uncertainty in trying to aid people to improve their own skills of practical autonomy, rather than categorizing them in terms of preconceived theories with resulting automatic formulas for treatment.

In a humanistic approach to health promotion, the main task of health promotion is to build consensus on values that matter, the best ways of living in accordance with those values, and the capabilities people need to pursue their life plans and live a life worth living. We gain confidence in the validity of such ends to the extent that more and more people share and support an emerging common vision. Specific activities for implementing a humanistic approach to health promotion in practical terms are described and discussed in two chapters, on the Center for Education, Promotion and action (Chapter 13) and the final chapter, Looking Forward, of this book.

Overview

The book is composed largely of essays originally published as peer-reviewed articles that span a twenty-five year period. Broadly speaking, the thirteen articles in the core of the book are different takes at articulating my concerns over the current direction of the field of health promotion and laying out a more promising direction. Each addresses different aspects of these paired themes. As each chapter was originally published as a free-standing article on its own, virtually all cover the relationship between epistemological and ethical concerns in order to provide a context for the particular focus or emphasis of each essay. I hope the reader will find that each illuminates different pieces of the broader argument and that the reader may see a progression or maturation in my thinking as I have wrestled with these issues over time, drawing on different literatures, making different analogies and using different case examples. On the other hand, because each article was originally produced as a free-standing article, the reading order is not essential, and the reader is free to dip into chapters that appear more relevant to one's interests. The original articles have been edited only slightly, mainly to reduce any redundancies as much as possible. Reflecting the different emphases of each chapter, the book is organized into two parts, with two sub-sections in each. The first part focuses on a critique of the currently dominant scientific approach to health promotion, subdivided into two sections: the first consisting of articles focusing on the epistemological issues at stake, and the second on the ethical problems raised by making certain epistemological and ontological assumptions about the human condition. The second part of the book lays out a positive humanistic alternative to the mainstream instrumental framework, where the first sub-section focus on the ethical warrant for humanistic approach, and the second on the characteristics, distinctive challenges, and case studies of a humanistic approach to health promotion.

After this opening introduction and overview, the next three chapters address the epistemological issues entailed in applying the model of the natural sciences to the study of human affairs. Chapter 2, "Reflections on the Relationship between Theory and Practice in Health Promotion," presents an analysis of the problems that have created a gulf between theory and practice in health promotion. Drawing on the classical distinction made by Aristotle between *theoria* (natural processes) and *praxis* (social practices), it traces the poor fit between the results of experimental, hypothesis-testing research and the guidance that practitioners need in developing programs in communities. It describes an alternative conceptualization of theory and concludes with the implications of this alternative model for closing the gap between theory, research and practice in health promotion. Chapter 3, "Beyond positivism: Humanistic Perspectives on Theory and Research in Health Education," aims to expand the set of ideas about what constitutes "theory" in health promotion research. It reviews seven functions of theory: prediction, explanation, making assumptions explicit, understanding, sense-making, sensitization and critique. The first two fall under the domain of positivist research; the latter five are drawn from theorizing conducted in the humanities. The critique argues that a broader conception of theory and research, one that moves beyond the bounds of the positivist paradigm, will aid public health professionals better navigate the challenges of working with creatures endowed with free will. Chapter 4, "An Uneasy Alliance: Combining Qualitative and Quantitative Research Methods," describes several difficulties that may arise when trying to combine qualitative and quantitative research methods. From my own field research, four problems that arose in attempting to translate qualitative into quantitative data are described: (1) making analytic sense of singular responses; (2) the mistaken logical inference that demands that each pattern of judgment should have discrete behavioral indicators; (3) the construction and use of ideal types; and (4) making analytic sense of universal responses. The chapter concludes with the implications of the different goals, assumptions, and standards of evaluation that inform each of the respective methods for future research.

The second section also has three chapters, shifting in emphasis to the ethical concerns at stake in the choice of research paradigm. Chapter 5, "Social marketing: a critical appraisal," presents a critical analysis of social marketing, a framework touted to be highly effective in achieving health promotion goals and objectives. In reviewing a representative and widely-cited article by Hastings and Haywood, three questions are asked about each of the proposed tenets of social marketing: are these ideas new? are they more effective than current health promotion practices? and do they raise any particular ethical concerns? On each of these counts, the analysis shows that the purported benefits of social marketing might not be as great as proponents claim. Several problematic unintended consequences that arise from the use of social marketing methods are discussed. The narrow focus on individual behavior change and the potentially manipulative techniques for inducing behavior change are of particular concern. It concludes with a call for further discussion about the limits and potential iatrogenic side-effects of adopting allegedly (more) effective social marketing strategies in health promotion. Chapter 6, "Promoting justice and autonomy in public policies to reduce the health consequences of obesity," examines potential ethical problems involved in adopting a social determinants of health framework uncritically. Public policies to reduce rates of obesity in the United States have generated considerable public controversy. The chapter examines the implications of proposed policies for the principles of justice and autonomy and key assumptions underlying the major contending positions with respect to the relative weight that should be assigned to them in balancing their respective claims. The analysis traces the crux of the debate regarding the ethical warrant for policies to restrict access to calorie-dense foodstuffs to two key issues: the appeal to different and conflicting theories of justice, and the conflation of autonomy with negative liberty in public debates. After clarifying the ethically relevant characteristics of autonomy that merit defense, the chapter concludes with a description of how the capabilities approach to justice may offer a more coherent ethical framework for developing and evaluating policies to address the obesity epidemic. Chapter 7, "What Types of Public Health Proposals Should Agencies Be Funding and What Types of Evidence Should Matter? Scientific and Ethical Considerations," describes how the established hierarchy of research designs poses practical, political, economic and other constraints that press towards the study of individuals rather than populations, which results in a bias towards clinical medical investigations instead of research on the effects of an intervention on the population as a whole. It concludes with recommendations for redressing the imbalance between research on individuals and research on populations in setting fair standards to guide NIH funding priorities.

The third section presents different models of a positive alternative, a humanistic approach to health promotion. Chapter 8, "Moral reasoning as a model for health promotion," describes the model of moral reasoning used by researchers to address ethical issues raised by different research design and recommends that this same model of normative reasoning be applied in health promotion. When faced with ethical dilemmas about the most appropriate course of action in health research, investigators conduct normative analyses to identify good reasons for choosing one option over another. These reasons provide grounds for determining what one should do, and for changing past practices in light of new moral considerations. Since researchers appear to think that this type of analysis is a good way to guide and change their own behavior, this model of moral reasoning has relevance and potential application to the field of health promotion, which engages in analogous processes of seeking to inform and guide changes in the behaviors of the lay public. It presents two case examples to illustrate the process of moral reasoning, which readers should find quite familiar. Chapter 9, "Assuring adequate protections," takes up the question of community autonomy, as distinct from individual autonomy, and lays out the ethical warrant for requiring community oversight of health research conducted in international settings. It reviews inadequacies in current standards of individual informed consent and research ethics committee reviews and shows how a broader population-based public health perspective raises new demands on justice involving due consideration of the rights, harms and benefits to the community as a whole. An ethical standard that requires community oversight of health research is justified on three principled grounds: respect for community autonomy and their right to self-determination; due consideration of the consequences of the research for the community as a whole; and, a more complete understanding of human autonomy. The chapter concludes with practical recommendations regarding the composition of Community Advisory Boards to ensure that they have legitimate decision-making authority in diverse socio-cultural contexts. Chapter 10, "Autonomy, Paternalism and Justice: Ethical Priorities in Public Health," recalls the significant time and effort devoted by public health professionals to identifying a sound ethical justification for paternalistic interventions that aim to prevent people from adopting unhealthy behaviors, but do so by overriding individual autonomy. It goes on to suggest that, on both empirical and ethical grounds, public health professionals should seek instead to expand individual autonomy to improve population health. To promote autonomy, the field should redirect current efforts toward clarifying principles of justice. Although public health's most visible stance is associated with an egalitarian conception of "social justice," it is imperative that public health professionals address gaping divisions in public understandings of justice. It closes with recommendations for initiating this process. Chapter 11, "A New Ethic for Health Promotion," describes two models for thinking about the purposes of health promotion–a medical model and an education model–and traces how concerns about the validity of different types of research have driven preference for the medical model. In the medical model, health promoters are expected to replicate the methods identified by researchers to effect targeted changes in the dependent variable of interest, health behaviors. The report then describes one familiar alternative way of thinking about the purposes of health promotion, namely, the educational processes involved in higher education. In pursuing a philosophy of liberal higher education, the purpose of research and practice would be to strengthen people's faculty for making value judgments. The analysis concludes with a discussion of the implications of the higher education model for the future of the field.

The fourth and final section of the book presents case studies of the application of a humanistic model for research and practice in health promotion. Chapter 12, "Ethical Issues in Community-Based Participatory Research," identifies potential sources of tension between the values of scientific rigor and community participation in CBPR. As explained there, CBPR lies at the nexus of two major underlying ethical concerns–respect for community autonomy and the fair allocation of limited public resources–which have generated considerable controversy about appropriate criteria for evaluating CBPR grant proposals. The complexity of evaluating CBPR proposals is compounded by the multiple purposes that it serves: (1) an ethical function of demonstrating respect for community autonomy; (2) a research method for eliciting ideas for interventions to improve population health; and (3) an intervention in itself, seeking to enhance the capacities of community participants. The growing use of CBPR thus raises two new ethical issues that deserve greater public attention: first, the issue of demonstrating respect for community autonomy when the locus of research shifts from the individual to community level and hence the problem of securing informed consent; and second, the fair distribution of scarce public resources when practical constraints make the most rigorous research designs for assessing the effects of community interventions virtually impossible. Chapter 13, "The CEPA Project: A New Model for Community-Based Program Planning," describes a new model of community-based program planning for HIV prevention developed by *El Centro de Educación, Prevención y Acción* (CEPA) project. Based on models of critical thinking, empowerment and participatory education, the guiding philosophy of CEPA is to narrow the gap between program developers and program recipients to the greatest extent possible. The report discusses the successes and challenges encountered in approaching this ideal. It concludes with recommendations for public health professionals to consider the full range of ways to engage and enlist community members in addressing public health issues. Chapter 14, "Promoting Dignity: The Ethical Dimension of Health," critiques a strict scientific account of the causes of unhealthy behaviors, based on the standards promoted in evidence-based medicine, where randomized controlled trials are upheld as providing the gold standard for establishing the validity of different explanations. By denying human autonomy, the scientific paradigm also denies the possibility of human dignity. In contrast, this chapter explains why dignity is an essential dimension of human health and well-being and describes key research challenges in moving the field of health promotion in a more humanistic direction. It concludes with the call to expand the scope of health promotion to embrace research and practice aimed at articulating values that matter and promoting human dignity.

The book concludes with a chapter on "Looking Forward." In it, I weave the various strands of the larger argument articulated in the different chapters into a single summary case. From there, I draw out the implications of the analysis in three critical areas: recommendations for improving population health; the skills and training needed for a new generation of health promotion professionals; and reflections on the struggle for creating a just society. I conclude with a call for assuming individual responsibility for engaging in democratic deliberations with fellow citizens towards the goal of assuring that all community members are raised in institutional contexts that provide the essential capacities needed to survive and thrive in the modern world today.

References

Altieri, Charles. 2015. *Reckoning with the Imagination: Wittgenstein and the aesthetics of literary experience*. Ithaca, NY: Cornell University Press.

Anderson, Charles. 1993. *Prescribing the Life of the Mind: An essay on the purpose of the university, the aims of liberal education, the competence of citizens and the cultivation of practical reason*. Madison, WI: University of Wisconsin Press.

Antonaccio, Maria. 2000. *Picturing the Human: The Moral Thought of Iris Murdoch*. New York: Oxford University Press.

Beauchamp, Thomas. 1980. "The foundations of ethics and the foundations of science." In *Knowing and Valuing*, edited by Hugo Tristram Engelhardt and Daniel Callahan, 260-268. Hastings-on-Hudson, NY: The Hastings Center.

Beecher, Henry K. 1966. "Ethics and Clinical Research." *New England Journal of Medicine* 274, 1354–1360.

Bellah, Robert. 1983. "Social Science as Practical Reason." In *Ethics, The Social Sciences, and Policy Analysis*, edited by Daniel Callahan and Bruce Jennings, 37-64, New York: Plenum Press.

Brock, Dan. 1995. "Public Moral Discourse." In *Society's Choices: Social and Ethical Decision Making in Biomedicine*, edited by Ruth Bulger, Elizabeth Bobby, and Harvey Fineberg, 215-240. Washington DC: National Academy Press.

Callahan, Daniel. 2002. Ends and Means: the goals of health care. In *Ethical Dimensions of Health Policy*, edited by Marion Danis, Carolyn Clancy, and Larry Churchill, 3-18, Oxford: Oxford University Press.

Carroll, John W. 2016. "Laws of Nature." *The Stanford Encyclopedia of Philosophy* (Fall 2016 Edition), edited by Edward N. Zalta, Available at: <https://plato.stanford.edu/archives/fall2016/entries/laws-of-nature/>.

Clayton, Philip. 2004. *Mind and Emergence: From Quantum to Consciousness*. New York: Oxford University Press.

Daniels, Norman. 1996. *Justice and Justification: Reflective Equilibrium in Theory and Practice*. New York: Cambridge University Press.

Doyal, Len and Ian Gough. 1991. *A Theory of Human Need*. London, UK: MacMillan Press.

Dworkin, Gerald. 1988. *The Theory and Practice of Autonomy*. Cambridge, UK: Cambridge University Press.

Ellis, Fiona. 2014. *God, Nature and Value*. New York: Oxford University Press.

Emanuel. Ezekiel, David Wendler, Jack Killen, and Christine Grady. 2004. "What makes clinical research in developing countries ethical? The benchmarks of ethical research." *Journal of Infectious Diseases* 189:930-7.

Ferreira, Paola, Manuela Ferreira, Christopher Maher, Kathryn Refshauge and Herbert R, Latimer J. 2002. "Effect of applying different 'levels of evidence' criteria on conclusions of Cochrane reviews of interventions for low back pain." *Journal of Clinical Epidemiology*; 55(11):1126-9.

Food and Drug Administration. 2014. *Deeming Tobacco Products to be Subject to the Food, Drug, and Cosmetic Act, as Amended by the Family Smoking Prevention and Tobacco Control Act; Regulations Restricting the Sale and Distribution of Tobacco Products and Required Warning Statements for Tobacco Product Packages and Advertisements.* Economics Staff Office of Planning Office of Policy and Planning Office of the Commissioner. Economics Staff Office of Planning Office of Policy and Planning Office of the Commissioner. Department of Health and Human Services. April 2014. Available at: https://www.regulations.gov/document?D=FDA-2014-N-0189-20877.

Frankfurt, Harry G. 1971. "Freedom of the Will and the Concept of a Person." *Journal of Philosophy* 68 (1): 5–20.

Giddens, Anthony. 1976. *New Rules of Sociological Method.* London: Hutchinson Library.

Glanz, Karen, Frances Lewis, and Barbara Rimer, eds. 1997. *Health Behavior and Health Education: Theory, Research and Practice.* Second Edition. San Francisco: Jossey-Bass Publishers.

Griffin, James. 1986. *Well-being: its meaning, measurement and moral importance.* Oxford, UK: Clarendon.

Griffin, James. 1998. *Value Judgement: Improving our Ethical Beliefs.* New York: Clarendon Press.

Holland, John H. 1998. *Emergence: From Chaos to Order.* New York, NY: Perseus Books.

Kenny, Anthony. 1992. *Aristotle on the Perfect Life.* Oxford: Clarendon Press.

Macdonald, Cynthia, and Graham Macdonald, eds. 2010. *Emergence in Mind.* New York: Oxford University Press.

Marmot, Michael, and Richard Wilkinson. 1999. *Social determinants of health.* New York: Oxford University Press.

Medical Research Council. 1948. "Streptomycin treatment of tuberculous meningitis." *Lancet* 1: 582-96.

Metzl, Johnathan M., and Anna Kirkland, eds. 2010. *Against Health: How Health Became the New Morality*. New York: New York University Press.

Michaels, David and Celeste Monforton. 2005. "Manufacturing uncertainty: Contested science and the protection of the public's health and environment." *American Journal of Public Health*, 95(Suppl 1), S39–48.

Mischel, Walter, Yuichi Shoda, and Monica L. Rodriguez. 1989. "Delay of Gratification in Children." *Science* 244: 933–38,

Michie, Susan, Robert West, Kate Sheals, and Cristina A. Godinho. 2018. "Evaluating the effectiveness of behavior change techniques in health-related behavior: a scoping review of methods used. *Translational Behavioral Medicine*, 8(2): 212-224,

Montagu, J. D. 1994. "Length of life in the ancient world: a controlled study." *Journal of the Royal Society of Medicine* 87:25-26.

Neubauer, Deane, and Richard Pratt, R. 1981. "The Second Public Health Revolution: A critical appraisal." *Journal of Health Politics, Policy and Law* 6(2): 205–228.

Nussbaum, Martha. 1992. "Human Functioning and Social Justice: In Defense of Aristotelian Essentialism." *Political Theory* 20(2): 202-246.

Olshansky, S. Jay, Bruce A. Carnes and Christine Cassel. 1990. "In Search of Methuselah: Estimating the Upper Limits to Human Longevity." *Science* 250(4981): 634-640.

Porter, Roy. 1997. *The Greatest Benefit to Mankind: A Medical History of Humanity.* New York: W. W. Norton and Company.

Rawls, John. 1988. "The Priority of Right and Ideas of the Good." *Philosophy and Public Affairs* 17(4): 251-276,

Rosen, George. 1993. *A History of Public Health*. Expanded Edition. Baltimore, MD: The Johns Hopkins University Press.

Searle, John. 2004. *Freedom and Neurobiology: Reflections on Free Will, Language and Political Power*. New York, NY: Columbia University Press.

Sullum, Jacob. 1998. *For Your Own Good: The Anti-Smoking Crusade and the Tyranny of Public Health.* New York: The Free Press.

Taylor, Charles. 1985. "What is Human Agency?" In Charles Taylor, *Human Agency and Language: Philosophical Papers, Volume 1*, 15-44. Cambridge: Cambridge University Press.

Tavernise, Sabrina. 2014. "In New Calculus on Smoking, It's Health Gained vs. Pleasure Lost." *New York Times,* Aug. 6, 2014.

Veatch, Robert. 2005. *Disrupted Dialogue: Medical Ethics and the Collapse of Physician-Humanist Communication.* New York: Oxford University Press.

Wilkinson, Richard and Michael Marmot. 2003. *Social determinants of health: the solid facts.* 2nd edition. Copenhagen, Denmark: WHO.

World Health Organization. 2008. *Primary Health Care: Now more than ever.* The World Health Report, 2008. Geneva, Switzerland: WHO Press.

2. Reflections on the Relationship between Theory and Practice

The subject of the relationship between theory and practice is a perennial topic of discussion at health education conferences, meetings and classrooms. The gulf between the work of academics in conducting social scientific research and the efforts of practitioners in developing and implementing programs is frequently lamented. Among the many reasons suggested to account for this gap are: a presumed lack of familiarity and understanding of theories on the part of practitioners; an apparent failure on the part of practitioners to see the relevance of various theories to resolving the health problems they face; the potential isolation of researchers from "real world" limitations–the confounding and compounding factors and generally uncontrolled messiness of the social and political exigencies that affect health problems; and, the difficulty in translating theoretical constructs into lived experiences, and *vice versa* (Burdine and McLeroy, 1992; D'Onofrio, 1992).

This chapter traces the difficulties in integrating theory and practice to yet another possibility: misunderstandings about the nature of "theory" and the type of theory that is most appropriate for understanding human behavior. It begins by describing the most broadly disseminated and accepted understanding of theory and clarifies its relationship to practice. This conceptualization of theory is then critiqued and an alternative model of theory and its relation to practice is described. To draw out the differences between the two perspectives, the essay builds on the classical distinction made by Aristotle about the different types of human experiences. Aristotle termed these different types of experiences *theoria* and *praxis*.

The central thesis of this chapter is that the current gap between theory and practice arises because theories based on the model of *theoria* are not well suited for understanding human behavior. This model has been imported from the natural sciences and is based on the tenets of logical positivism. In studying human behavior, however, theories based on this paradigm may be inadequate and inappropriate, for reasons developed here. Clearly, they have had at best only modest success in trying to live up to their claim of explaining and predicting human behavior. According to their harshest critics, they in fact do little more than dress up common sense in esoteric jargon. Practitioners thus may find that this type of theorizing provides little help in program development.

The piece concludes with an alternative type of theorizing based on an Aristotelian understanding of *praxis.* In the domain of *praxis,* knowledge is contingent and contextual rather than universal, determinate and invariable. Hence, theorizing here is more appropriately modeled on the type of understandings and truth gained in the humanities–history, philosophy and literature. The implications of this model for bridging the gap between research, theory and practice are then described

What is theory?

The most widely disseminated definitions of theory used in public health education are derived from the philosophy of logical positivism (Ayer, 1952; Glanz *et al.,* 1990). According to proponents of this school of thought, there are no differences between theories generated in the natural sciences and those in the social sciences. While it is a common (yet often unstated) assumption in most introductory health promotion textbooks, one of the more outspoken advocates of this position is the sociologist Homans, who writes: "As an ideal, the nature of theory, of explanation, is no different in the social sciences from what it is in the physical sciences" (Homans, 1970, p. 59). Theorizing here is characterized by three major features: testability, generalizability and power (Homans, 1970; van Ryn and Heaney, 1992; see Table 1.3 in Chapter One).

In the positivist perspective, the most important feature of theory is that it must conform to the tenets of the verification principle (or "testability"). The verification principle states that the *only* form of valid and reliable knowledge is that which can be empirically tested. Conversely, any belief that cannot be subjected to empirical confirmation is meaningless metaphysical speculation (Ayer, 1952). Theories are statements about the hypothetical relationships among various factors thought to cause some phenomenon of interest. The most important feature of this form of theorizing is that it must enable the researcher to deduce hypotheses and make predictions. Researchers test hypotheses by predicting the changes in the dependent variable that will occur as a result of changes in the independent variable(s). Despite considerable controversy about the status of the verification principle in philosophical circles today, it is this predictive, hypothesis-testing paradigm that now dominates the conduct of social scientific and behavioral health research.

The positivist definition of theory gives rise to one particular perspective regarding the relationship between theory and practice. When social scientific theories are based on the model of the natural sciences, practitioners are expected to use theory in precisely the same way that researchers do.

To illustrate the prescribed relationship, we may start with an example from the natural sciences. Chemists had a theory–now a law–that describes the relationships among the pressure, volume and temperature of gases in closed containers. Boyle's Law is stated mathematically as $PV = nRT$. Working deductively, chemists hypothesized that, by changing the pressure or the volume, they could predict and control the resulting changes in the temperature. After establishing the precise relationships, the link between theory and practice then becomes clear: if anyone wants to raise the temperature, they know they can increase the pressure and/or volume to achieve this goal.

Based on this hypothesis-testing paradigm, public health practitioners are likewise expected to manipulate identified independent variables in order to bring about desired changes in the dependent variable of interest. Any of the most commonly used theories in health education, such as the Health Belief Model or Social Learning Theory, may be used to illustrate this prototypical relationship.[1] Some theories, such as the Theory of Planned Behavior (Aizen, 1988), are even stated in mathematical formulas, further emulating the model of the natural sciences. Like chemists applying pressure to increase the temperature of enclosed gases, health educators are supposed to design programs to modify the independent variables to effect changes in the dependent variable. So, they try to increase the target population's sense of susceptibility, or their sense of severity, or their sense of self-efficacy, etc. This point needs to be emphasized: in the positivist perspective, intervening to change theoretically specified independent variables to bring about desired changes in dependent variables is the ideal and expected relationship between theory and practice.

Generalizability

A second critical feature of theory in the positivist perspective is generalizability. Based on its generalizability, a "good" theory can be applied to a variety of health problems in a variety of situations. Boyle's ideal gas law, for example, shows why underlying principles are the same for explaining why the pressure in car tires rises as the tires heat up while driving as those that explain why pressure cookers work. This characteristic has straightforward implications for practice too.

For example, the Health Belief Model may not only be used to address health problems ranging from vaccinations to mammograms to

AIDS prevention, but also may be used with adolescents and adults, men and women, and people from all races and socio-economic backgrounds. In the positivist perspective, the value of theory is directly proportional to its potential for application across all these diverse circumstances. In contrast, an alternative conceptualization of theory, described below, asserts that the value of theory is proportional to its ability to stimulate awareness, discernment and sensitivity to the unique features of each particular situation.

Power

Finally, a third defining characteristic of theory is power (Homans, 1970). Generalizability is one facet of power, but in broader terms, the power of a theory derives from its capacity to reveal the underlying dynamics of phenomena. Theory enables us to see how superficially unrelated events are alike, or even more powerfully, how they are identical. To borrow another example from the natural sciences, the laws of physics reveal the identity of forces at work in apples falling and moons orbiting. This quality, the power to reveal, is perhaps the most attractive feature of theorizing. The promise of positivist theory is a parsimonious statement that will lay bare the underlying unity of an immense diversity of phenomena.

Unfortunately, it is difficult, if not impossible, to identify comparable examples from the health promotion or social science literatures. On the contrary, perhaps the most striking feature about the social scientific theorizing today is the lack of powerful explanatory models that reveal deep insights into human behavior. For example, the idea that "people who think they are susceptible to disease X will be more likely to take preventive actions than those who think they are not as susceptible" does not take us very far in understanding people's health behaviors. Likewise, it is not particularly revealing to find out that people who feel confident they can do something will be more likely to do it than those who do not feel so confident. An exploration of the reasons for this paucity of powerful social scientific theories will be used to introduce the differences between *theoria* and *praxis* described by Aristotle. In more modern terms, problems arise with the positivist paradigm because of its failure to take into account the differences between *natural processes* and *human practices* (Oakeshott, 1975; Berlin, 1980; Postman, 1988). (See Chapter 3 for further discussion.)

The limits of positivist theory

A starting point for discussing the limits of positivism is to acknowledge the conspicuous lack of success of the social sciences have had in developing theories with explanatory power even remotely comparable to those found in the natural sciences. The point seems self-evident, but some social scientists are still reluctant to countenance the idea. Some assert that the social sciences have in fact achieved comparable successes. Others suggest that social scientists simply have not had sufficient time or resources (e.g. "the field is still relatively young," Glanz *et al.,* 1990, p. 22), but with more time and resources, they will produce comparable theories. The political scientist and professor emeritus at Yale, Charles Lindblom (1990), captures the concerns of those who are not convinced:

> Although [natural] science may overreach itself in genetic engineering or some other heady ambition, the whole world continues to need science and engineering for one task after another: building bridges, protecting the fertility of soils, and harnessing energy among others. Not only helpful, they are indispensable and unmistakably so. Without science and engineering, there would be no heart bypass, no moon shot, no high speed organization and retrieval of information, and no nuclear destruction. Not so for social science. The centuries have given it abundant opportunities. Practiced as long a natural science, it goes back at least to ancient Greece. In the last century thousands of social scientists trying to practice the methods much like those of the natural sciences have swarmed over institutions and social processes to try to extract propositions hidden to the lay mind. For all that effort and for all its presumed usefulness, I cannot identify a single social science finding or idea that is undeniably indispensable to any social task or effort. Not even one, I suggest. (Lindblom, 1990, p. 136.)

It is notable that the critique of the current direction of social scientific research transcends ideological persuasions. Similar observations have recently been made by liberal (Smith, 1990), radical (Giddens, 1976) and conservative (Sykes, 1988) critics.

If one accepts the idea that the social sciences have not been able to develop theories of human behavior with the same precision, parsimony and power as natural sciences, then the question arises as to why this is so (Brown, 1984). As pointed out by Lindblom, the idea that this failure is due to insufficient time or resources appears untenable. There are differences between natural processes and human practices that make the positivist model inadequate and inappropriate for understanding human action.

What makes social practices different

The most critical difference between natural processes and social practices has been identified in the works comprising the "linguistic turn" in modern philosophy (Wittgenstein, 1972; Bernstein, 1978; Taylor, 1985a). All of the differences that follow derive in large measure from their fundamental insight.

Language and human action

The linguistic turn in philosophy brought to light an essential, ontological distinction between natural processes and human practices. This difference rests on the fact that natural processes are independent of the language used to describe them, but human practices are *not* independent of language. That is, however human beings choose to describe the orbiting of the moon, it has no effect on its orbit. Whether we say it is due to "gravity" or due to "phlogiston," the moon still goes on orbiting just the same. However, not so with human practices. How we describe people's behavior influences their behavior. More precisely, social practices are partially *constituted* by the very language that is used to describe them.

The practice of "voting," for example, can be used to illustrate how human activities are dependent on language (Taylor, 1985b). The act of raising one's hand has no intrinsic meaning–or "cause"–outside of the linguistic conventions used to define a given social practice. That is, the "cause" of people raising their hands depends on the meaning people assign to that act. To highlight this dependence, we need only think of other contexts: school children raise their hands to get called upon by their teacher, football players raise their hands to signal a fair catch, other people raise their hands to say hello. What is the "cause" of their hand-raising behavior? It depends on what they are doing, but what they are doing can only be known through the words used to describe and give meaning to the act.

To take another example, "well-being" is understood by some people to be a state that is achieved through proper diet and exercise. For others, "well-being" is understood to be a state that is achieved through acting on one's social conscience: being courageous, living modestly, pursuing justice and aspiring to wisdom. There is no third-party, neutral, objective (for positivists, preferably mathematical) language that can reconcile these differences and tell us what well-being "really" is. Meanings are created, challenged, changed and fought over during the course of human events.

Here is the critical point. Unlike the moon, people are influenced by the meanings that are attached to these concepts. What sorts of prescriptions health educators give to people depend on what one means by "well-being." In short, unlike natural processes, the essence of human practices does not lie in the structure of matter but in a shared social world of meaning, a world created by the language and culture of a people.

The instability of interpretations

With natural processes, because events are not influenced by their descriptions, relationships between causes and effects have a certain fixity (except perhaps at the extremes, as Heisenberg reminds us). For social practices, because of their dependence on language, accounts of phenomena are relatively fluid and subject to multiple interpretations. From this essential difference, a number of other interesting differences follow. If social practices are open to multiple interpretations and multiple meanings, then the study of human action can never achieve the level of certainty to which positivists aspire. Cumulatively, these differences undermine the ability of the positivism to offer any better explanations of human behavior than the commonplace generalities they already have.

One way of cutting into the issue of what makes social practices different is to illustrate how the interpretation of events may change over time. Starting with events in the recent past, the categories that follow show how the human capacity to generate alternative interpretations of events gives rise to uncertainties and ambiguities that subvert linkages between purported causes and effects. This list is not meant to be exhaustive, but illustrative of the problems besetting positivism.

Short-term past: Childhood events, for example, are commonly thought to cause certain patterns of behaviors later in life. However, the same events take on different meanings at different times. Adolescent rage at the absence of a father may give way to a more mature appreciation of his dedication and commitment to supporting the family through hard work and long hours. The act remains the same, but the interpretation has changed. What was once a "cause" of anger is transformed in a different light into a "cause" of pride. With the fluidity in interpretation, the precise meaning of events (and hence the ability to establish cause-and-effect relationships) always remains unsettled and open to revision.

Long-term past: In a longer historical perspective, concepts that inform behavior (and even entire worldviews) get transformed. The sociologists Berger *et al.* (1973), for example, offer a thought-provoking analysis of why concepts like "chivalry," "chastity" and "honor" have become obsolete in the modern world. Unlike natural processes, the factors that motivate social practices are not eternally constant. While there is every reason to believe that the force of gravity has been exactly the same ever since the big bang, this stability is not true for concepts describing the social world. The things that inspire and motivate people nowadays are not the same as those that moved people in medieval times. Hence, another element of uncertainty is introduced into the attempt to explain social practices.

Present: The multiplicity of meanings and interpretations extends into the present as well. Current events yield different interpretations from different actors, a phenomenon sometimes referred to as the Rashomon Effect. In Kurosawa's film, six eyewitnesses to an encounter in the woods offer startling different accounts of what transpired between the couple.

Similarly, the actions of a group of armed soldiers are seen by some people as terrorists, but by others, as the heroic struggles of freedom fighters. Which view is the truth? It depends on one's perspective. The point here is that how people react to events depends on how they interpret those activities. If the events themselves have no fixed determinate meaning independent of the language used to describe them, then people's reactions become more difficult to predict.

Future: The difference between natural processes and social practices is seen even more clearly when considering the future. Natural processes are not influenced by the future; the temperature of a gas does not change because of what the pressure might do later. However, the same is not true for social practices. Here, the significance of language is unmistakable. In contrast to the previous issues discussed, the future has none of the empirical properties of past and present events. The future influences behavior only as people care to speculate about it through words and language. These words affect the choices people make, but the ideas themselves are generated by the human creative imagination. Hence, even more so than in the previous cases, indeterminacy is inherent. The influence of different ideas about the future is undeniable, but the future is undeniably subject to many possible interpretations too.

The recursive nature of human intelligence

Another factor that contributes further elements of unpredictability to social practices is the recursive nature of human intelligence. Whenever any factor is found to correlate with human behavior, people can–and do–act on that information, *either* to upset its governing capacity *or* to insure its occurrence (as in self-fulfilling prophecies). A person's awareness of a factor changes her interpretation of the situation in which it formerly (may have) had an influence. If a theory then tries to take into account a new factor like "awareness-of-the-independent variable(s)," the subject can still escape its law-like predictability by acting on that information (i.e., the theory's incorporation of our knowledge of the original variable), and so on, into infinite regress.

In sum, each of these categories of problems adds significant and ineradicable elements of uncertainty, contingency, ambiguity and instability to any attempt to establish theories or laws about human practices. The cumulative effect of all of these differences is to make the positivist paradigm inadequate for understanding human behavior. More precisely, whenever positivist methods are applied, the results are going to be theories exactly like we have now, i.e. ones that can account for approximately 10-40% of the variance at best and that recite the obvious.

From an epistemological standpoint, there is nothing wrong with factors identified through the positivist methodology; it is only that they are not especially insightful. Do we need "theory" to tell us that people who think getting disease X is very severe are more likely to do something about it than people who think it is not so bad? Or that people who say they intend to do something are more likely to do it than people who say they do not intend to do it? At best, these factors may be helpful to novitiates who can sometimes be overwhelmed about where to get started. However, beyond the most rudimentary level, positivist theory provides little help to experienced practitioners.

Given the failure of a positivist methodology to discover social laws, social researchers have turned in recent years to a re-examination of the differences between natural processes and human practices recognized by Aristotle a long time ago. Drawing on observations about different types of experiences, Aristotle thought a different type of knowledge, one that could acknowledge and adapt to the uncertainties and ambiguities of social life, was needed to understand and guide human conduct.

What is practical reason?

In Book Six of the *Nicomachean Ethics,* Aristotle distinguishes three types of human experiences47 and the types of knowledge that are appropriate to each. These types of knowledge have been termed theoretical knowledge, practical reason and technical skills. For brevity's sake, this essay will address only the first two.

The first type of experience Aristotle called *theoria.* Theoria refers to the experience of events that are absolute, invariant, eternal and universal. Aristotle termed knowledge about these events, *episteme,* or theoretical knowledge. Episteme is concerned with the order and structure of the natural universe and it corresponds to what we call modern science.

The second type of experience that Aristotle identifies is *praxis.* Praxis refers to the changing, variable and contingent relationships in the socio-historical domain. Aristotle called knowledge about these experiences *phronesis,* or practical reason. Praxis refers to the sphere of moral and political conduct, and knowledge regarding these experiences corresponds to what we might call wisdom today.

Because it has to take into account the contingent, ever-changing, endless variety of historical situations, Aristotle recognized that universal laws could never adequately capture this type of experience or convey understandings that would suffice for people to be able to function well in the social world. Hence, in contrast to theoretical knowledge, practical reason focuses on developing sensitivity and insight into the unique features of each situation.

What is practical reason? Given that each social situation is in certain respects unlike any other (e.g., a new cast of characters, a fresh context, a peculiar set of circumstances, unforeseen challenges, surprises, etc.), practical reason is the ability to recognize, acknowledge, pick out and respond to the singular salient features of a complex and unique situation (Cooper, 1975; Berlin, 1980; Bellah, 1983; Engberg-Peterson, 1983; Nussbaum, 1986). It is not deduction from abstract generalizations. Most importantly, "*phronesis* or practical reason involves an irreducible element of perception of the particular, that just here and now, this is the right thing to do, which cannot be articulated fully in any set of general features that this situation bears" (Taylor, 1988, p. 810).

Practical reason is the thinking process involved in deciding what to say or how to do that which best suits the particular situation at hand. Practical reason is involved in weighing which of the available courses of action is most appropriate given the specific circumstances (Larmore, 1987). However, because of the complexity and distinctiveness of each social situation, this can never be reduced to a general formula. Rather, in Aristotle's words, "the decision lies with the perception" (Aristotle, 1962, p. 1109b23). Thus, the essence of practical reason is sensitivity and discernment. Practical reason is the exercise of the faculty of judgment. Practical reason involves tact, as we think about how the other(s) will react and the reaction that will be most helpful in the situation at hand.

Some examples will help to illustrate the use of practical reason. The chapter concludes with the implications of this type of knowledge for theory, research, and practice.

Examples of practical reason

The examples below will be familiar to practitioners and are illustrative of common situations in which positivist theory is remarkably unhelpful. The examples are intended to name and to legitimate practitioners' use of non-theoretical modes of reasoning.

Community organizing/community development: There has been a resurgence of interest in recent years in intervention activities falling under the broad rubric of community organizing and community development strategies (Chavis and Florin, 1990; Lorion and Ross, 1992). This type of intervention offers many potential examples of the use of practical reason, two of which follow.

The first instance concerns the process for determining which approach to take: the more militant, confrontational approach of community organizing, or the more consensual, "bottom-up" approach of community development, or, as is more often the case, some mixture of the two (Rothman, 1979)? How does the practitioner decide? A good practitioner will base her decision on knowledge of the history of the community, the demographic composition of the community, the players and personalities involved, their history of working together, the issue at hand (especially as it relates to other community concerns), potential political resistance from different stakeholders and a host of other considerations. As a brief perusal of this list suggests, there is no calculus–no equivalent of Boyle's Law–that is going to give the practitioner an answer to her question. Everything depends on a sensitive, perceptive assessment of the local situation, its unique features, and the specific context. Her deliberations are the essence of practical reason.

Say, then, the health educator decides to use a community development approach. Is she now in a position to set about manipulating a set of identified independent variables? Again, the answer is no. Typically, the practitioner will be faced with trying to find the right balance between exerting leadership (Gardner, 1984) and fostering community ownership (Fawcett, 1993). When should she speak out and when should she bite her tongue? Finding the right balance will depend on her remaining attuned to the ebb and flow of the singular, salient features of a complicated situation with all of its own distinct characteristics. Practical reason enables her to act in sync with the dynamic flow of events and to improvise as needed.

AIDS prevention: Another critical issue facing the field of public health education today is preventing the spread of HIV infection. Freudenberg (1989), in his review of current programs, identifies a typical problem, in this case, in working with the Latino community. As Freudenberg puts the problem,

> Machismo, for example, includes the concept that men are responsible for women and children. Tapping into this belief, rather than personal health protection, may help increase the effectiveness of messages designed to encourage Black and Latino men to use condoms. (At the same time, however, . . . the double standard for sexual conduct must be challenged by AIDS educators.) (Freudenberg, 1989, p. 148.)

So, on the one hand, it may be effective to appeal to the existing value of "machismo" as it extends to the protection of women to encourage the use of condoms. However, on the other hand, the educator does not want to reinforce sexist power relations. What should he do? How should he counsel his clients? The educator wants to build on a powerful and highly salient value, but he does not wish to perpetuate oppression. His course of action is thus a matter of tact. He will walk a fine line, reinforcing the value at some points, challenging it at others. His emphasis will depend on his assessment of the particular person at the particular time and place.

Another example may be seen in needle exchange programs. Outreach workers want intravenous drug users to make use of the exchange program, but they want to encourage this population to seek out treatment programs too. So, they do not want to come on too heavy, but they do want to advocate treatment. How do they know when someone is ready to hear the treatment message? They get to know the individuals, their stories, their situation. Then, based on their own best judgement, they decide when, and how, and what approach to take to bring up treatment options.

Media advocacy: Despite its appearance in several textbooks on theory, media advocacy may be better described as a quintessential example of practical reason (Advocacy Institute, 1989; Wallack, 1990). There are no factors or independent variables identified in descriptions of this strategy. The only way for health promoters to employ media advocacy techniques is to be ready to take advantage of current events and to recognize immediate opportunities as they arise.

For example, two major tools of media advocacy are the use of "creative epidemiology" and press conferences. The effective use of either depends on practical reason. Creative epidemiology is exactly that–creative. To develop a press release using creative epidemiology takes insight into what will grab the attention of the intended audience and inspiration to avoid having the re-packaged information fall flat, sound corny, or obfuscate the point. Likewise, press conferences take presence of mind. Typically, reporters ask surprising (off-the-wall?) questions that could not possibly have been anticipated. It takes a quick wit to reframe question to make the points one wants to make. Theory will not deliver the pithy "sound bites" that make the evening news. They are a product of practical reason.

Implications for theory, research and practice

If there is a fundamental, ontological distinction between human practices and natural processes, then it may seem reasonable to suggest that we need a different approach to studying human beings. The dearth of robust positivist theories in the social sciences suggests that current efforts may be quixotic. Based on the distinction between *theoria* and *praxis,* the preceding analysis lays the foundations for re-defining theory, research and practice.

Theory

In contrast to the position put forth by Homans, the sociologist Blumer (1970) has identified an alternative conceptualization of theory. As Blumer states,

> . . . its aim is not to form scientific propositions but to outline and define life situations so that people may have a clearer understanding of their world. In every society, particularly in a changing society, there is a need for meaningful clarification of basic social values, social institutions, modes of living and social relations. (Blumer, 1970, p. 84.)

As Blumer continues, rather than making statements about hypothesized relationships between independent and dependent variables, theories might instead be statements that put forth and elaborate "sensitizing concepts."

Examples of sensitizing concepts might be ideas like "institutional embeddedness" and the "burden of individual responsibility" from my own work (Buchanan, 1991, 1992). The value of such statements derives not from their capacity to yield predictions about people's behavior, but from their ability to stimulate awareness and discernment. They are *not* exploratory or pre-operationalized variables. Their value lies in yielding a richer, fuller, more complete understanding of a situation, an understanding that can be shared with others in an effort to shed new light on potential blind spots, opaque stirrings, confusing turns of events, and so on.

Research

With a re-orientation of the purposes of theory development, the focus of research could shift too. The purpose of research need no longer be to test deductive hypotheses. Its purpose could be defined, instead, to foster the development of practical reason. Thus, the type of research that would be most valuable would be that which seeks to deepen one's sensibilities.

Fortunately, this mode of research is well known. It is precisely the type of research that scholars in the humanities–in history, literature and philosophy–conduct all the time. For those engaged in social research, acknowledging the difference between *theoria* and *praxis* would entail a shift away from hypothesis-testing experimental designs and towards case studies, ethnographies, participatory and qualitative research. The purpose of such studies would be to sensitize researchers, practitioners and the lay public to the broadest range of nuance and complexities of human involvements. The purpose of this type of research is to refine people's capacity for perceiving more subtle distinctions.

Practice

Finally, the preceding suggests two points about bridging the gap between theory and practice. First, the analysis presented here is intended to explain the reasons for the gulf in the first place. To wit, the model of the natural sciences is ill-suited for studying human behavior. However, with an appropriate re-conceptualization of theory, practitioners may find the results of the research and theorizing proposed here more helpful in guiding and informing their work.

While a shift in the orientation of research will be helpful, it probably will not be sufficient in itself to cultivate the development of practical reason. On this point, Aristotle was unequivocal. As Larmore (1987) writes:

> Judgement itself, [Aristotle] stressed, is not an activity governed by general rules; instead, it must always respond to the peculiarities of the given situation. Thus, no one can acquire judgement by being imparted some kind of formal doctrine. It can be learned only through practice, through being trained in the performance of right actions. (Larmore, 1987, p. 15)

According to Aristotle, practical reason is gained only through active participation and involvement in public life.

Conclusion

There have been a number of recent reports that have called attention to the mismatch between the training provided by academic institutions and the needs of practitioner in public health departments. The Institute of Medicine (1989) report, *The Future of Public Health,* notes the "potential isolation" of academic programs. Similarly, the recent additions of "Practice" or "Program" sections to leading health education journals offer another tacit acknowledgement of the poverty of positivist theory and research. To address these problems, the Public Health Faculty/Agency Forum (1991) has called for a renewed emphasis on practicums as part of public health training. It is time to realize that the practice of health promotion will improve through stronger support for mentoring programs with our finest practitioners and the development of theory more befitting the wisdom and humanity of their experience. The analysis presented here provides both a partial diagnosis of the problem and a justification for supporting their recommendations.

A key purpose of this chapter has been to provide those who have felt stifled by the hegemony of positivism with stronger arguments to support a change in direction. To be sure, researchers in public health will face formidable barriers in challenging the dominant natural sciences model. Unlike topics and areas of interest in the bulk of the pure social sciences, the factors affecting a person's health belong properly to both the natural and social science realms. For certain aspects of a given health problem, the natural sciences model is perfectly appropriate for explaining, predicting. controlling and bringing about desired outcomes, as evidenced by the significant advances made in modern medicine. Given the preponderance of medical doctors staffing NIH review panels and the high esteem with which such science is held, the prospects for replacing the positivist model in the near future appear dim. Private foundations, where "pure research" is often viewed with a more jaundiced eye, probably offer the strongest hope for funding the new directions for health education research proposed here.

Notes

*. Many textbooks make a distinction between "theories" and "models" where models are usually, although far from consistently, defined as simplified, schematic representations of a set of variables, and theories as a broader, more abstract, more all-encompassing set of propositions (confirmed hypotheses). (See, e.g., Black and Champion, 1976; Reading, 1979; Miller and Wilson, 1983.) That is, "a model is like a mini-theory" (Simon and Burstein, 1985, p. 53). Equally, many texts acknowledge

that the terms are often used interchangeably, as I do in this piece. I do not think my criticisms of the Health Belief Model constitute a "straw man" argument, however, since the major point is precisely to explore the reasons the field has not been able to put forward other, better, genuine theories.

References

Advocacy Institute. 1989. *Smoking Control Media Advocacy Guidelines.* National Cancer Institute. Bethesda. MD: National Institutes of Health.

Aizen, Icek. 1988. *Attitudes, Personality and Behavior.* Chicago: The Dorsey Press.

Aristotle. 1962. *Nicomachean Ethics.* Translated by Martin Oswald. Indianapolis: Bobbs-Merrill.

Ayer, Alfred J. 1952. *Language, Truth and Logic.* New York: Dover.

Bellah, Robert N. 1983. "Social science as practical reason." In *Ethics, the Social Sciences and Policy Analysis*, edited by Daniel Callahan and Bruce Jennings, 37-64. New York: Plenum Press.

Berger, Peter, Brigitte Berger, and Hensfried Kellner. 1973. "Excursus: on the obsolescence of the concept of honor." In Peter Berger, Brigitte Berger, and Hensfried Kellner, *The Homeless Mind: Modernization and Consciousness.* New York: Vintage Books.

Berlin, Isaiah. 1980. "The divorce between the science and the humanities." In Isaiah Berlin, *Against the Current.* New York: Viking Press.

Bernstein, Richard. 1978. *The Restructuring of Social and Political Theory.* Philadelphia: University of Pennsylvania Press.

Black, James and Dean Champion. 1976. *Methods and Issues in Social Research.* New York: John Wiley.

Blumer, Herbert. 1970. "What is wrong with social theory?" In *Sociological Methods: A Sourcebook,* edited by Norman Denzin, 84-95. Chicago: Aldine.

Brown, Robert. 1984. *The Nature of Social Laws: Machiavelli to Mill.* Cambridge: Cambridge University Press.

Buchanan, David. 1991. "How teens think about drugs: insights from moral reasoning and social bonding theories." *International Quarterly for Community Health Education* 11:315-332.

Buchanan, David. 1992. "An uneasy alliance: combining quantitative and qualitative research methods." *Health Education Quarterly* 19(1): 117-135.

Burdine, James and Ken McLeroy. 1992. "Practitioners' use of theory: examples from a working group." *Health Education Quarterly,* 19, 331-340.

Chavis, David and Paul Florin. 1990. *Community Development, Community Participation, and Substance Abuse Prevention.* Santa Clara County, CA: Bureau of Drug Abuse Service, Department of Health,

Cooper, John. 1975. *Reason and Human Good in Aristotle.* Cambridge, MA: Harvard University Press.

D'Onofrio, Carol. 1992. "Theory and empowerment of health education practitioners." *Health Education Quarterly* 19, 385-404.

Engberg-Pedersen, Troels. 1983. *Aristotle's Theory of Moral Insight.* Oxford: Clarendon Press.

Fawcett, Stephen, Adrienne Paine, Vincente Francisco, and Marni Vliet. 1993. "Promoting Health through Community Development." In *Promoting Health and Mental Health: Behavioral Approaches to Prevention,* edited by David Glenwick and Leonard Jason, 233-55. New York: Haworth Press.

Freudenberg, Nicholas. 1989. *Preventing AIDS.* Washington, DC: American Public Health Association.

Gardner, John W. 1984. *Excellence.* New York: W.W. Norton.

Giddens, Anthony. 1976. *New Rules of Sociological Method.* London: Hutchinson Library.

Glanz, Karen, Frances Lewis, and Barbara Rimer. 1990. "Theory, research and practice in health education: building bridges and forging links." In *Health Behavior and Health Education: Theory, Research and Practice*, edited by Karen Glanz, Frances Lewis, and Barbara Rimer, 17-32. San Francisco: Jossey-Bass.

Homans, George. 1970. "Contemporary Theory in Sociology." In *Sociological Methods: A Sourcebook,* edited by Norman Denzin, 51-69. Chicago: Aldine.

Institute of Medicine. 1989. *The Future of Public Health.* Washington, DC: National Academy of Sciences Press.

Larmore, Charles. 1987. "The centrality of judgment." In Charles Larmore, *Patterns of Moral Complexity*, 5-13. Cambridge: Cambridge University Press.

Lindblom, Charles. 1990. *Inquiry and Change: The Troubled Attempt to Understand and Shape Society.* New Haven: Yale University Press.

Lorion, Raymond and James Ross. 1992. "Programs for change: Office for Substance Abuse Prevention demonstration models." *Journal of Community Psychology* 3-9, OSAP Special Issue.

Miller, P. McC. and Michael Wilson. 1983. *A Dictionary of Social Science Methods.* New York: John Wiley.

Nussbaum, Martha. 1986. "Non-scientific deliberation." In Martha Nussbaum, *The Fragility of the Good*, 290-317. Cambridge: Cambridge University Press.

Oakeshott, Michael. 1975. *On Human Conduct.* Oxford: Clarendon Press.

Popper, Karl. 1959. *The Logic of Scientific Discovery.* New York: Hutchinson and Company.

Postman, Neil. 1988. "Social Science as Moral Theology." In Neil Postman, *Conscientious Objections: Stirring Up Trouble about Language, Technology and Education,* 3-19. New York: Alfred Knopf.

Public Health Faculty/Agency Forum. 1991. *Final Report.* Washington, DC: Bureau of Health Professions, Health Resources and Services Administration.

Reading, Hugo. 1979. *A Dictionary of the Social Sciences.* London: Routledge and Kegan Paul.

Rothman, Jack. 1979. "Three models of community organization practice." In *Strategies of Community Organization: A Book of Readings,* 3rd ed., edited by Fred Cox, John Erlich, Jack Rothman, and John Tropman, 25-45. Itasca, IL: F. E. Peacock.

Simon, Julian and Paul Burstein. 1985. *Basic Research Methods in Social Science.* 3rd ed. New York: Random House.

Smith, Page. 1990. "The social non-sciences." In Page Smith, *Killing the Spirit: Higher Education in America*, 223-252. New York: Viking Press.

Sykes, Charles. 1988. "The pseudo-scientists: the social sciences." In Charles Sykes, *Profscam: Professors and the Demise of Higher Education*, 202-223. Washington, DC: Regnery Gateway.

Taylor, Charles. 1985a. "Interpretation and the Sciences of Man." In Charles Taylor, *Philosophy and the Human Sciences*, 15-57. Cambridge: Cambridge University Press.

Taylor, Charles. 1985b. "Self-Interpreting Animals." In Charles Taylor, *Human Agency and Language*, 45-76. Cambridge: Cambridge University Press.

Taylor, Charles. 1988. "Critical Notice." *Canadian Journal of Philosophy* 18, 805-814.

van Ryn, Michelle and Catherine Heaney. 1992. "What's the use of theory?" *Health Education Quarterly* 19, 315-330.

Wallack, Lawrence. 1990. "Media advocacy: promoting health through mass communication." In *Health Behavior and Health Education: Theory. Research and Practice*, edited by Karen Glanz, Frances Lewis, and Barbara Rimer, 370-386. San Francisco: Jossey-Bass.

Wittgenstein, Ludwig. 1972. *Philosophical Investigations.* Translated by G.E.M. Anscombe. Oxford: Basil Blackford.

3. BEYOND POSITIVISM: HUMANISTIC PERSPECTIVES ON THEORY AND RESEARCH IN HEALTH EDUCATION

The purpose of this chapter is to expand the set of criteria used to define "theory" in public health education. Based on a broader understanding of the definition and uses of theory, a wider range of research strategies will become available to the field, as the purpose of research has frequently been said to develop and to test theory. One major goal in seeking to expand the scope of theory and research is to make them more relevant to health education practitioners (Burdine and McLeroy, 1992; Hochbaum and Lorig, 1992; McLeroy *et al.,* 1993).

Currently, theory and research in public health education are based virtually exclusively on the tenets of logical positivism. In one widely used textbook, Glanz *et al.,* for example, state, "In health education and health behavior, as well as in this text, the dominant perspective that supports the largest body of theory and research is that of logical positivism" (Glanz *et al.,* 1990, p. 23). For the purposes of this essay, positivism can be equated with the experimental, hypothesis-testing paradigm used in the natural sciences.

While a full critique of the positivist paradigm lies beyond the scope of this piece (see Bernstein, 1978; Lindblom, 1990; Toulmin, 1990; Buchanan, 1992, 1994), three points will help lay the foundation for the discussion that follows. In brief, the epistemological and ethical shortcomings of positivism give rise to serious reservations about its suitability for the field of health education.

First, where positivism assumes there is no essential difference between natural and social phenomena, scholarship in the humanities sees a fundamental, critical distinction between them (Polkinghorne, 1983). While there are many ways of broaching the distinction, one of the more salient differences is based on the fact that human beings have agency: the ability to choose on the basis of their intention to bring about an intended state of affairs.

The conservative philosopher Oakeshott (1975) makes the distinction between *processes* in the natural world and human *practices.* Natural processes are embedded in the very structure of nature; they are the inherent product of the composition and configuration of the component elements. Think, for example, of the processes involved in chemical reactions. In contrast, human practices require intelligence; they need to be learned, understood and granted one's assent. As Oakeshott (1975, pp. 13-14) states, "An apple does not need to have learned a 'law' of gravitation in order to fall . . . its determinateness or indeterminacy is not a result of its components having learned or understood their parts well or ill." However, manners, customs, religious observances, taboos and any other complex behavior need to be learned. Therefore, Oakeshott concludes, human practices are a categorically different kind of phenomena than natural processes. Hence, human practices require a different approach in order to understand their meaning, morality and motivation. From an epistemological standpoint, critics suggest that these differences may account for the limited success of the positivist methodology in explaining human behavior (Weed, 1995; Lawson and Floyd, 1996). Second, many scholars see positivism as part and parcel of an instrumental, utilitarian trend in the modem world, which they argue lies at the heart of the growing sense of alienation, moral malaise and social disintegration (Sullivan, 1982, 1995; Haan, *et al.,* 1983; Taylor, 1992). It is a frame of mind that views the world as if ends and means were independent *(a la* cause-and-effect), and hence, fosters an outlook primed for treating human beings as a means to achieve goals not of their own choosing (Buchanan *et al.,* 1994). While space precludes going into detail, Sullivan (1995, pp. 165-166), for example, writes:

> The dimensions of the challenge [of resolving social problems] become clearer as we ask what stands in the way of an effective response. The answer is disturbing, though manifest. Beside, or rather behind, the inertia of entrenched interests there is also an ideal and a regime of knowledge which is strongly resistant to the stance of social engagement and moral inquiry demanded of today's challenges. This is the epistemic regime of positivism . . . The continuing hold of positivistic dogma over the thinking and practice of higher education is a key problem which must be confronted by anyone who concludes that the needs of our time demand a reshaping of professional knowledge.

In this view, positivism is not only not the only method for gaining valid knowledge, but it is a powerful ideology that thwarts the field's interests in alleviating suffering and promoting social justice. Critics assert that ethical concerns about the ideological impact of positivism make countenance of the soft "we need both kinds" position (Steckler, *et al.,* 1992) pleaded by many researchers today untenable (Davies, 1996).

Finally, a shift from an instrumental positivist framework towards a more humanistic outlook would have major implications for the practice of health education. In the positivist perspective, a beguiling metaphor for the field is the practice of medicine. Just as doctors and nurses measure high blood pressure and prescribe medications that effectively reduce this risk factor, so the analogy for health education is a science with the same precision and efficacy of being able to measure a behavioral antecedent (say, outcome beliefs) and to prescribe educational interventions that will cause a comparable change in behavior. A large part of the continuing appeal of positivistic methods is its promise to provide the same power to achieve control over human behavior as medical providers now have over human physiology.

Table 3.1: Seven functions of theory

Paradigm	Function
Positivist	
Prediction	To hypothesize in advance about the strength and direction of relationships among independent variables or about the results of experimental interventions
Explanation	To give or show the cause of a phenomenon
Humanistic	
Making assumptions explicit	To develop or formulate direct, publicly available statements about states of affairs previously taken for granted
Understanding	To grasp or uncover the meaning and significance of events
Sense-making	To put forward an interpretation of events to stimulate a discerning awareness and appreciation of their significance
Sensitization	To stimulate a more receptive, more responsive and more delicate awareness of the nuances of a given situation through thorough analytic descriptions
Critique	To evaluate and analyze the merits and demerits of extant and potential states of affairs

In contrast, in a point developed further in the conclusion, humanistic research promotes the advance of *phronesis,* or practical reason (see Buchanan, 1994; Taylor, 1995). The purpose of developing practical reason is not to predict, control or change anyone, but to deepen our understanding of what it is to live a human life, to contribute to human self-understanding and decency.

With that background, the body of the chapter starts with a description of the most common definition of theory used in the field today. This definition is based on the principles of logical positivism. It then discusses two functions of theory in the positivist mode: prediction and explanation. It goes on to present an alternative definition of theory, based on values and purposes guiding humanistic research. With an expanded definition of theory, the chapter then develops five additional functions of theory to guide research. A summary description of the seven uses of theory is presented in Table 3.1. I conclude with a discussion of the implications of this expanded conceptualization for bridging the gap between theory and practice in health education today.

Two functions of theory from a positivist perspective

At the core of positivism is the verification principle. According to verification principle, one can distinguish valid knowledge from mere personal opinion if and only if there is a means to confirm (i.e., verify) the truth of any given statement. To test their validity, statements need to be re-cast as cause-and-effect hypotheses of the 'If-Then' form: if *X* occurs, then *Y* will result. For example, to test whether attitudes are related to behaviors, we need to re-frame the statement as a hypothesis, like "If attitudes change (become more positive), then behaviors will change (become more frequent)." We can then test whether attitudes are, *in fact,* related to behaviors.

In the positivist perspective, theories must therefore be in the form of statements about relationships among different variables from which hypotheses can be deduced. Hypotheses make predictions about the effect of changes in the independent variables upon the dependent variable of interest. Thus, the first and most common use of theory is to make predictions.

Prediction

Virtually all health education textbooks today use some variation on this standard positivist perspective on the form and function theory is supposed to take. For example, Glanz *et al.,* (1990), citing Kerlinger (1986), present the following characteristic definition:

> [Theory is] a set of interrelated constructs (concepts), definitions and propositions that present a systematic view of phenomena by specifying relations among variables, with the purpose of explaining and predicting the phenomena. (p. 21)

To test predictions, researchers conduct experiments by modifying the independent variables and observing whether the expected effect on the dependent variable occurs. For example, researchers predict that increases in perceived susceptibility will lead to changes in health behaviors, such as the adoption of protective behaviors. Conducting experiments constitutes the most rigorous and ultimate standard through which the validity of theory is established. It is the ideal to which all positivist research strives.

This experimental, hypothesis-testing model has been hugely successful in the natural sciences (where it is absolutely appropriate, as Oakeshott suggests). Although it has not nearly achieved the same degree of success in studies of human behavior, positivists believe there are no irresolvable differences between the natural sciences and the social sciences. As Kerlinger (1979) writes elsewhere, “The general approach to knowledge and understanding of physics and psychology is the same.”

The positivist paradigm dominates the field of health promotion today. When the function of theory is to make predictions, then the purpose of research is to develop and to test theories of the form of “a set of interrelated constructs (concepts), definitions and propositions that present a systematic view of phenomena” by specifying relations among variables. This type of theorizing and its associated research program are currently the most commonly accepted and defended approach towards scholarship, grant support and publication in the field.

Putting theory into practice is straightforward here. After theories have been validated, practitioners are expected to know (usually through academic training programs) which factors they need to modify in order to achieve the desired results. For instance, to increase condom use, health educators now know that they need to design activities that will instill a sense of susceptibility to infection in their target audience, and so on.

Explanation

A second function of theory is explanation. This use of theory follows from a positivist epistemology too. Indeed, prediction and explanation are sometimes regarded as identical processes of scientific thinking (von Wright, 1971). That is, it is the ability to make accurate predictions that enables one to explain the relationships among variables.

One distinction between prediction and explanation is that explanation is used to make events intelligible after the fact (von Wright, 1971). Where prediction is forward-looking, explanation is *post-hoc.* The function of theory in this sense is not to anticipate events, but to account for what has already happened. For example, health educators may predict that an educational intervention will lead to an increase in protective behaviors, such as condom use to protect against HIV infection. However, when the results show little change in behaviors, we may invoke theory to explain that the lack of perceived susceptibility among youth explains the low level of resultant behavior changes.

In short, because of the standard set by the verification principle, positivist theory must take a highly specific form. The goal for researchers is to develop theories from which testable hypotheses can be deduced. Unless theory yields verifiable hypotheses, positivist principles hold that researchers cannot provide the kind of demonstrative evidence that separates potentially erroneous beliefs from scientifically validated facts. Hence, formulating theories from which testable hypotheses can be deduced is the standard setting the field's research agenda.

Five functions of theory from a humanistic perspective

For the sake of argument, let us now assume there is an intrinsic critical distinction to be made between social *practices* and natural *processes,* and that the methods used in researching things in the natural world are not necessarily the only ones that can provide valuable, valid information. If we bracket for the time being the idea that theory must take the particular form defined by the verification principle, then a number of new possibilities for defining the form and function of theory open up. For now, let us say social "theory" can tentatively be considered any answer to the question, "Why?" as in "Why do people act this way?" Where positivism specifies that intelligible answers must identify the *causes* of behavior, humanistic research, in contrast, seeks to uncover the *reasons* that people do the things that they do.

Making assumptions explicit

To begin, we may start with a function of theory that can be defined in either positivist or humanistic terms. In addition to prediction and explanation, another potential function of theory is to make one's assumptions explicit.

Many, if not most, public health promotion programs are developed and implemented without an identified theoretical basis (Burdine and McLeroy, 1992; Hochbaum, *et al.,* 1992). The field has devoted considerable energy towards pondering this state of affairs, but for whatever reasons, practitioners rarely set out designing programs based explicitly on any of the field's familiar theories. More often than not, practitioners call on their experience and common sense in developing programs. I think this is what people mean when they say there is a gap between theory and practice in the field. However, if we can expand our set of ideas about what constitutes theory, we may see that these programs are not atheoretical.

When theory is broadened to include any answer to the question, "Why?" then, in those instances where the more well-known theories are not invoked, it may not be that the programs are atheoretical, but rather it is more likely the case that the underlying theory has not been explicitly articulated. From a broader perspective, it is virtually impossible to develop a program without some theory, however implicit, some rationale about why the proposed activities will lead towards the desired result. Each of us carries a large set of assumptions that are "always already" there about why people do the things they do (Schutz, 1967). Unless practitioners are doing program planning capriciously, they pick strategies based on why they think people are behaving in a particular way and what may lead them to re-consider their current behavior.

For example, a popular exercise in youth development programs is to draw a "life map," a pictorial representation of an individual's significant life events. If one looks for an explicit theoretical basis for this exercise, looking for something like Social Learning Theory, the Theory of Protection Motivation, Transtheoretical Theory, and so on, it cannot be found. However, if one were to press the practitioner about why she decided to conduct this exercise, a wealth of ideas would inevitably emerge. The exercise builds trust, which may be lacking in these youths' lives. It creates an open atmosphere, a space where they can feel safe to disclose problems that are bothering them. It is cathartic: the opportunity to talk about problems in and of itself releases some of the pain they are carrying. It is fun and engaging, engrossing otherwise bored youth. Behind each of these ideas are implicit theories about why youth get into trouble these days: they are isolated, with no one they can trust or turn to for support, they have been hurt, they are bored.

From a positivist perspective, each of these ideas needs to be transformed into testable hypotheses to determine their validity. Researchers seek to develop operational definitions to measure social isolation, painful life events and boredom, and then look for correlations with identified public health problems (substance abuse, unprotected sex, etc.). If they find a correlation, then the most powerful test of the validity of these factors is to conduct an experiment, with random assignment to treatment and control groups. An intervention (like the Life Map exercise) is conducted to see if it lowers the treatment group's sense of isolation, boredom, etc., and then observe whether these changes in turn lead to reductions in problem behaviors. After conducting these experiments, then and only then would one know for sure that boredom, etc., are valid risk factors that should be targeted for intervention.

However, from a humanistic perspective, one could take a different approach. The reason for this is that, from a humanistic perspective, the causal significance of these issues pales before their significance in terms of meaningfulness. Boredom does not *cause* youth to do anything. It is a feeling and a way of experiencing the moment about which one may choose to do something or not. It may mean one needs to learn to recognize, name and deal with the discomfort. It may mean it is time to take up a hobby. However, it may also only require an act of re-interpretation, as in reveling in the glory of idle summer days.

In the positivist perspective, the condition is viewed instrumentally, as a risk factor, something to be reduced or eliminated in order to solve social problems. In this perspective, the task of health education is to design activities that will lower the identified risk factors. But, from a humanistic perspective, these ideas are the stuff of life, where means and ends are inextricably intertwined. How we think about them (e.g. boredom as risk factor versus boredom as potentially treasured time free of demands) gives shape to how we lead our lives. The role of boredom in people's lives raises questions: questions about the degree to which life should be filled with constant stimulation and distractions; about how much we should demand of ourselves and others that these times be committed to constructive, elevating uses; questions about the shape of the life that we want to live, as all of us grope for ways to make meaningful use of our short time on earth. Here, the practitioner can problematize the issues, raising questions for discussion and deliberation to which all parties can be invited to respond. Making assumptions explicit creates an opportunity to open a dialogue about formerly implicit, unexamined suppositions about the reasons people do things (like taking drugs). Together, people can then decide whether they want to do something about the situation or not.

For researchers, a change in perspective would have many implications. Rather than viewing practitioners as ignorant or negligent about the benefits of using proven theories, researchers could come to see them as a primary source for theory development (Burdine and McLeroy,

1992; Green, 2006). Rather than trying to come up with a single standardized operational definition, researchers would seek out as many dimensions as possible regarding the ways in which people experience these subjective states, trying to uncover rich and variegated descriptions that explore all of the lived nuances, shades of meaning and paradoxa. These studies would be helpful to practitioners in helping them to become more articulate about their own assumptions, to diagnose the diverse situations that they face better and to recognize when people are having trouble making their assumptions more explicit.

A change in perspective would also create an opportunity for opening the field up to discussions about how these issues have been treated in other fields, such as literature (Spacks, 1995) or philosophy (Russell, 1935), breaking down the unfortunate barriers that have arisen between the humanities and the social sciences. By moving back and forth between empirical data and subtle, creative portraits, philosophical reflections and historical developments, researchers could provide the kind of knowledge that would help practitioners bring new insights, new ways of looking at the issue and additional food for thought to the discussions.

Understanding

The most frequently stated alternative function of theory, beyond prediction and explanation, is understanding. Extensive discussions of the differences between explanation and understanding have been put forward, including Von Wright's *Explanation and Understanding* (1971), Apel's *Understanding and Explanation* (1984) and Taylor's "Explanation and practical reason" (1995). In brief, where explanation seeks to make events predictable through knowledge of their causes, understanding seeks to make phenomena intelligible through knowledge of their *telos*: their aim, intention, purpose and meaning (von Wright, 1971). The inclusion of understanding would expand the boundaries of theory and research to include not only the search for causes of behavior, but also the task of seeking to grasp its underlying rationale (Anderson, 1993; Steinberg, 1993). From a humanistic perspective, the search for independent, antecedent causes will never be sufficient to explain behavior because a more complete understanding depends on comprehending the aims, purposes and intentions of the individual. While intentions may be influenced by past events, their formation principally takes shape in a creative process of picturing how one would like to exercise one's agency, one's willpower, to change the course of future events. They are unpredictable precisely to the degree that people are free to make choices about what they want to do. However, being unpredictable does not mean that people's behavior is unintelligible or indecipherable. To understand the meaning of behavior, researchers must look beyond prior causes to search for the protagonist's purposes. These purposes are expressed as reasons, the underlying rationale, for the choice of one course of action over another. People are not prisoners of the past, inexorably driven by antecedent causes. People *act,* not just react.

At this point, we can offer a well-known alternative definition of theory. The anthropologist Geertz (1973, p. 5) states:

> Believing, with Max Weber, that man is an animal suspended in webs of significance he himself has spun, I take culture to be those webs, and the analysis of it to be therefore not an experimental science in search of law but an interpretive one in search of meaning.

Rather than seeking to develop theory in the form of "a set of inter-related constructs . . .", theory as understanding is often presented in the form of narratives (Coles, 1989). Narrative is an integral way in which human intelligence organizes experience to grasp its meaning (Appleby *et al.,* 1994). Narrative connects the past and the present to the future. The value and validity of this type of theorizing is frequently experienced as revelation, the "Ah-Ha" experience, as in "now I get it, now I understand what is going on in this situation."

If this type of theorizing were to be more widely accepted and available in the field, practitioners could turn to theory not for prescriptions about what to do but for insight. If the definition of theory were enlarged, we could better appreciate the value of reading, for example, a narrative description of the pervasive influence of "individualism" in American life (Bellah *et al.,* 1985). The value of this type of research comes not from some conclusion about whether individualism is a risk factor that needs to be eliminated but to see more clearly the ways in which we unconsciously and unintentionally reinforce this value and recognize better its many permutations as we listen to others struggle to figure out what is going in our society (see, e.g. Buchanan, 1991a, on its relationship to substance abuse). Through the research and theorizing of these scholars, features of situations that were formerly opaque, puzzling or unacknowledged are made more salient, transparent and less confusing.

Sense-making

The next function of theorizing is "sense-making." The distinction here is that "understanding" is usually viewed as a process of discovery, whereas "sense-making" involves an act of creation.

The sense-making function of theory introduces the notion of the social construction of reality (Berger and Luckman, 1966) or, as Searle (1995) re-phrased it, the construction of social reality. Here, the contention is that, in the social world, the principles and values by which we lead our lives are not "out there" embedded in the structure of the universe waiting to be discovered, but they are corrigible products of the human intellect subject to constant revision and re-thinking. As theory is used here, researchers do not deny that the act of explicating a situation is a creative act in which the researcher–"values, warts and all"–actively molds how events are to be interpreted (Appleby *et al.,* 1993, p. 249). The process of conducting research and developing theory is more one of making, rather than finding, creating, rather than uncovering (Lindblom, 1990). Or as Anderson (1993, p. 69) puts it, researchers are "not discovering meaning but bravely imputing meaning to a universe, which, more likely than not, has none."

Buchanan (1996) provides an example of the applicability to health education of this particular use of theory. In a case study of community coalition building, Buchanan tries to make sense of the constant tensions and frequent breakdowns in communication between community members and university academics. Using the community organizing typology developed by Rothman, he attempts to show how the actions of community members can be interpreted to fall under the principles of "locality development," whereas the actions of academics can be better described in terms of the characteristics of a "social planning" approach. Because community members and academics operate using different goals, assumptions, basic change strategies, etc., the two parties frequently talk past one another, fail to see the significance of issues voiced by the other side and fail to understand why the others do not share their concerns.

The point here is that I am not claiming to have discovered that community members are inherently "locality developers" or academics "social planners" in a way that leads them invariably to act in certain ways. The point is that this type of research and theorizing may help those involved (and other readers) get a handle on potential sources of confusion and frustration. It gives people points of reference to discuss to see if they can work out their differences. The test of its validity is whether it does, *in practice,* help people to make sense of their situation.

Sensitization

Yet another function of theory is sensitization. The sensitizing function of theory serves to heighten people's awareness of a broader range of the particular contingencies bearing on a specific situation. Here, theory and research are used to sharpen, highlight and bring to the foreground as many aspects as possible that make the situation at hand unique, distinct and different from other situations (in direct contrast to the search for common, generalizable features sought in positivist research).

Recalling Geertz's definition of theory, he suggests that the way researchers "analyze webs of significance" is through "an interpretive [approach] in search of meaning." Examples of this type of theorizing are the analytic themes, frameworks and ideal types that emerge in ethnographies, field work, case studies and the like. One such example is the theoretical construct of "institutional embeddedness" (Buchanan, 1991b). Through in-depth interviews, Buchanan found that some youth frame decisions about drug use in terms of their roles within their families, schools, church and community (e.g., "I don't think I should because Baptists are not allowed to"), whereas others think about the decision largely in terms of their individual desires (e.g., "I don't feel like it"). Through these types of studies, we become more sensitive to what is going on in a situation, where without them certain features would pass unnoticed.

The value of these types of studies is that people can develop a more perceptive, more discerning appreciation of their unique circumstances when they have these constructs available to them. When one reads a good (precise, authentic, accurate, persuasive) ethnography, aspects of a situation about which one was formerly blind, puzzled or unawares become more apparent. The warrants for the validity of sensitizing concepts are the felt capacities of the reader for acting more lucidly/less blindly, more cognizantly/less obliviously, with a keener, more refined sense of discrimination in functioning in the singular situations they encounter as they move through the world.

Critique

The final use of theory presented here is critique (Fay, 1987). Gitlin (1991) reminds us that social theory was historically conceived in terms of social criticism in the service of social change. Theory as critique traces its roots to the emancipatory project of the Enlightenment, particularly as it focused on the problematics of existing power structures (Habermas, 1988). Sociology began as an attempt to find footing for social critique. If one thinks of the works of Marx, Durkheim or Weber, all were deeply concerned about the contemporary state of society. Each in his own way was trying to flesh out ideas for alternative forms of social organization as a way of calling attention to the problems and deformations in the extant mode.

The purpose of theorizing here is to challenge a going concern by holding it up to a more ideal image (Anderson, 1993). This form of theorizing confronts the *status quo* by asking the questions that need to be asked, raising the issues that need to be raised and offering counterfactuals to claims about the inevitability of current conditions (Lindblom, 1990). In its most provocative form, researchers in this mode write about piercing the veil of ideological hegemony to root out false consciousness. In its less strident forms, theory as critique is an effort to re-think assumptions by postulating different possibilities.

While the decline of this type of theorizing has recently been lamented (Jacoby, 1987), the tradition lives on in numerous works, such as Bellah *et al.'s, The Good Society* (1991), and Boyte's (1989), and Etzioni's (1993) respective versions of communitarian society. The most well-known critical theorist in health education is, of course, Freire (1968, 1973). In its own way, this piece is a theoretical account critiquing current practices in the field of health promotion research and offering an outline of other possibilities.

Conclusion

The purpose of this chapter has been to sketch out humanistic alternatives to the form and functions of theory in health education. It is hoped that broader criteria for defining theory will open the door to a broader range of research strategies and thereby make research more relevant to practitioners. To conclude, a common concern, which needs to be addressed, is the standards by which the validity of humanistic research should be assessed.

One part of the continuing appeal of positivist research is its declaration of clear, precise, unequivocal criteria for distinguishing scientific fact from personal opinion. The historians Appleby *et al.* (1994) suggest that indeed the principal legacy of positivism today is an enduring belief in the dichotomy between objective knowledge and subjective opinion. Throughout this analysis, I have made numerous references to the ways in which the validity of humanistic research is evaluated. It is time to bring these thoughts together to summarize.

To cut to the chase, there are no criteria in humanistic research that offer the same degree of certainty as those used in the natural sciences. Humanistic researchers accept that their interpretations are always "essentially contestable" (Geertz, 1973, 29). However, in Taylor's (1985, p. 18) analysis, this is not a methodological failure but rather something inherent in the nature of social phenomena: "such uncertainty is an ineradicable part of our epistemological predicament." In its starkest terms, the ultimate guarantor of the truth of assertions about the social realm is, therefore, the mutual assent of those affected by the claims. At first sight, this may seem frightening, especially for a field that has struggled for legitimacy, growing up in the shadow of the biomedical sciences where positivist approaches are appropriate and highly efficacious. What then can we offer as collateral warrants for the value and validity of humanistic research?

Challenging the positivist legacy, most scholars today acknowledge the necessity of establishing a third option: something in-between experimental, scientific proof and the perception that anything less is inherently suspect (Polkinghorne, 1983; Chandler *et al.,* 1991). It is possible to conduct social research that is supported by evidence, but corrigible, inherently in need of constant revision and correction (Schama, 1991). We gain confidence in the quality of humanistic research the more closely it is tied to specific concrete material events and the more closely it builds on prior research (even while pointing out its inadequacies and proposing subsequent refinements and amendments). We look to assess its quality by the degree to which it is precise (sharply detailed in its descriptions), accurate (neither omissions nor fabrications; corroborated from multiple perspectives), authentic (documented; free of distortions; aware of its limits) and persuasive (it makes a compelling case; Geertz, 1995). However, make no mistake, the assessment of humanistic research inescapably requires judgment, the same kind of judgment earlier labeled practical reason.

In the end, this is what I think it is all about. The field needs the kind of research that can help all of us–researchers and practitioners alike–become more sensitive, critical, articulate, constructive, less oblivious to those subtle yet important dynamics that sway public debate, less blind to unconscious assumptions and more understanding of the complexities of modern political life. For researchers, the program outlined here suggests three immediate directions.

First, researchers need to work more closely with practitioners, but turning the tables, to see what we can learn from them, rather than the usual other way round: what are the theories they are putting into practice? This type of research is dialogical, going back and forth, give and take, as both researcher and practitioner struggle to articulate tacit assumptions and make sense of the swirl of events anytime one engages the community. Second, researchers need to write up more ethnographies, case studies, policy analyses, historical reconstructions, thought pieces, analyses of overarching themes from focus groups, critiques, field work, oral histories, key informant interviews, assessments of public opinion and much more comprehensive literature reviews. (In a telling indicator of the enduring legacy of positivism, one of the rare ethnographies to reach print was published in the "Commentary" section of public health's masthead journal; see Eckert, 1983.) Third, public health education researchers need to incorporate the work of researchers in philosophy (e.g. Hyland, 1981; Nussbaum, 1994), history (e.g. Whorton, 1982; Green, 1986; Baur, 1988) and literature (e.g. Zeh, 1988; Burke, 1969; Downie, 1994) into their analyses of how theory can be put into practice.

In an alternative mode, the real test of the value and validity of health education theories would lie in their ability to provoke discussion and action. Supported by research of a different kind, practitioners could make public health truly public, raising questions for discussion for all concerned community members to deliberate. The power of this type of research derives from its ability to inspire others to see things in a new light so that they might change their minds. Ultimately, the success of this approach relies on the cultivation and flourishing of people's capacity to discern excellence from nonsense, to judge good from bad ideas and to rectify efforts to live together decently (Anderson, 1993). Relative to prediction and control, I submit that the alternatives to theory and research outlined here lie closer to health education's most cherished principles.

References

Anderson, Charles. 1993. *Prescribing the Life of the Mind: An essay on the purpose of the university, the aims of liberal education, the competence of citizens and the cultivation of practical reason*. Madison, WI: University of Wisconsin Press.

Apel, Karl-Otto. 1984. *Understanding and Explanation: A Transcendental-Pragmatic Approach.* Cambridge: MIT Press.

Appleby, Joyce, Lynn Hunt, and Margaret Jacob. 1994. *Telling the Truth about History.* New York: W. W. Norton.

Baur, Susan. 1988. *Hypochondria: Woeful Imaginings.* Berkeley, CA: University of California Press.

Bellah, Robert. 1983. "Social Science as Practical Reason." In *Ethics, The Social Sciences, and Policy Analysis*, edited by Daniel Callahan and Bruce Jennings, 37-64, New York: Plenum Press.

Bellah, Robert, Richard Madsen, William Sullivan, Ann Swidler, and Steve Tipton. 1985. *Habits of the Heart: Individualism and Commitment in American Life.* Berkeley, CA: University of California Press.

Bellah, Robert, Richard Madsen, William Sullivan, Ann Swidler, and Steve Tipton. 1991. *The Good Society.* New York: Alfred Knopf.

Berger, Peter and Thomas Luckman. 1966. *The Social Construction of Reality.* New York: Doubleday.

Bernstein, Richard. 1978. *The Restructuring of Social and Political Theory.* Philadelphia, PA: University of Pennsylvania Press.

Blumer, Herbert. 1970. "What is wrong with social theory?" In *Sociological Methods: A Sourcebook*, edited by Norman Denzin, 84-95. Chicago: Aldine.

Boyte, Harry. 1989. *Commonwealth: A Return to Citizen Politics.* New York: Free Press.

Buchanan, David. 1991a. "A social history of American drug use." *Journal of Drug Issues* 22: 31-52.

Buchanan, David. 1991b. "How teens think about drugs: insights from moral reasoning and social bonding theories." *International Quarterly of Community Health Education* 11: 315-332.

Buchanan, David. 1992. "An uneasy alliance: combining quantitative and qualitative research methods." *Health Education Quarterly* 19(1):7-135

Buchanan, David. 1994. "Reflections on the relationship between theory and practice." *Health Education Research* 9: 273-283.

Buchanan, David. 1996. Building Academic-Community linkages for health promotion: a case study in Massachusetts." *American Journal of Health Promotion* 10: 29-36.

Buchanan, David, Zafar Hossain, and Sasiragha Reddy. 1994. "Social marketing: a critical appraisal." *Health Promotion International* 9(1): 49-57.

Burdine, James and Ken McLeroy. 1992. "Practitioners' use of theory: examples from a workgroup." *Health Education Quarterly* 19: 331-340.

Burke, Kenneth. 1945. *A Grammar of Motives.* Berkeley, CA: University of California Press.

Chandler, James, Arnold Davidson, A. and Harry Harootunian (Eds.). 1991. *Questions of Evidence: Proof, Practice, and Persuasion across the Disciplines.* Chicago, IL: University of Chicago Press.

Coles, Robert. 1989. *The Call of Stories: Teaching and the Moral Imagination.* New York: Houghton-Mifflin.

Davies, John B. 1996. "Health research: need for a methodological revolution?" *Health Education Research* 11(2): i-iv.

Downie, Robin S. 1994. *The Healing Arts: An Oxford Illustrated Anthology.* Oxford: Oxford University Press.

Eckert, Penelope. 1983. "Beyond the statistics of adolescent smoking." *American Journal of Public Health* 73: 439-441.

Etzioni, Amitai. 1993. *The Spirit of Community: Rights, Responsibilities, and the Communitarian Agenda.* New York: Crown Publishers.

Fay, Brian. 1987. *Critical Social Science.* Ithaca, NY: Cornell University Press.

Freire, Paulo. 1968. *Pedagogy of the Oppressed.* New York: The Seabury Press.

Freire, Paulo. 1973. *Education for Critical Consciousness.* New York: The Seabury Press.

Geertz, Clifford. 1973. *The Interpretation of Cultures.* New York: Basic Books.

Geertz, Clifford. 1996. *After the Fact.* Cambridge: Harvard University Press.

Gitlin, Todd. 1991. "The politics of communication and the communication of politics." In *Mass Media and Society*, edited by James Curran and Michael Gurevitch, 329-342. London: Edward Arnold.

Glanz, Karen, Frances Lewis, and Barbara Rimer. 1990. *Health Behavior and Health Education: Theory, Research and Practice.* San Francisco, CA: Jossey-Bass.

Green, Harvey. 1986. *Fit for America: Health. Fitness, Sport and American Society.* Baltimore, MD: The Johns Hopkins University Press.

Green, Lawrence. 2006. "Public Health Asks of Systems Science: To Advance Our Evidence-Based Practice, Can You Help Us Get More Practice-Based Evidence?" *American Journal of Public Health* 96(3):406-9.

Haan, Norma, Robert Bellah, Paul Rabinow, and William Sullivan (Eds.). 1983. *Social Science as Moral Inquiry.* New York: Columbia University Press.

Habermas, Jürgen. 1988. *On the Logic of the Social Sciences.* Cambridge: MIT Press.

Hochbaum, Godfrey and Kate Lorig. 1992. "Foreword to the roles and uses of theory in health education practice." *Health Education Quarterly* 19: 291-294.

Hochbaum, Godfrey, James Sorenson, and Kate Lorig. 1992. "Theory in health education practice." *Health Education Quarterly* 19: 295-314.

Hyland, Drew. 1981. *The Virtue of Philosophy: An Interpretation of Plato's Charmides.* Athens, OH: Ohio University Press.

Jacoby, Russell. 1987. *The Last Intellectuals: American Culture in the Age of Academe.* New York: Basic Books.

Kerlinger, Fred N. 1979. *Behavioral Research: A Conceptual Approach.* New York: Holt, Rinehart and Winston.

Kerlinger, Fred N. 1986. *Foundations of Behavioral Research,* 3rd ed. New York: Holt, Rinehart and Winston.

Lawson, John and Jerald Floyd. 1996. "The future of epidemiology: a humanist response." *American Journal of Public Health* 86: 1029.
Lindblom, Charles. 1990. *Inquiry and Change: The Troubled Attempt to Understand and Shape Society.* New Haven, CT: Yale University Press.
McLeroy, Ken, Allan Steckler, Bruce Simons-Morton, Robert Goodman, Nell Gottlieb, and James Burdine. 1993. "Social science theory in health education: time for a new model?" *Health Education Research* 8: 305-312.
Nussbaum, Martha. 1994. *The Therapy of Desire: Theory and Practice in Hellenistic Ethics.* Princeton, NJ: Princeton University Press.
Oakeshott, Michael. 1975. *On Human Conduct.* Oxford: Clarendon Press.
Polkinghorne, Donald. 1983. *Methodology for the Human Sciences: Systems of Inquiry.* Albany, NY: State University of New York Press.
Russell, Bertrand. 1935. *In Praise of Idleness, and other Essays.* New York: W. W. Norton.
Scharma, Simon. 1991. *Dead Certainties (Unwarranted Speculations).* New York: Alfred Knopf.
Schutz, Alfred. 1967. *The Phenomenology of the Social World.* Evanston, IL: Northwestern University Press.
Searle, John. 1995. *The Construction of Social Reality.* New York: The Free Press.
Spades, Patricia. 1995. *Boredom: Literary History of a State of Mind.* Chicago, IL: University of Chicago Press.
Steckler, Allan, Ken McLeroy, Robert Goodman, Sheryl Bird, and Lauri McCormick. 1992. "Toward integrating qualitative and quantitative methods: an introduction." *Health Education Quarterly* 19: 1-8.
Steinberg, Peter. 1993. *The Concept of Political Judgment.* Chicago, IL: University of Chicago Press.
Sullivan, William. 1982. *Reconstructing Public Philosophy.* Berkeley, CA: University of California Press.
Sullivan, William. 1995. *Work and Integrity: The Crisis and Promise of Professionalism in America.* New York: Harper Business.
Taylor, Charles. 1985. "Interpretation and the sciences of man." In Charles Taylor, *Philosophy and the Human Sciences,*15-57. Cambridge: Cambridge University Press.
Taylor, Charles. 1992. *The Ethics of Authenticity.* Cambridge: Harvard University Press.
Taylor, Charles. 1995. "Explanation and practical reason." In Charles Taylor, *Philosophical Arguments,* 34-60. Cambridge, MA: Harvard University Press.

Toulmin, Stephen. 1990. *Cosmopolis: The Hidden Agenda of Modernity*. New York: The Free Press.

von Wright, Georg. 1971. *Explanation and Understanding*. Ithaca, NY: Cornell University Press.

Weed, Douglas. 1995. "Epidemiology, the humanities and public health." *American Journal of Public Health* 85: 914-918.

Whorton, James. 1982. *Crusaders for Fitness: The History of the American Health Reformers*. Princeton, NJ: Princeton University Press.

Zeh, Juli. 1988. *The Method*. London: Harvill Secker.

4. An Uneasy Alliance: Combining Qualitative and Quantitative Research Methods

Any health professional who has tried to use the results of social scientific research to guide the planning or evaluation of health promotion programs is undoubtedly well acquainted with the limitations of both qualitative and quantitative research (Krenz and Sax, 1986; Borman, LeCompte, and Goetz). On the one hand, the results of quantitative research often seem shallow and abstract. In the quest for a parsimonious explanatory model, quantitative researchers try to identify independent variables that are generalizable to the population as a whole. By definition, these variables have been found to correlate with the dependent variable of interest in sample populations composed of people who may differ by socioeconomic status, race, gender, age, religion, etc. It is not surprising therefore that any factors that hold up are usually both banal and not particularly powerful predictors of behavior.

On the other hand, the results of qualitative research almost invariably raise questions about its objectivity and representativeness. In an effort to provide thick, rich descriptions, qualitative researchers rely on a relatively small number of case studies. One cannot help but wonder whether (or in what ways) both the selection of the case in hand and the particular observations pertaining to it are idiosyncratic. Even if several examples are cited to illustrate an emergent theme, nagging doubts remain about how representative they are of anyone or any situation other than the one under consideration. One also wonders whether different researchers would have found the same results and arrived at the same conclusions. If not, what does that say about the status of the report?

Given the strengths and weaknesses of each, the prospect of combining qualitative and quantitative methods would seem on the surface to be a particularly promising research design. But in practice, this usually means that qualitative research is relegated to an epistemologically subordinate role. Qualitative research is regarded as an exploratory, descriptive, or hypothesis-generating method. Results from qualitative studies must await the true test of valid and reliable knowledge that is gained only through quantitative, hypothesis-testing, experimental research designs.

This chapter describes one attempt to integrate these approaches. Its major purpose is to present an analysis of the difficulties encountered in trying to reconcile the different goals, assumptions, and standards for evaluation of qualitative and quantitative research.

Description of the Research

The research described here (and elsewhere; Buchanan, 1991) was designed to gain a better understanding of the processes that put adolescents at risk for substance abuse. Based on the foregoing considerations, an approach that could combine the depth of qualitative research with the breadth of quantitative research seemed the most sensible way to proceed. To take advantage of the strengths of each and make them mutually informative, the respective methods were linked in a two-stage research design.

In the first stage of the research, 255 eighth grade students from five junior high schools in the San Francisco Bay Area volunteered to participate in the study. Students filled out a six-page survey questionnaire that covered the following four areas: (1) demographic information; (2) personal experience with drugs; (3) perceptions of different social issues as moral, social-conventional, or personal events (Turiel, 1983; Nucci, 1985) (including drug use and standardized controls); and (4) use of leisure time.

To link the quantitative and qualitative results and still protect confidentiality, the research design made use of a "quasi-anonymous" data collection procedure. Before distribution, each questionnaire was coded with a five-digit letter/number code. These codes were listed on a separate roster with the names of the participating students. Questionnaires were distributed by calling student names and handing them the appropriately numbered questionnaire. Student names thus did not appear on the questionnaires. But, by referring to the rostered code numbers, the questionnaire results for each individual student were known to the researcher.

The second stage of the research consisted of in-depth, follow-up interviews. Students were selected for interviews based on their questionnaire results. In a nod to the tacit hierarchy of quantitative and qualitative research methods, the sampling frame for selecting interviewees was set up so that simple statistical tests could be conducted on the interview results. Interview participants were selected on the basis of their: (1) drug use status–to obtain equal numbers of nonusers, experimenters, and experienced drug users; and (2) demographic characteristics–to obtain equal numbers of students from two different socio-economic groups and by gender. With roughly equal numbers of students in each cell, the results of the interviews could be used to test whether the responses of nonusers, experimenters, and experienced drug users were significantly different. The

Table 4.1: Proposed Interview Sample Characteristics by SES* and Drug Use Experience

	Nonuser[a]	Experimental[a]	Experienced[a]	Total
Low SES[b]	15	15	15	45
Middle SES[b]	15	15	15	45
Total	30	30	30	90

* – SES = Socioeconomic Status
[a] – Nonuser defined as someone who had never tried any illegal drug; Experimental user defined as someone who had tried marijuana but no other illegal drug; Experienced used defined as someone who had tried marijuana and some other illegal drug or someone who had sold an illegal drug
[b] – Low socioeconomic status (SES) defined as someone attending a school where over 60% of students were on AID to Families with Dependent Children (AFDC); Middle SES defined as attending school where less than 1% of students were on AFDC

Table 4.2: Actual Interview Sample Characteristics by SES* and Drug Use Experience

	Nonuser[a]	Experimental[a]	Experienced[a]	Total
Low SES[b]	15	16	7	38
Middle SES[b]	19	21	17	57
Total	34	37	24	95

* – SES = Socioeconomic Status
[a] – Nonuser defined as someone who had never tried any illegal drug; Experimental user defined as someone who had tried marijuana but no other illegal drug; Experienced used defined as someone who had tried marijuana and some other illegal drug or someone who had sold an illegal drug
[b] – Low socioeconomic status (SES) defined as someone attending a school where over 60% of students were on AID to Families with Dependent Children (AFDC); Middle SES defined as attending school where less than 1% of students were on AFDC

proposed interview sample and the actual final interview sample are shown in Tables 4.1 and 4.2. The results of the interview analysis could also be linked to the questionnaire results through the code-numbered student rosters.

Two examples illustrate how quantitative and qualitative methods could be used to augment one another. In a simple example of the anticipated process, analysis of the interviews revealed that a number of students expressed concerns about current U.S. drug laws. They found them irrational, confusing, and hypocritical. Figure 4.1 provides some representative examples.

Figure 4.1: Perceived Irrationality of Drug Laws

Elliot: [I: Do you think there should be laws against smoking marijuana?] Not–not really, because it's like saying–if they made a law, what would the law be? . . . That's like saying that coffee, they'd have to put a law on coffee 'cause coffee can be harmful to you if you drink too much. Like coffee's a chemical. It's like saying, well, "Is it dangerous for people to drink coffee?" I mean you *know* the effects that it's gonna cause, and if you want to do it, you just do it.

Jack: To me, alcohol is also a drug. So, I mean, I don't see why they make alcohol legal, but marijuana not 'cause more people die from being drunk than having marijuana . . . They say alcohol's alright, so I don't see what the difference is.

Kristine: It's the same, you know, it's just the same. I mean, if people can drink, why not marijuana? And that is one thing that people say, is, like marijuana, is it just the same as alcohol and I do agree with that. I mean, if alcohol's legal, you know, why isn't marijuana? It does the same amount of damage.

Donny: Drinking, that's bad. I think drinking's worse. I mean, marijuana, you can control yourself, but when you're drunk or something, you don't know what you're doin', you can't control yourself. It's [marijuana] less dangerous. When you get high on weed, you can stop yourself, like if something happened. When you're drunk, you can't.

Ellen: [I: Do you think it should be against the law to smoke marijuana?] No, I think if it's gonna be against the law to smoke marijuana, it should be against the law to smoke cigarettes . . . I mean, they've done all those tests and everything saying that marijuana's equal to five cigarettes and this kind of stuff, but I mean, what are those things funded by, the American Tobacco Society? Of course, they're gonna make it look like tobacco's better for you . . . And alcohol, I think alcohol's scary, because it seems like it's a lot more addictive than a lot of things . . . Because if they're doing these tests saying, "Oh, marijuana's as bad as five cigarettes," well, if cigarettes are so bad that you compare them to marijuana, why can't they both be illegal? I think alcohol should be illegal. It's just as dangerous a drug as anything else. I mean, if they're gonna outlaw one, they should outlaw 'em all. Alcohol is a very dangerous drug. I don't see how they can possibly justify legalizing something like that. I think it's because so many rich people drink. I think they're just prejudiced, you know, like I've already said, alcohol and tobacco, the government has money in those things, that's why they're legalized. I don't think they really care whether or not people are getting hurt.

As noted above, the problem with this type of presentation is that one immediately wants to know how widespread these views are. If all of the young people interviewed think our laws are fundamentally irrational, then there is cause for immediate and serious concern. On the other hand, if these views are relatively rare, then we need not get overly excited about them. As it turned out, 25 of the 95 students interviewed (26%) said they thought marijuana was either less harmful or no more harmful than legal drugs like alcohol, nicotine, and caffeine. More interestingly, the percentage was only modestly higher (31%) among experienced and experimental drug users than among nonusers (19%), a non-significant difference.

Turning now to a more complex example, the questionnaire included a series of questions about student perceptions of certain social behaviors. These questions were designed to tap the psychological domain that they use to understand and classify these events: do they regard them as moral, social-conventional, or personal issues? The question and the results for the item on marijuana use are seen in Table 4.3.

The results in Table 4.3 show that 79% of nonusers think it is wrong to smoke marijuana whether or not there are laws against its use. One potential interpretation of this finding is that these students perceive marijuana use to be a moral issue. It is subject to universal, principled sanctions, irrespective of various national legal codes. Conversely, 60% of the experienced users think it is okay to smoke marijuana whether or not there are laws against it. A potential interpretation is that these experienced drug users perceive marijuana use to be a personal matter. Its use is outside the domain of legitimate social sanctions. But, for reasons to which we now turn, cognitive-developmental psychologists argue that the validity of these interpretations can only be confirmed through in-depth interviews.

Table 4.3: Questionnaire Responses to Marijuana Issue by Drug Use Status

CHOOSE the answer that best describes your thinking.

_____ a) It is wrong to smoke marijuana whether or not there are laws against it. [Wrong]

_____ b) It is wrong to smoke marijuana *because* there are laws against it. [Wrong because]

_____ c) It is okay to smoke marijuana whether or not there are laws against it. [Okay]

_____ d) It depends: ______________________________

	Wrong	Because	Okay	Depends	Total
Nonuser	110 (79%)	23 (16%)	4 (3%)	2 (1%)	140 (55%)
Experimental	45 (50%)	28 (31%)	11 (12%)	6 (7%)	90 (35%)
Experienced	5 (20%)	3 (12%)	15 (60%)	2 (8%)	25 (10%)
Total	160 (63%)	54 (21%)	30 (12%)	10 (4%)	255

After collapsing Experimental and Experienced Users due to small cell sizes, thus creating a dichotomy between Users vs. Nonusers, and dropping "Depends" and one non-response (left blank), Chi-square results (N = 244) show $\chi^2 = 74.56$, $df = 2$, $p < .05$

There is a long history of debate about the validity of standardized psychological tests. Piaget objected to the use of the standardized Stanford-Binet IQ test because he thought that it did not capture or reflect the test-takers' reasoning process. Students could get the right answers for the wrong reasons. Currently, the debate continues about whether such tests are discriminatory, biased by class and race, or at best measure only one type of intelligence.

Likewise, in studies of moral reasoning, researchers can determine how students interpret different questions only through conducting in-depth interviews. The interviews allow the researcher to see the process through which they arrive at their answers. Do the students who checked response (a) to question #6 in fact think that marijuana use is a principled, moral issue? One can make sense of their response only through a thorough exploration of the reasons they give to explain their choice.

After the interviews, the process can then come full circle, from quantitative data, to qualitative, and back to quantitative. Based on the sampling frame described above, simple statistical tests can be used to see whether there are significant differences between users and nonusers in the interview data. Such tests would determine the internal validity of the study. The subsample of interviews could then also be used to check the validity of the questionnaire results. If the interview and questionnaire data are consistent (i.e., not significantly different), the questionnaire results would then allow one to make claims about the generalizability and external validity of the results.

With the growing sophistication in techniques for content analysis, protocol analysis, coding manuals, and so on (Ericsson and Sion, 1984; Miles and Huberman, 1984), it might then seem that qualitative data can readily be assimilated to a quantitative framework to good purpose. The intensity of labor required in qualitative research may always be a limiting factor, especially in analyzing sufficiently large samples. But, as these examples suggest, the respective methods appear to complement one another well. At least that was what was expected in selecting the original research design. The final analysis, however, turned out to be more complicated.

Integration Dilemmas

During the course of the analysis, a number of problems arose in trying to reduce the qualitative data to a quantitative form. This section describes four examples of the types of problems encountered. The next section relates these problems to underlying philosophical differences separating the qualitative and quantitative research paradigms. The conclusion draws out the implications of these differences for future efforts to integrate the respective approaches in social research.

Singular Responses

The first example concerns the problem of making analytic sense of single cases. In quantitative analysis, if only one person out of nearly 100 expresses a particular opinion, it is typically regarded as either an outlier (and dropped from the final analysis) or an extremely weak correlate of little or no significance. It is considered unrepresentative of the population sampled.

In qualitative research, the systematic move to discount the significance of single cases is not considered warranted. The question that arises is: if only one person expresses a certain point, does that mean it is unrepresentative of others' thinking? Or, is it possible that this person is perhaps more sensitive and perceptive than others? Perhaps more articulate and better able to give expression to others' half-formed, as yet inchoate thought? The following excerpt provides an example of this type of case:

> [Can you tell me why wearing black is so popular?] Black is just like, well, it's just like, I don't know. I always feel like the people who are wearing it, it's like they're making a statement like, you know, it's like the world, it's like you're having a funeral for society. It's like the world is dead, you know, and that's how I feel a lot of the time. It's just like everything, you know, everything's so messed up, you know. I might as well just wear black, like it's a funeral for the world. People ask you that, "Are you going to a funeral or something?" "Ha! Ha!" It's like, you know, that color. It's like a funeral 'cause it's really *sad* that we've gotten so, I guess, it's just that we've gotten so into society, we've lost view of a lot of things, you know. It's like we're so into what other people think, and, you know, our government, and so many complicated things, giving money to a government that's killing people because we're supposed to be helping that country, and, you know, it's just like so, everything's so complicated now, you know. It's like the idea of being a person is just like totally gone. Everything has just gotten so hectic. Everybody talks about, "Oh my God! A nuclear war!" It's like, what's so bad about that, you know. I mean, we might as well start all over again. You look at all the teenage suicides, you know. I mean, parents and suicides, killings, murders, you know, everything. It's like, why would people do that unless they're really messed up. It's not normal. It's like nobody cares, I don't know. It's just, like, a statement, I guess.

The response reflects a deeply nihilistic view of modern American culture. In qualitative research, extraordinary statements like this are not methodically disregarded. Instead, the researcher must pause to consider the meaning and significance of such statements. Where do such sentiments come from? Is it, for example, perhaps a pure case of certain tendencies or underlying social trends?

The issue raised by this example is determining the most appropriate criteria for assessing the significance of singular instances. Should their relevance be measured solely on the basis of brute strength in numbers? Or are there other ways of gauging their import? Alternate criteria might include things like where or how such statements fit in the historical context, their relationship to sociocultural themes reflected in literature and other art forms, or their resonance with current philosophical debates or modes of ethical discourse.

For quantitative researchers, a common retort is that statements like the above can at best provide "hypothesis-generating" material. New items can then be developed and tested in a survey questionnaire format.

For a variety of reasons, this option does not appear viable either. Outlooks such as the above may not easily be tapped by standardized questionnaires. Well known obstacles include things like ego defensives, the social desirability of responses, and different coping mechanisms. The example also touches on issues more germane to our concerns here, such as different assumptions about the nature of human action, as discussed in the final section.

Logical Inferences

The second example of the problems encountered in this hybrid research design relates to questions of logical inference. The primary focus of the research was to examine how teens think about how they ought to decide about whether or not to try drugs. In the analysis of the interview data, three themes emerged regarding this question (Buchanan, 1991). For the sake of this discussion, let us take a look at the second theme.

The second theme identified two distinct patterns differentiating the teens' perceptions of drug use. These patterns are distinguished by whether they see drug use as a matter of personal choice or not. Some students say the decision about using drugs is theirs and theirs alone to make. It is simply a matter of personal choice. Each individual has a right to decide for him- or herself. For others, there are a range of additional considerations that they feel they need to take into account beyond their own personal individual desires: they think about things like their age, the law, what their parents would say, and so on. Two problems came up here in the translation of qualitative to quantitative data.

As mentioned above, to assess the significance of a relationship between independent and dependent variables, the methods of quantitative research most commonly look at the strength of the correlation. In this study, the relationship of interest is that between student perceptions of the issue of drug use (as a matter of personal choice or not) and their drug use status (as nonuser, experimental user, or experienced user).

The first problem encountered concerns coding. Forcing each of the students into one or the other of the dichotomous categories (e.g., "defines issue as matter of personal choice" or "not") would have done a disservice to the data. It is simply truer to reality to acknowledge that it was not a matter of students believing one way or the other. Rather, it was more often the case that students held conflicting beliefs about which they were deliberating. For example, on a question about whether parents have any say over their offspring's drug use, one student responded, "To a certain extent, I don't think they should be, um, it's really not, it's none of–well, it's sort of their business." The response vividly captures the nature of the struggle that almost all of the teens seemed to feel.

The second and more serious problem is that there is no logical reason to expect a one-to-one correspondence between judgment and action. The apparent lack of a set, fixed relationship between different stages of moral reasoning and discrete behavioral indicators is an oft-cited criticism of Kohlberg's theory of moral development (Kurtines and Grief, 1974). But, as Kohlberg and others have frequently replied (Turiel, 1983), the relationship between judgment and action may be more complex.

For example, just because someone thinks drug use is a matter of personal choice, it does not follow that s/he will be a drug user. Even if they think everyone has the right to choose, any number of people obviously could decide that they personally simply do not want to try drugs. Quantification in this case would therefore be misleading. The appearance of a number of nonusers who think drug use is a matter of personal choice weakens the strength of the correlation. But it does not then follow that how teens think people ought to decide is only marginally related or has little to do with behavior. The logic of quantitative design would lead us to infer that judgment is only weakly related to action. The logic of qualitative design leads us to pursue the relationship in greater depth: how do these deliberations fit together with other psychological and sociological factors? How do they mesh with the larger context of their decision-making?

Ideal Types

The third example of the problems encountered in trying to integrate qualitative and quantitative methods concerns the construction and use of ideal types (Weber, 1949; Burger, 1987). During the analysis of qualitative data, often the researcher will hear partial statements of emergent themes. These fragments may run through a large number of interviews, yet constantly be intricately intertwined with other themes. Ideal types allow the researcher to extract a cleaner, more demonstrative presentation of a particular way of thinking about an issue. Ideal types are constructed by piecing together the related fragments from different points in an interview and from interviews with different people.

One well known example of this method of analysis is the identification of four "ethical styles" (authoritarian, principled, utilitarian, and expressive) in a number of recent sociological works (Potter, 1972; Tipton, 1982; Bellah *et al*, 1985). As these researchers note, people rarely operate in one single mode. More typically, people shift back and forth among these styles as they try to make moral sense of their situation. The creation of ideal types, such as these ethical styles, serves to clarify the different ways people think about issues.

In this study, the tendency to view drug use as a matter of personal choice was rooted in a deeper understanding of one's sense of individual identity. For some young people, their sense of who they are is filled with social referents: they feel connected to their family, they belong to a religious community, they are part of the team as athletes, they want to be good students. For others, their self-understanding reflects a sense of radical individualism: they are free from the encumbrances of any social ties. "It's my life and I'll do whatever I want to do" without reference to or interference from anyone else who might just happen to occupy the same lifespace.

This atomized vision of their lives creates a disturbing problem for them. Since (for them) individuals act in isolation, the burden of responsibility for any decision rests squarely on the individual. In contrast, for the others, a strong sense of social identity results in a shared sense of responsibility (e.g., I acted this way because all Catholics act this way). But for the radically free individual, one must accept personal responsibility for any choices. As the following interview excerpts indicate, this sense of responsibility is apparently a heavy burden. Drug use then appears to ease the burden of personal responsibility. It provides a form of release from the onerous weight that comes with having to accept total responsibility for one's decisions. The example has been pieced together from a number of different subjects to bring out in sharp relief the frequent, yet fragmentary references to the phenomenon.

> Yeah, because you can't depend on anybody. You feel that nobody understands you except you. It's just kinda stupid the way they try to make it [drug use] so simple and it's not. It's a major choice. Because you want to know. It's like the choice between just not doing it at all and always worrying about it, not doing it and not worrying about it, doing it and worrying about it, or doing it and not worrying about it. It's a major thing because you're gonna be worrying one way or the other. Nobody can–you should believe in yourself to be able to think that you're gonna make the right choice for you. And so, if you're strong enough to do that–and I don't know if you can tell from the beginning–then, then it's your decision.
>
> It's like you have *so* many problems and you're tired of facing problems and it gets to be a bother. You want to get away from it all, you know, just forget everything that's happening. I mean, I guess it's like I wish society wasn't made so you felt you had to be out of control to be, you know, stupid for a while. But if society's gonna be this uptight, might as well, you know. It's just kinda funny 'cause it's like you're acting below your level, but it's fun anyway, just that you act like a fool and not feel dumb.

> You know, I mean, just act like a total ignoramus, just act like a total fool and it's okay. You just don't worry about it, and if they think, well, you're dumb, it's just like . . . I don't care.

The repeated references make a theme like this difficult to ignore, but its use as any kind of scoreable coding category is not feasible. The constructed category does not have an exact empirical referent. Except as an ideal type, the code "Burden of Individual Responsibility" does not exist. Yet without this method of analysis, it seems valuable data would be lost.

Universal Themes

Finally, the last example concerns the problem of how to incorporate universal themes into the analysis. The epidemiologist Rose (1985) has identified the crux of the problem found in the most commonly used types of quantitative analysis. As the title of his article suggests, the problem lies in recognizing the difference between "Sick Individuals and Sick Populations." As he explains,

> The whole basis of the case-control method is to discover how sick and healthy individuals differ. Equally the basis of many cohort studies is the search for 'risk factors' . . . [which] leads to the use of relative risks as the basic representation of etiological force: that is, 'the risk in exposed individuals relative to the risk in non-exposed individuals' . . . [The problem with these] individual-centered, within-population comparisons [is that] if the exposure to a necessary agent is homogeneous within a population, the case/control and cohort methods will fail to detect it . . . [For example,] if everyone smoked 20 cigarettes a day, then clinical case-control and cohort studies alike would lead us to conclude that lung cancer was a genetic disease; and in a sense that would be true since, if everyone is exposed to the necessary agent, then the distribution of disease is wholly determined by individual susceptibility.

As Tesh (1988) and Held (1980) have pointed out, the methods of analysis drive the way that we frame research questions, and hence, the answers we are likely to find. Rather than asking "Why do large numbers of people in our society take drugs?", the tools of quantitative research lead us to ask instead "Why do these particular individuals take drugs?"

In this study of the relationship between moral reasoning and teenage drug use, one of the major conclusions was that the ascendancy of an ethical code of utilitarian individualism puts *all* teenagers in our society at risk for drug use. Figures 4.2a and 4.2b provide two examples of this mode of ethical evaluation.

Figures 4.2a: Examples of Utilitarian Individualistic Ethos
[p. 3] 1 don't think anyone should, um, smoke or do any drugs because it makes you really stupid. And you're never gonna get really well educated, or if you're a kid doing this, it takes your mind off what your schoolwork is really. Drugs are gonna make it worse, and you may never, you know, if you decide you want to become a doctor, you're not going to be able to become a doctor because you never got a very good education. [p. 6] When you're, when you smoke marijuana as a little kid and then move on and you don't have a very good education, you're gonna get stupid jobs, like sweeping floors. [p. 7] They have to think of their future. If they want, if they want to be real successful, then it doesn't make sense to do drugs. Like when I grow up, I'm gonna be, you know, successful, and successful people are gonna have to deal with those stupid people. But if you don't do drugs, you're saying, "I want to live life. I want to make it the most successful thing I can, you know, in my power that I can do." [p. 15] You gonna waste your life and, you know, get bad grades, but I'm gonna get a college degree and I'm going to be really successful. [p. 22] I want to be really successful when I grow up. I want to be really, really wealthy. I want to be the most successful person I could ever be and that's why–[I: What does success mean to you?] Uh, money. [pause] And, uh, I would say popularity, because, um, I know a lot of people that are really rich, but they don't have popularity. And it's okay if you don't want popularity, I guess, because, uh, then you got to do a lot of speeches, and I'm not good at getting in front of a lot of people, and um, you have to, you have to get pictures all the time. You gotta deal with the, deal with the, uh, public. And I want to be really successful and not have to deal with them. In my job, I don't want to have anything to do with the public. [p. 31] The most important thing to think about is their future. If they care about their future, then they gotta consider the fact that, maybe that, drugs can take their mind off what, their education, and their education's what, what, it all depends on their education what their future is.

Figure 4.2b: Examples of Utilitarian Individualistic Ethos
[I: What do you think about people who sell cocaine? Does that seem all right to you?] I don't know. To me it is. Just making them some money, that's about it. Ain't nothing wrong with making a little money. But if they get caught with it, they gotta do some time. Everybody have to do some time if they get caught with it. [So, does that make a difference to you, going to jail?] I can see it if they makin' a lot of money, that's worth going to jail over. I can understand if they goin' for a lot of money. Then I'd go for a lotta money, not over twenty or forty dollars. That ain't worth it. [Well, does that seem worth it to you, to make a lot of money, but maybe go to jail?] If I make a lot of money? Like how much? [I don't know, you tell me.] 'Round two thousand, that's worth it, goin' for. Two or three thousand. [So, if you could make that kind of money, even though you might go to jail, it'd be worth it to you?] Yeah, if they don't catch it on me. I could just put it up somewhere, and when I get out, I just go to it. That's worth it to me. Some people are makin' that much money. A heck a people making that much money. [So, do you think it's all right to sell cocaine?] Yeah. If they're tryin' to make some money, you can sell it if they want it. And if people that's sellin' wants the money, it's all right. [So, do you think the laws are doing any good?] No. You catch 'em, catch 'em sellin' it, they'd be out in a couple of months. [Well, what do you think about sending people to jail for selling cocaine, does that do any good?] Yeah, if they in there for a long time. 'Cause, when they in jail, they get bigger. [What do you mean, they get bigger?] They get bigger, stay in there for a long time, make 'em–In the penitentiary, they get bigger, they lift weights. They can't get it in there. [So, you think it's good for people to go to jail for a while?] Yeah, if they get caught. If they get caught, they should stay in there at least two years, a year and a half. If there's a lot of it, they should go to jail and stay there for a year and half. They get unhooked off it. [So why do you think we have laws against selling and using drugs?] Don't ask me. I don't know that answer. There ain't nothing I can say about 'em. I don't care, (that's) my opinion. If they want to smoke it, let 'em. That's my opinion.

Despite their diametrically opposed views on drug use, the examples are more revealing for their similarities than their differences. For both Elisa and Alfred, their goals in life (the measure of success, happiness, and fulfillment) are defined in terms of utilities: money and material rewards.

The means to achieve these ends are strictly instrumental. They may go by different routes (education vs. drug dealing), but the activities themselves have no intrinsic merit. Education, like drug dealing, is just a means to an end. This calculative, self-interested, utility-maximizing attitude was pervasive in this study–not entirely unmitigated–but by far the most salient ethos of the young people interviewed. As the study concluded, when the pursuit of material self-interests becomes the ideal of the good life, when life has no larger purpose other than the maximization of personal gratifications, people will turn to drugs because they are so effective in fulfilling that purpose.

But these arguments and the evidence presented here can only be made in a qualitative fashion. As Rose points out, if we tried to assimilate this factor into a quantitative analysis, the significance of this universal theme would wash out. Once again, the findings do not lend themselves to quantitative analysis.

Given the problems identified here, what do they suggest about the prospects for integrating qualitative and quantitative research? In a sense, the problems encountered above are artifactual and arise only because the research design attempted to quantify qualitative data. An easy out would be to suggest that the data collected and analyzed through the respective methods should stand side-by-side and let each speak for itself. But because quantitative methods have come to dominate the processes of social science so completely, the resort to a banal "we need both kinds" would simply perpetuate the subordinate, ancillary role now given to qualitative research. Before ceding the terrain, a better understanding of the issues at stake in accepting the current hierarchy is in order. A brief review of the different goals, assumptions, and standards of evaluation of the respective approaches may also be helpful to clarify their differences.

Distinct Goals, Assumptions, and Standards of Evaluation

Over the years, a major debate about the nature and purposes of the social sciences has erupted. It is often couched in terms of qualitative versus quantitative research but is more accurately identified as a debate between positivist and hermeneutic ("interpretive") epistemologies. The different approaches have given rise to different goals, assumptions, and standards of evaluation in social research.

Both the goals and standards of evaluation of positivist research derive from the verification principle. According to the verification principle, the only statements that can lead to true knowledge are ones that can be empirically tested (Ayer, 1946; Popper, 1959; Bernstein, 1978). The archetype of positivist research is the natural sciences, and for many, the natural sciences are now the model for the social sciences. In day-to-day practice, this has meant that testing hypotheses and collecting evidence demonstrating the ability to effect changes in dependent variables are the quintessential tasks of social research. The ability to predict outcomes has thus become both the goal and the standard of evaluation of positivist research. This view of research is commonplace in any standard research textbook. In a classic expression of the positivist position, the psychologist Bandura (1977), for example, writes, "The value of a theory is ultimately judged by the power of the procedures it generates to effect psychological changes . . . Theories must demonstrate predictive power."

Assumptions

The appropriateness of using the goals and standards of the positivist paradigm for social research is dependent on one major assumption. That assumption is that there are no essential differences between human behavior and the behavior of chemicals in a test tube, gases in a bubble chamber, or planets in space. Human behavior may be more complex, but in principle, it is no different from any (other) natural process. It is governed by immutable laws that are determined by the very structure of the universe. Based on this assumption, positivists claim the methods and "language" (i.e., mathematics) of physics and chemistry are not only the best, but even more strongly, the only valid and reliable means to explain human behavior.

This assumption has not gone unchallenged. Since Wittgenstein and the "linguistic turn" in philosophy, social theorists have called attention to essential differences between the natural and social sciences. As suggested by the phrase, the most critical difference is the different relationship that natural processes and human practices have to human language. Specifically, where processes in nature are *independent* of the language that we use to describe them, human actions and practices are *not* independent of the language we use to describe them. That is, unlike processes in nature, human practices are in part created and constituted by the very language we use to make sense of them. An example will help to clarify the difference.

In the natural sciences, gravity is a term used to describe the attraction between physical bodies. Gravity can be defined in terms of the mathematical equation, F = ma. In natural processes, this relationship holds no matter how human beings choose to describe it. How we talk about gravity has no influence on the orbiting of planets. The force of gravity is independent of human language. In adopting this model for the social sciences, an analogy that positivists have been trying to make work for some time now is that of motivation. The most common attempt to describe human motivation today is some sort of expectancy-value equation, like M = EV.

But the essential difference that linguistic philosophers have been calling to our attention is that human motivation is not independent of how we choose to describe it. Motivation is shaped and informed by the way we talk about it. The meaning of an event is inextricably linked to its webs of significance, how it ties to past, present and future experience, taking on greater significance the larger the number of connections and their inter-relatedness. In one community, people learn that they should not defile their bodies because they are sacred gifts from God. People in another community tell one another that they should not smoke, or drink, or eat too much because they want to be rewarded with pleasurable experiences and avoid aversive consequences. The motivations of the people in these two communities are different. Each is partially shaped, informed, and transformed by the language that is used to describe their experience.

Unlike the orbiting of planets, how we talk about our motivations influences how we experience it. There is no independent, objective standpoint from which we can say what motivation "really" is. If we choose to speak about the sources of human behavior in terms of freedom and dignity, then people will act on the basis of their understanding of what it means to be a free and dignified human being. If we choose to describe human behavior in terms of positive and negative reinforcement contingencies, then human beings will begin to act almost as predictably as pigeons. As Iris Murdoch (1997) once said, "Man is a creature who makes pictures of himself, and then comes to resemble the picture."

To put this in a slightly different way, we distinguish ourselves from objects in nature through our ability to articulate and to will ideals of the good life for human beings. But these ideals do not exist outside of the human creative capacity to give voice to them. They are not "out there" (or "in there," depending on which metaphor you prefer) waiting to be discovered, like gravity. In interpretive research, human behavior is thus seen to be more than the sum of past causes propelling us in some inexorable direction. For interpretive researchers, human thought and action are also understood–at least in part–to be a striving to articulate these ideals and bring into being new ways of living. Human behavior is not just the result of brute, empirical, antecedent causes. It is also inspired by ideals about how we ought to live.

Goals

Based on a different set of assumptions, interpretive researchers have a different set of goals, methods, and standards for social research. Positivists want to test hypotheses that will enable them to predict and control human behavior; the goals of a positivist social science are achieved through experiments. Interpreters say their goal is to contribute to human understanding and decency. The ends of an interpretive social science are achieved in the process itself of engaging people in dialogue. Ends are achieved through mutual discussion and reflection on the most appropriate ways of living the ethically good life (Bellah, 1983; Postman, 1988). The value of positivist research derives from its ability to predict, control, and change people's behavior. This capability enables positivists to effect goals pre-determined by the funding agency. The value of an interpretive social science derives from its ability to aid people in improving their own skills of autonomy and participation in community life.

Positivist research is instrumental. It does not concern itself with questions about the goals or ends of human life, but only with the means to achieve goals set outside the research process. Ends and means are seen to be separate. The process of determining that *how* eliminate drug use is unrelated to the process of deciding whether it *should* be. Research focuses on discovering the most effective or efficient means to an established end. Questions about whether or not the target population shares that goal are not part of the research process.

Under a different set of goals and assumptions, interpretive researchers suggest that the ends and means are inseparable. Instead of seeking to identify presumed causal variables, interpretive researchers engage people in dialogue about the relationship between chosen behaviors and their understanding about what they want out of this life. In the process of trying to articulate this relationship, both the researchers and the participants become more aware of what is appealing and what is detracting about their respective conceptions of the good life. In the process of mutual discussion and reflection, we become clearer about how our current practices move us toward–or away from–that which would make our lives more fulfilled, less impoverished, more coherent, less fragmented, more integrated, less alienated.

For example, in the research described here, the interviews were not only a means, or method of research, but they were also an end in themselves. In the exercise of their imagination (through the anticipation of events, sympathy with others engaged in such activities, or based on their own experiences), students had the opportunity to reflect and refine their perceptions of morally complex situations. Freed from the urgency for an immediate decision to act, the interviews created an occasion for students to discuss, elaborate, reconsider, and possibly change their minds about potential responses to situations that they are likely to encounter. If the goal of the research is to enhance the self-understanding of the participants, then the interviews were an essential and inextricable part of that process. To the extent that presentations of the results of the research stimulate further public discussion, then the goals of this research will more than be met.

Standards

Granted their differences in goals and assumptions, the problem remains about how to evaluate the results of qualitative research. In quantitative research, the standards are clear and specific: have the variables been operationally defined with distinct empirical indicators? Are the variable categories mutually exclusive and exhaustive? Is the sampling procedure biased in any way? Are the statistical tests appropriate to the types of variables measured? Has the null hypothesis been rejected at a p-value indicating that it is unlikely the differences between treatment and control groups are due to random error?, and so on. In short, have all the proper procedures been followed correctly?

In qualitative research, there are no analogous procedures. The results are evaluated substantively, not procedurally. It is the difference between form and content. In qualitative research, good research is recognized by the degree to which it provides insight into human action. Does knowing the results of the research help us to see more clearly what was before obscure and opaque? Does it enable us to get in closer touch with our deepest motives or the entire range of our oft conflicting motives? Do we live more lucidly, less blindly, more clairvoyantly, less compulsively after reading the report? Does it reduce our puzzlement about the lifeworlds of people from different walks of life and different cultures? Do the results provide food for thought, new ideas, and new ways of looking at things that challenge formerly accepted conclusions? Or for that matter, do they enhance our admiration and respect for the profundity of traditional wisdom?

The bald assertion of a lack of systematic criteria for evaluating qualitative research sounds disturbing. It needs further explanation. A number of qualitative researchers have in fact been struggling to define a set of comparable standards in recent years. There are two possible responses to this pursuit.

From a strong hermeneutic position, the idea that there could be definite, absolute criteria is untenable. Just as human practices are historically contingent and mutable, so too the criteria for evaluating research. Many social theorists now accept the idea that there are no final formal standards (Morgan, 1983; Bernstein, 1983). As Taylor (1985), states, uncertainty, unfortunately, is ultimately an irresolvable epistemological problem in studies of the human condition (Taylor, 1985). It is a position the anthropologist Geertz (1973) has figuratively described:

> There is an Indian story–at least I heard it as an Indian story–about an Englishman who, having been told that the world rested on a platform which rested on the back of an elephant which rested in turn on the back of turtle, asked (perhaps he was an ethnographer; it is the way they behave), what did the turtle rest on? Another turtle. And that turtle? "Ah Sahib, after that it is turtles all the way down."

Still, not everyone (including Geertz) is comfortable with the "work of art"–either it moves you or it does not–conception of interpretive research. Thus, in a process very much akin to the conduct of qualitative research itself, many researchers have been trying to articulate the reasons why we think one study is better than another. The ongoing effort to identify these reasons is worthwhile. But the proposals thus far (and I think there is no getting beyond this point) are not absolute, incontestable criteria, like those defined in positivist research. They are more like a series of provisional recommendations for increasing the audience's confidence in the interpretations presented. They help to reassure the reader that the analyses are not seriously misinformed. They are not absolute or final in the same way that methods are in quantitative research. In positivist research, if you do not take a random sample, you absolutely cannot draw certain conclusions. There are no equivalent checklists in qualitative research.

For example, one proposed "standard" is prolonged engagement (Guba and Lincoln, 1989). It means studying a situation over a longer rather than shorter period of time. Prolonged engagement will probably reduce the likelihood of distortions, but not necessarily. It is certainly not a precondition for producing good research. Some of the most brilliant works in anthropology–one thinks of Tylor or Sir James Fraser–were written by people who spent very little time actually in the cultures they were writing about. Another proposed criterion is triangulation. It means getting information from more than one source. Again, triangulation may be a sound recommendation, but one can collect information from all of the relevant sources in the world and still produce vapid research.

The position described here comes closest to what Guba and Lincoln (1989) call "ontological authenticity," or, "improvement in the individual's (or group's) conscious experiencing of the world." It is difficult, however, to see how they think this standard is supposed to be applied other than in the substantive sense stated above. It is hardly an external, objective criterion that can be applied by neutral referees.

In interpretive research, the quality cannot be assessed by following prescribed formulas. Rather, its quality lies in the power of its language to display a picture of the world in which we discover something about ourselves and our common humanity. To paraphrase Geertz (1973), progress in qualitative research is thus marked less by a perfection of consensus than by a refinement in the debate. There are no definitive conclusions, only a discussion to be sustained.

Conclusion

There are a number of reasons why the use of quantitative/positivist research methods has become so prominent. Among these are: (1) the outstanding and unquestionable success of the "scientific method" in gaining control over the natural world; (2) the psychological comfort offered by having firm, immutable standards ("hard" science) in an age of relativistic uncertainties; (3) the interest in the government and other funding agencies in gaining access to the means to control behaviors they deem undesirable (drug use, for example); (4) a certain Faustian dream on the part of some social scientists that, if only they could set up the right experimental conditions, then they could provide indisputable evidence – solid empirical data beyond reproach–to direct policymakers in resolving difficult social problems; (5) a sincere concern on the part of others that, if we do not uphold objective scientific standards, then we will be left with only subjective opinion, which will inevitably lead to skepticism, cynicism, apathy, and despair; and finally (6) a lack of familiarity with the different goals, assumptions, and standards of qualitative, interpretive social research.

The many reasons reinforcing support for quantitative methodologies create the uneasy alliance between qualitative and quantitative research methods. Because of these strong beliefs, quantitative methods constantly threaten to overwhelm the use of qualitative data. It is more demanding to ask people to grapple with uncertain judgments about whether a particular interpretation does justice to the complexity of human interaction. People prefer the reassurances that come from knowing the exact size of a percentage, p-value, or correlation coefficient. Hence, when combined, qualitative themes never seem quite to measure up to "scientific" certitude offered by quantitative research.

It has been the intent of this analysis to illustrate some of the difficulties encountered in translating qualitative data into a quantitative framework for analysis. Four types of problems have been presented to help identify their incongruities. Because of the current disparities in their acceptance, future proposals to combine qualitative and quantitative research need to be carefully considered and only cautiously undertaken.

Against the grain of current trends, I would like to see the current hierarchy reversed and priority given to qualitative, interpretive research. On both ethical and epistemological grounds, the goals and assumptions of quantitative, positivist research need to be reexamined and their shortcomings recognized. Human beings are not like chemicals in a test tube. Unless or until the limitations of applying the model of the natural sciences to understanding human practices are addressed, the problem with quantitative research is that it too readily lends itself into treating them as if they were. Alternatively, we may discover, as the ethicist Pincoffs (1986) once said, "Truth is stranger than prediction."

References

Ayer, Alfred J. 1952. *Language, Truth and Logic.* New York: Dover.

Bandura, Albert. 1977. *Social Learning Theory.* Englewood Cliffs, NJ: Prentice-Hall, Inc.

Bellah, Robert N. 1983. "Social science as practical reason." In *Ethics, The Social Sciences, and Policy Analysis*, edited Daniel Callahan and Bruce Jennings, 37-64. New York: Plenum Press.

Bellah Robert N, Richard Madsen, William Sullivan, Ann Swidler and Steve Tipton. 1985. *Habits of the Heart: Individualism and Commitment in American Life.* Berkeley, CA: University of California Press.

Bernstein, Richard. 1978. *The Restructuring of Social and Political Theory.* Philadelphia, PA: University of Pennsylvania Press.

Bernstein Richard. 1983. *Beyond Objectivism and Relativism: Science, Hermeneutics, and Praxis.* Philadelphia, PA: University of Pennsylvania Press.

Borman, Kathryn, Margaret LeCompte, and Judith Goetz. 1986. "Ethnographic and qualitative research design and why it doesn't work." *American Behavioral Scientist* 30:42-57.

Buchanan, David. 1991. "How teens think about drugs: Insights from moral reasoning and social bonding theory." *International Quarterly of Community Health Education* 11:315-332.

Burger, Thomas. 1987. *Max Weber's Theory of Concept Formation: History, Laws, and Ideal Types.* Durham, NC: Duke University Press.

Ericsson, K. Anders and Herbert Simon. 1984. *Protocol Analysis: Verbal Reports as Data.* Cambridge: The MIT Press.

Geertz, Clifford. 1973. "Thick description: Toward an interpretive theory of culture." In Clifford Geertz, *The Interpretation of Cultures*, 3-36. New York: Basic Books, Inc.

Guba, Egon and Yvonna Lincoln. 1989. *Fourth Generation Evaluation.* Newbury Park, CA: Sage Publications.

Held, David. 1980. *Introduction to Critical Theory: Horkheimer to Habermas.* Berkeley, CA: University of California Press.

Krenz, Claudia and Gilbert Sax. 1986. "What quantitative research is and why it doesn't work." *American Behavioral Scientist* 30:58-69.

Kurtines, William and Esther Grief. 1974. "The development of moral thought: Review and evaluation of Kohlberg's approach." *Psychological Bulletin* 81:453-470.

Miles, Matthew and A. Michael Huberman. 1984. *Qualitative Data Analysis: A Sourcebook of New Methods.* Beverly Hills, CA: Sage Publications.

Morgan, Gareth. 1983. *Beyond Method: Strategies for Social Research.* Newbury Park, CA: Sage Publication.

Nucci, Larry. 1981. "Conceptions of personal issues: A domain distinct from moral or societal concepts." *Child Development* 52:114-121.

Pincoffs, Edmund. 1986. *Quandaries and Virtues: Against Reductivism in Ethics.* Lawrence, KS: University of Kansas.

Popper, Karl. 1934/1959. *The Logic of Scientific Discovery.* New York: Hutchinson and Company.

Postman, Neil. 1988. "Social science as moral theology." In Neil Postman, *Conscientious Objections: Stirring Up Trouble about Language, Technology and Education*, 3-19. New York: Alfred Knopf.

Potter, Ralph B. 1972. "The logic of moral argument." In *Toward a Discipline of Social Ethics*, edited by Paul Deats, 93-114. Boston, MA: Boston University Press.

Rose, Geoffrey. 1985. "Sick individuals and sick populations." *International Journal of Epidemiology* 14:32-38.

Taylor, Charles. 1985. "Interpretation and the sciences of man." In Charles Taylor, *Philosophy and the Human Sciences*,15-57. Cambridge: Cambridge University Press.

Tesh, Sylvia. 1988. *Hidden Arguments: Political Ideology and Disease Prevention Policy.* New Brunswick, NJ: Rutgers University Press.

Tipton, Steve. 1982. *Getting Saved from The Sixties: Moral Meaning in Conversion and Cultural Change.* Berkeley, CA: University of California Press.
Turiel, Elliot. 1983. *The Development of Social Knowledge: Morality and Convention.* Cambridge: Cambridge University Press.
Weber, Max. 1949. *The Methodology of the Social Sciences.* Glencoe: The Free Press.

5. Social Marketing: A Critical Appraisal

By David R. Buchanan, Sasiragha Reddy, Zafar Hossain

In a widely cited article in *Health Promotion International,* Hastings and Haywood (1991) make a provocative case for the application of marketing principles to the field of public health promotion. They argue that key concepts in social marketing may help health promoters become more effective in achieving public health goals. According to these authors, the three major tenets of marketing are a "consumer orientation, an integrated approach and the pursuit of profitability or other predetermined objectives rather than volume of sales" (p. 135).

While carefully avoiding the suggestion that social marketing promises a unique and universal panacea for health promotion (p. 136), Hastings and Haywood make the more modest claim that marketing, like other disciplines such as education and social psychology, can contribute "in some way" to the work of health promoters. Specifically, they suggest that the use of social marketing principles will lead health promoters to "communicate more effectively" (p. 135).

Social marketing has gained widespread currency and has been highly influential in many public health campaigns, such as the AIDS campaigns in America, Great Britain, Australia and South Africa (Baggaley, 1989; Rhodes and Shaughnessy, 1989; Woods *et al.,* 1991). While any benefits are certainly welcome, we must also ask if there are any costs inherent in the use of these new strategies. The purpose of this chapter is to articulate more explicitly concerns that have arisen about the use of marketing principles in the health field.

Since the term "social marketing" was first coined by Kotler and Zaltman (1971), it has generated controversy within the marketing field itself and in other disciplines, especially among health professionals. This chapter examines the three major strategies of social marketing proposed by

Hastings and Haywood. With respect to each of these, three questions are posed. First, are these principles offering anything new, or are they familiar ideas re-packaged in marketing jargon? Second, are these principles more effective than standard health promotion practices? Finally, does their application raise any ethical concerns?

The Novelty of Social Marketing

Hastings and Haywood state that the three major strategies of marketing are a consumer orientation, an integrated approach and the pursuit of profitability. Of these, they state that consumer orientation is the more important principle. It is an idea that has also been an essential part of the field of public health education since its inception.

Consumer orientation

Consumer orientation means that one "must understand and empathize with the perceptions, motivations, behavior, and above all, needs of the consumer in order to produce effective health communication" (p. 137). In practice, consumer orientation is achieved through market research (e.g. focus groups), market segmentation and target marketing. Communications are then tailored to the specific needs and motivations of target groups differentiated by sociodemographic, psychographic, and behavioral characteristics.

Being responsive to the needs of various sub-groups of the general population is critical to the success of public health campaigns. Yet this principle is often shortchanged in public health. In particular, when health promotion programs are designed on the basis of social scientific theories, the principle of attending to sub-group needs and differences is often neglected. The bulk of social scientific research seeks to identify a parsimonious set of causal factors, common across the broadest range of demographic categories, to fit into a generalized model of human behavior. Theories such as the Health Belief Model, for example, provide the lowest common denominator; the distinctive features of specific sub-populations are not incorporated into the model. Thus, the emphasis on "consumer orientation in social marketing may serve as a refreshing antidote to the application of positivist social scientific research to health promotion problems.

Granted its importance, we question whether this insight has been lost on health promoters. On the contrary, writing as early as 1945, Derryberry recognized that people had to be actively involved from the outset of any program (Derryberry, 1945, 1949). Likewise, in the oft-cited words of the noted US health educator, Dr. Dorothy Nyswander, health education must "start where the people are" (Nyswander, 1967). Based on these public health principles, the first step in any public health campaign in widely accepted practice is a needs assessment.

There are several major health promotion planning documents, such as the Planned Approach to Community Health (PATCH) (Centers for Disease Control, 1991), the Assessment Protocol for Excellence in Public Health (APEX) (National Association of County Health Officers, 1991) and Healthy Communities 2000 (American Public Health Association, 1991), which describe different strategies for identifying community members' needs and for gaining their input into program development. Likewise, the process of conducting a needs assessment merits a chapter in virtually all introductory public health textbooks (see, for example, Green, 1990; Breckon *et al.*,1989; Braucht, 1990). These documents describe a process directly comparable to a consumer orientation yet have done so without reference to marketing terminology.

But if we examine these ideas more closely, there is one important point on which they differ. In marketing, as Hastings and Haywood note, a consumer orientation is recommended to obtain "competitive advantages" (p. 135). In health promotion, a needs assessment is conducted both to make programs more effective and because it is the right thing to do. The imperative is based on a principled understanding of the nature of the relationship to the population in need. Involving the community in program development reflects health promoters' respect for the dignity, autonomy and right to self-determination of the populace. We return to this point in the final section.

Integrated approach

The second major tenet of marketing is an integrated approach. The components to be integrated in the "marketing mix" are the "four Ps": promotion, product, price, and place. Although promotion often receives the most attention, proponents of social marketing are emphatic that it is not enough to focus on promotion alone. Social marketers must take into consideration the effects of product, price and place in developing market campaign. Once again, questions arise about whether these ideas are new or simply a change in terminology.

A comprehensive approach to health problems is the bedrock of public health. The public health model is founded on the familiar triad: agent, host and environment. The need for multi-sectoral strategies was strongly re-affirmed in the 1978 Declaration of Alma Ata (World Health Organization, 1978). The call for intersectoral collaboration could indeed be considered the cornerstone of the current health promotion movement.

There are also substantial problems with the translation of marketing's "integrated approach" into the health field. Product, price and place are usually not as easily manipulated in the health field. Stopping smoking (product) is difficult (price). Health promoters would be more effective *if* people did not have to suffer the pain of withdrawal, but people do. Clean needle exchanges (product) are an effective means of preventing HIV infection, but programs remain controversial. Distributing condoms in schools (place) may be the most logical choice from the perspective of "channel analysis" of "life path points," but calling for an integrated approach does not overcome community resistance. The "four Ps" are a catchy mnemonic, but the issues are not new to public health professionals. Nor are the obstacles any more easily overcome by labeling them with the idiom of marketing.

Pursuit of profitability

Finally, the most innovative component of social marketing with regards to health promotion is undoubtedly the pursuit of profitability. As we discuss in the final section, the concept of "profitability" is both deeply flawed and harbors potentially adverse consequences if it were to be taken seriously as a "major tenet" or guiding principle for the field. For now, suffice to say that the pursuit of profitability would indeed be a radically new idea compared to health promotion's current goals, which have been identified as the pursuit of equity and social justice (Beauchamp, 1979; Epp, 1986).

The Effectiveness of Social Marketing

Whether or not we believe that social marketing has something innovative to offer, we may still ask if using social marketing concepts might make health promoters more effective. A number of questions have been raised both from within marketing circles and from without.

Hastings and Haywood point out that the push towards applying marketing principles to sell a social cause, idea, or behavior has been met with some skepticism by marketers themselves. As friendly critics suggest, it is not clear that the situation in health promotion is comparable to true market conditions. Two issues stand out: whether social marketers act like commercial marketers in seeking to identify and respond to unmet consumer needs or wants ("fill a market niche") and whether there is a true exchange of values in the social marketing situation.

Commercial versus social marketing

The driving force guiding commercial markets is supply and demand. In true markets, entrepreneurs produce products to satisfy unmet consumer needs or wants. But in social markets, producers are generally not responding to consumer demand. On the contrary, a good case could be made that social marketers largely try to persuade people to give up things (cigarettes, alcohol, fatty foods, etc.) that commercial markets have delivered all too successfully.

In true markets, there is a great deal of flexibility in the types of products and services that are produced. They are constrained only by the consumers' virtually limitless desires. But in health promotion, funding priorities are set by epidemiological trends on the burden of disease. Hence, the types of products and services are constricted in significant ways. Health promoters must "sell" non-smoking, whether or not the "consumer" feels the need. It is a different task to respond to unmet consumer demand than to prevent inherent problems brought about through misfortune or through individual or social irresponsibility.

Exchange versus altruism

Turning to the next issue, the nature of the exchange in commercial markets is well defined: products or services are exchanged for money. From the producer's point of view, the incentive for entering the market is to earn monetary profit. Hastings and Haywood state that the third pillar of marketing is the pursuit of profitability.

Other authors have weighed in on this point, as it goes to the essence of what "marketing" means. For some, the pursuit of profitability is not essential because non-profit agencies can (and in their opinion, should) engage in marketing activities (Kotler, 1975; Rados, 981; Lovelock, 1984). For non-profit agencies, the bottom line is a balanced budget, not profits (Coffman, 1986). Here, the apparent absence of a profit motive may be true in the technical sense that the resources generated by a non-profit enterprise remain with the corporation rather than being garnered by private individuals. But the idea of non-profit marketing fails to distinguish the vast differences among, for example, the multi-million dollar merchandising enterprise of Educational Television Services (*Sesame Street*), the solicitation of donations to support United Way services, and government-sponsored, tax-supported programs such as Women, Infants and Children (WIC).

To accommodate such a wide range of activities, a definition of marketing must become so broad that it becomes meaningless. For example, Rados (1981) stated that "Marketing, then, deals with two of the many methods [persuasion and adaptation] by which A tries to get B to do his will, where B has freedom to act as he chooses" (p. 17), a definition that could encompass social interactions ranging from love to blackmail. Kotler and Clarke (1987) go as far as to say that "A societal marketing orientation holds that the main task of an organization is . . . to adapt the organization to delivering satisfactions that preserve and enhance the consumer's and society's well-being" (p. 32). If "marketing" is about changing institutions to improve social well-being, then we can hardly be against it. But "marketing" in this sense seems to have abandoned the economic for the political; we must ask whether these authors have strayed too far in their efforts to make marketing a universal outlook.

In his more sensible moments, Kotler (1975) states "The core concept of marketing is . . . the exchange of values between two parties" (pp. 22-23). Rados (1981) expands on this point, noting "The idea of exchange penetrates economics . . . Before an exchange, a person has one set of goods, after it he has another" (p. 18). He goes on to contrast this economic definition of marketing with philanthropy, which is characterized as the "one-way transfer of resources," which means "the donor receives nothing in exchange" (p. 19, emphasis his).[1] These latter notions appear to be much closer to a standard dictionary definition of marketing as "the act or process of selling or purchasing" (Webster's , 1977).

If "marketing" is essentially about the process of buying and selling ("exchanging values"), then one wonders whether the incentives for health promoters are equivalent or even comparable to those of manufacturers. What exactly is being exchanged on social markets, and what is the nature of the incentive for the social marketer? Are social marketers truly in the health promotion business to make a profit? On this point, Hastings and Haywood suggest that the notion of "profit" might have to be expanded to include things like "better quality of life" or "improve[d] public health" (p. 137). Yet the highly altruistic quality of these motivations is more commonly understood to stand in direct contrast to the pursuit of self-interests characteristic of the market. Moreover, the distant, often unlikely, realization of these "returns" belies the idea that something is truly being exchanged. The "exchange" does not look like any true *quid pro quo* and would not be understood as such, but for the attempt to fit this social practice into marketing terminology.

In sum, there are significant differences between true commercial markets and social markets, according to people in the marketing field themselves. These differences have led sympathizers to question whether marketing principles can be effectively applied to social situations. Hastings and Haywood acknowledge these concerns but suggest that the weight of opinion is now in favor of proceeding despite the differences. Researchers in public health have raised other questions about the effectiveness of applying marketing principles to health promotion.

Commercial versus health communications

At the outset, Hastings and Haywood assert that "communication is a central aspect of health promotion" (p. 135). The value of marketing principles, they declare, emerges from the development of more effective communications. These principles include acquiring better knowledge of the audience, developing better message strategies, assuring better message placement and media mix, and finding better ways of monitoring audience responses. In commercial marketing, this corresponds to the development of the advertising campaign. The implicit assumption for social marketing is that health status will improve with more effective communications.

If the assumption is that people's health status is poor because they lack specific information, or that the relevant information has been ineffectively communicated, then the assumption is certainly suspect. Examples of the tenuous link between knowledge and behavior abound in the health field. Smoking is the most obvious case. Smokers are well aware of the dangers of smoking, yet they continue to smoke. As Wallack (1989) points out, "Information is necessary but not sufficient to alter the determinants of health." But then again, rarely is advertising used to convey information (Clarke, 1989).

The more likely, and more disturbing, assumption underlying social marketing campaigns is that people's health is poor because they have not been sufficiently motivated. By "effective" communications, marketers mean that the information has not been packaged to appeal to the specific interests and motivations of the target audience. As two of the leading proponents of social marketing, Kotler and Roberto (1989, pp. 32-33) put it,

> The social marketer will initiate activities that motivate the target-adopter to act now, rather than later. In sales parlance, this is called "closing the sale."

The first assumption here is that people become ill because they do not want (enough) to be healthy. The second assumption is that existing social conditions do not present serious (enough) barriers to attaining good health. People just need to get the right message at the right time in the right way and any obstacles can be overcome.

In contrast, the field of health promotion is marked by its recognition of the critical effect that environmental conditions create in supporting or undermining health. Documents such as the Ottawa Charter have enumerated the following as *pre-requisites* to health: "peace, shelter, education, food, income, a stable ecosystem, sustainable resources social justice and equity" (Epp, 1986). In lieu of addressing these factors, social marketing concentrates on communicating messages to individuals liberated from their social context by the assumptions of the free market.

Integrated versus comprehensive approach

Social marketing, however, does not limit itself to mass media communication campaigns. It depends on an integrated approach. The "integrated approach" described by social marketing advocates, however, seems substantially different from the comprehensive approach used in health promotion. If Hastings and Haywood's discussion of "external environments" is a fair indication, then the social marketers' integrated approach appears to take extant environmental conditions as givens.

According to Hastings and Haywood, "The external environment, *which is often outside the health promoter's direct control,* includes technological, political, cultural and economic influences" (p. 137, emphasis added). The ensuing discussion provides several illustrations of the effect of these influences in constraining the work of social marketers. Significantly, the authors offer no examples of social marketers seeking to change these external influences.

Health promoters, on the other hand, know that political, technological, cultural and economic influences must be addressed if we are to improve the overall level of public health. In this context, the omission of any discussion of the impact of economic influences on health in Hastings and Haywood's article is conspicuous. By advocating an approach that takes these influences as sheer constraints, and not as legitimate targets of change, social marketing strategies cannot possibly be more effective than current health promotion programs.

The Ethics of Social Marketing

In the preceding sections, we identified two ethical concerns: the first concerns the types of motivational appeals that result from using marketing strategies in program development; the second, the effect of using a marketing framework on the ways in which health promoters think about their relationship with the public. At bottom, we are concerned about the increasing encroachment of technical and economic modes of reasoning into social and political spheres of human experience.

Importing social marketing principles into the field of health promotion might make sense if we assumed that means and ends are independent. That is, the idea that social marketing principles are suitable and appropriate for health promotion rests on the assumption that these particular means will have no effect on desired ends. Under the assumption of independence, we can freely substitute any means or method without influencing the final goal. This type of reasoning is typical of technical, economic logic; it may be contrasted with socio-political reasoning where means and ends are seen to be inextricably intertwined (Dumont, 1977; Sullivan, 1982).

In the discussion at hand, there is a presumed consensus on the goal (health promotion) and the only issue for deliberation is determining the most efficient means to achieve that end. Proponents of social marketing claim to offer a more effective or more efficient means of attaining health goals. They imply that this will have no effect on the goals themselves. The issue deserves careful attention.

Distortions in social marketing's motivational appeals

In a brief vignette on the benefits of social marketing, Hastings and Haywood describe a campaign to encourage drinking alcohol in moderation. According to their marketing research, they found that girls [sic] think boys who control their drinking are more attractive. As the authors state, "This then has implications for the message content of a proposed television advertisement as the 'sexual attractiveness' of drinking in moderation could be promoted as a benefit" (p. 137). Based on marketing principles, they plan to use sex appeal to sell their product, moderate drinking.

As exemplified by their illustration, we are concerned that the methods of social marketing may cause us to lose sight of our destination. There is already widespread concern about the effects of the constant barrage of sexual innuendo in the mass media, especially on young people (Kilbourne, 1986; Lowry and Towles, 1989). Although it is difficult to prove cause and effect, the public in general senses that inundating society with messages framed in terms of sexual attraction is related to the rise of irresponsible sexual behaviors, as evidenced in the early initiation of sexual activity, rates of STIs, teen pregnancy, and so on. Clearly, the omnipresence of sex in advertising is now an unavoidable part of the socialization process for people growing up in modern society. Hastings and Haywood are suggesting that the use of sex appeal should be expanded into ever more areas of social life.

So, even if this hypothetical campaign were successful in getting young men to drink in moderation, we might not consider it a success if at the same time the campaign denigrated women and promoted sexual promiscuity. It would be ethically irresponsible. Not only do the ends not justify the means, but the ends themselves have shifted. We started off wanting people to be healthier, one part of which was thought to be drinking in moderation. We end up with moderate drinkers whose images of women as sex objects have been reinforced.

Hastings and Haywood's example leads into a more explicit examination of the tactics used in marketing campaigns that purportedly make them more effective. While acknowledging that social marketing campaigns consist of more than promotion alone, we will focus on marketing communications here, as this is the area that Hastings and Haywood say has the most to contribute to health promotion.

Pollay (1986) has reviewed the works of scholars in the humanities and the social sciences for their thoughts on the social and cultural consequences of advertising. His article provides an overview of the major themes uncovered in various interpretations of the processes by which advertising has its influence. To which human motives does advertising most often make its appeals? Pollay (p. 33) summarizes the prevailing view:

> Greed, lust, sloth and pride were identified earlier as common ad themes. One might also consider the extent to which advertising encourages envy and gluttony. If anger were added to the list, we would have what are popularly known as the seven deadly sins.

The light tone of his summary should not diminish the gravity of his point. By and large, market communications pander to the basest, most ignoble of human motives. Advertising reinforces "materialism, cynicism, irrationality, selfishness, anxiety, social competitiveness, sexual preoccupation, powerlessness, and/or a loss of self-respect" (p. 18). While Hastings and Haywood criticize health promoters, conventional and coercive "do this and suffer" approach[2] (p. 137), Pollay makes explicit what marketers have to offer as alternatives. These are not the types of values health promoters wish to reinforce.

Problems with the social marketer's relationship to the public

The second ethical concern focuses on the relationship between public health professionals and the public that will be promoted by the ideas, terms and language of a marketing frame of reference. As mentioned earlier, we question whether "competition" and "profitability" are suitable and appropriate terms to characterize the methods and goals of health promotion. We would now like to expand on the difference in the contrasting perspectives.

For social marketing, Hastings and Haywood are clear, "The concept of exchange is crucial to social marketing" (p.136). We have two concerns with importing notions of exchange and related concepts into the field of health promotion. By promoting an exchange mentality, social marketing concepts propagate radical transformations in: (i) the types of motivations thought to characterize health promoters' work and (ii) the ways in which health promoters relate to the public. We wish to explore the implications of such a transformation. To anticipate, our concern is that such a transformation will both undermine health promoters' sense of commitment to the field and lead to a more antagonistic way of thinking about their relationship to the public.

In marketing, the nature of the relationship between two parties is characterized by the strategic pursuit of self-interests. It is an adversarial bargaining relationship. One aims to get the best deal possible for oneself. There is a mutual antagonism that is captured in the primordial marketing principle, *caveat emptor*. The two parties are drawn together by a cost-benefit calculus, and as soon as the costs are perceived to be too high by one or the other, the relationship is terminated.

In contrast, people have traditionally entered the health field out of a sense of caring for others, not to satisfy self-interests. The vast majority of public health professionals still feel that to be in public health means to have a vocation, a sense of calling (Sullivan, 1995). They strive to create a healthy society in which no one will be handicapped from participating due to unnecessary illness and suffering. They continue to work in the field out of feelings of sympathy and solidarity with those in need. The yardstick by which their work is measured is the realization of a collective good that flows from the elimination of disease, pollution, hunger, poverty and oppression.

A shift to the idea that it would be better to think of the purpose of health promotion in terms of exchange would mark a major transformation. If enough people can be talked around into thinking that the reason for doing health promotion is for the gains that health promoters get for themselves, we believe the field will be sapped of a major source of strength. If it ever comes to the point that people expect *quid pro quo* benefits as a condition of their continued provision of services, then a certain depth of character will have been closed off (Taylor,1985). With the growing intrusion of an exchange mentality, the values of altruism, self-sacrifice and concern for the common welfare are, and will continue to be, diminished. We believe the field is better off now, while health promoters still draw inspiration from role models who give freely of themselves without self-regard. Under the logic of exchange, such people can only be considered "suckers."

Finally, if health promoters conceive of their work in marketing terms, then the ways that they think about their relationship to the public will also be transformed. The uneasiness that many people feel about social marketing is that it constantly threatens to collapse into a manipulative relationship. Health professionals fear that the equivalent of the Willie Horton ads[3] will pop up in the health field. And when ends and means are regarded as independent, it is easier to slip into thinking that changing people's behavior is merely a means to an end and that any and all strategies are open for equal consideration.

In the social realm, however, ends and means are not independent. How we get there affects where we end up. When we treat people as a means to fulfill our ends, it diminishes their sense of agency and self-respect. People are an end in themselves and must be treated as such. Under a different set of assumptions, dialogue–the act of creating a public space for mutual discussion, deliberation and debate–is critical for health promotion. Health promoters are not in the business of trying to get the public to buy anything. The purpose of health promotion is to give the public control over the conditions that affect their lives and health (Epp, 1986). Thus, the process of participating in an enduring and reflective relationship with our fellow citizens to discuss and realize the conditions conducive to good health is at the core of health promotion. When ends and means are (re-) integrated, health promoters are more likely to think and act as though the attainment of good health is achieved through the process of treating people with dignity and respect. It is the erosion of this understanding that most concerns us about the increasing encroachment of social marketing into health promotion.

Conclusion

The field of health promotion is now faced with the prospect of adopting marketing principles to guide its work. Already, the claim that people are entitled to the health promotion services *on principle,* and not because they are cost-effective, is losing force. With the ascent of economic modes of reasoning, the field is being transformed. The terms of the debate are being shifted from whether certain approaches are morally right, ethically good social practices, to whether or not the cost/benefits are demonstrably compelling.

At this point in time, Hastings and Haywood's proclamation of the benefits of social marketing is hardly necessary. Social marketing is here and its increased use seems inevitable. The purpose of this analysis has been to raise questions about assumptions of social marketing and the effects of those assumptions on the field of health promotion. It has been our experience that many colleagues have expressed a vague discomfort with the enthusiasm for social marketing. Before the trend becomes entrenched, it is time to consider what is at the bottom of these intuitions.

We have tried to show that the basis of these concerns is primarily ethical. By pushing certain issues (product, price, place, and promotion) into the foreground, other issues–the justice of certain kinds of social arrangements, the quality of shared public life, the tolerance of poverty, the regard for the rights of minorities in democratic institutions–recede into the background. We think this is unacceptable. Based on the preceding analysis, further discussion of the suitability of using social marketing techniques for health promotion is critical.

Notes

1. In the end, Rados waffles, stating that "some marketing is exchange, but not all of it; and that readers are welcome to their own opinion" (p. 20).
2. The characterization of health education as based on fear appeals is misinformed; there is a long history of research and practice acknowledging the ineffectiveness of fear appeals.
3. The Willie Horton ad was a notorious commercial fanning racial fears used in the 1988 Republican re-election campaign in the USA.

References

American Public Health Association. 1991. *Healthy Communities 2000: Model Standards,* 3rd edn. Washington DC: American Public Health Association.

Baggaley, Jon. 1989. "The acquired immunity to ads syndrome." *Marketing Week* 12: 42-47.

Beauchamp, Dan. 1976. "Public Health as Social Justice." *Inquiry* 13: 3-14.

Braucht, Neil. (Ed.) 1990. *Health Promotion at the Community Level.* Newbury Park, CA: Sage Publications.

Breckon, Donald, John Harvey, and R. Brick Lancaster. 1989. *Community Health Education: Settings, Roles and Skills,* 2nd edn. Rockville, MD: Aspen Publications.

Centers for Disease Control. 1991. *The Planned Approach to Community Health.* Atlanta, GA: National Center for Chronic Disease Prevention and Health Promotion, Division of Chronic Disease Control and Community Intervention.

Clarke, Eric. 1989. *The Want Makers.* New York: Viking.

Coffman, Larry. 1986. *Public Sector Marketing: A Guide for Practitioners.* New York: John Wiley and Sons.

Derryberry, Mayhew. 1945. "Health education in the public health program." *Public Health Reports* 60(47): 1394-1402.

Derryberry, Mayhew. 1949. "Health is everybody's business." *Public Health Reports* 64(41): 1293-8.

Dumont, Louis. 1977. *From Mandeville to Marx: The Genesis and Triumph of Economic Ideology.* Chicago: University of Chicago Press.

Epp, Jake. 1986. *Achieving Health for All: A Framework for Health Promotion in Canada.* Toronto, Canada: Health and Welfare Canada.

Green, Lawrence. 1990. *Community Health,* 6th edn. St Louis, MO: Times Mirror/Mosby College Publishing.

Hastings, Gerard and Amanda Haywood. 1991. "Social marketing and communication in health promotion." *Health Promotion International* 6: 135-145.

Kilbourne, Jean. 1986. "The child as sex object: images of children in the media." In *The Educator's Guide to Preventing Child Sexual Abuse,* edited by Mary Nelson and Kay Clark, 40-46. Santa Cruz, CA: Network Publications.

Kotler, Philip. 1975. *Marketing for Non-Profit Organizations.* Englewood Cliffs, NJ: Prentice-Hall.

Kotler, Philip and Roberta Clarke. 1987. *Marketing for Health Care Organizations.* Prentice-Hall Englewood Cliffs, NJ.

Kotler, Philip and Eduardo Roberto. 1989. *Social Marketing: Strategies for Changing Public Behavior.* New York: Free Press.

Kotler, Philip and Gerald Zaltman. 1971. "Social marketing: an approach to planned social change." *Journal of Marketing* 35: 3-12.

Lovelock, Christopher. 1984. *Services Marketing.* Englewood Cliffs, NJ: Prentice-Hall.

Lowry, Dennis and David Towles. 1989. "Prime time TV portrayals of sex, contraception and venereal diseases." *Journalism and Mass Communication Quarterly* 66: 347-352.

National Association of County Health Officers. 1991. *Assessment Protocol for Excellence in Public Health.* Washington, DC: National Association of County Health Officers.

Nyswander, Dorothy. 1967. "The open society: its implications for health educators." *Health Education Monographs* 1: 3-13.

Pollay, Richard. 1986. "The distorted mirror; reflections on the unintended consequences of advertising." *Journal of Marketing* 50: 18-36.

Rados, David. 1981. *Marketing for Non-Profit Organizations.* Boston, MA: Auburn House Publishing.

Rhodes, Tim and Robert Shaughnessy. 1989. "Selling safer sex: AIDS education and advertising." *Health Promotion International* 4(1): 27-30.

Sullivan, William. 1982. *Reconstructing Public Philosophy.* Berkeley, CA: University of California Press.

Sullivan, William. 1995. *Work and Integrity: The Crisis and Promise of Professionalism in America.* New York, NY: Harper Collins, Inc.

Taylor, Charles. 1985. "What is Human Agency?" In Charles Taylor, *Human Agency and Language: Philosophical Papers, Volume 1*, 15-44. Cambridge: Cambridge University Press.

Wallack, Lawrence. 1989. "Mass communication and health promotion: a critical perspective." In *Public Communication Campaigns*, edited by Ronald Rice and Charles Atkin, 353-368. Newbury Park, CA: Sage Publications.

Webster's New Collegiate Dictionary. 1977. Springfield, MA: G and C Merriam.

Woods, Diana, David Davis, and Bonita Westover. 1991. "America responds to AIDS: its content, development and outcome." *Public Health Reports* 106: 616-622.

World Health Organization. 1978. *Alma-Ata 1978: primary health care.* "Health for All" Series no. 1. Geneva, Switzerland: World Health Organization.

6. Promoting Justice and Autonomy in Public Policies to Reduce the Health Consequences of Obesity

There is significant concern among health professionals today about the toll of overweight and obesity on the health of the American people, and indeed, the world population. According to data from the Centers for Disease Control and Prevention, in 2020, almost three-quarters (71.6%) of Americans ages 20 and up were overweight (defined as a body mass index (BMI) greater than 25 in adults), and fully 42.4% of all adults–more than 139 million Americans–met the clinical definition of obese (a subset of those who are overweight, defined by a BMI greater than or equal to 30) (Hales, Carroll, Fryar and Ogden, 2020). The prevalence of overweight and obesity continued to increase from 1999 to 2018, especially among men (National Center for Health Statistics 2020). Obesity contributes to a number of adverse health conditions, including heart disease, stroke, hypertension, type 2 diabetes, certain types of cancer, metabolic syndrome, and hypercholesterolemia. The CDC notes that the medical care costs of obesity in the United States are "staggering" (Hales, *et al.* 2020), citing a 2009 report that estimated total costs at $147 billion (Finkelstein, Trogdon, Cohen, *et al.* 2009). Epidemiologists say that obesity now vies with smoking as the leading preventable cause of death and disability in the United States (Jia and Lubetkin, 2010). Given the high level of concern, a number of public policies have been proposed to reduce the incidence and prevalence of obesity in the United States. This chapter examines the implications of proposed policies for the principles of justice and autonomy, towards the goal of clarifying ethical standards to guide future policy development to alleviate the significant burden of obesity on the health and finances of the American people.

Many proposals to prevent and reduce the prevalence of obesity have been put forward, from limits on portion sizes to workplace weight loss incentives, bans on school vending machines, pro-rated health insurance premiums, shame-based PSAs, and restrictions on the use of food stamps, to name but a few. The proposals by former New York City Mayor Michael Bloomberg to ban the sale of large sugary drinks and to impose new excise taxes on their purchase generated widespread public controversy and debate. A vocal group of public health activists supports their implementation; libertarians and like-minded supporters decry the intrusion of the nanny state into the sphere of private life and individual freedom. This chapter aims to clarify key moral, ethical, and political issues at stake in such disputes.

Implications for Justice and Autonomy in Obesity Regulations

As the issue has emerged in public debates, one heated point of contention is the extent to which restrictions on individual liberties can be justified by a counterbalancing increase in social justice. This terse statement contains a number of distinct issues that need to be carefully unpacked and examined, four points in particular. The first concerns the implicit theory of justice invoked by public health professionals in claiming that proposals like Bloomberg's advance the cause of social justice. Second, claims that restricting access to calorie-dense food products promotes justice–on the grounds that such policies will reduce health disparities between socioeconomic and racial/ethnic groups–can be challenged from the vantage point of other theories of justice. As discussed here, different theories of justice attach different weights to potential infringements on autonomy. Third, there has been a terribly unfortunate conflation in public discourse of the principle of autonomy with the absence of restrictions on individual freedom. It is important for anyone concerned about promoting health to recognize and advocate for a more robust public understanding of the ethically relevant characteristics of autonomy that merit defense. Finally, the significance of a more robust conception of autonomy can be justified and more coherently integrated into an account of justice generally referred to as the capabilities approach. In outlining the capabilities approach, my goal is to re-frame the currently perceived trade-offs between justice and autonomy and lay out their potential mutually reinforcing features. With greater clarity about both means and ends, I argue that the goal of improving the health of the population, including weight control, can be better achieved by expanding autonomy through promoting a conception of justice defined by the extent of human flourishing.

Clarifying the Claims of Social Justice

The term "social justice" is quite popular in the field of public health today, although many observers have commented that a specific definition or theory of justice is rarely cited and consensus far from established (Hofrichter, 2003). Although public health is often characterized as holding a fundamentally utilitarian outlook (Edwin Chadwick, author of the 1840 *Report on the Sanitary Condition of the Labouring Population*, was a professed disciple of Jeremy Bentham), the rise in popular professional interest in social justice *per se* is generally credited to the political scientist, Dan Beauchamp, and his 1976 paper "Public Health as Social Justice." Beauchamp explicitly cites Rawls as the source of his inspiration, while in the same paper, he coins the term "market justice" to characterize what he calls the rival and "dominant model of justice in the American experience" (citing Milton Friedman, Friedrich Hayek, and Irving Kristol as representative proponents of the contending view). Speculatively, I think that most progressive public health professionals these days loosely subscribe to a Rawlsian theory of justice, based on broad interpretations of his difference principle and his focus on the actions and effects of social institutions, rather than individuals, as the proper locus of attention for redressing injustices. Within this broad and largely tacit sphere of agreement, however, the terms "justice," "equity," and "equality" are used fairly indiscriminately and frequently interchangeably, which introduces my first concern.

In what was hailed as a progressive triumph at the time, the US Surgeon General's decennial *Healthy People 2000* report contained the first official statement of the goal of "reducing health disparities" (subsequently strengthened to "eliminating" health disparities in *Healthy People 2010*, and reiterated in *Healthy People 2020*). Proponents of bans and/or taxes on large soda pop drinks seek to justify restrictions on their availability on grounds that such policies will reduce health disparities between socioeconomic and racial/ethnic groups. Setting aside for the moment the empirical question of whether there is reasonable evidence regarding the effectiveness of this method for achieving the desired goal, it is evident that supporters of such restrictions hold and advocate an egalitarian conception of justice. To paraphrase Hofrichter (2003, 12), social justice is defined by an opposition to inequality. As Beauchamp and Childress (2001) explain, this understanding of justice can be described as one particular "patterned conception of distribution," succinctly stated as "to each, an equal share," where the "share" in question here is health status. In this view, in a just society, everyone should have the same health status. If the health problems associated with obesity affect the health of poor and minority people disproportionately, then an egalitarian outlook on justice demands that such differences be reduced and eliminated. There are at least two problems with this position.

Over the past decade, there has been growing recognition of the problems inherent in the sweeping goal of eliminating health disparities, specifically, in the increasing acknowledgement that differences in health status are due to many causes, only some of which can be considered unjust. Genetic diseases, for example, result in significant health disparities, but they are not within human power to control or the result of corrigible social arrangements. Sickle cell anemia is more prevalent in African-American populations, and while it is tragic, its distribution is not a matter of the justice of social institutions. As these incongruities have become more widely appreciated, there has been a recent shift in preference towards the term health equity, and hence, in eliminating health inequities (Baker, Metzler, and Galwa, 2005; Braveman and Grushkin, 2003). The disentanglement of terms marks a small but noteworthy step towards clarifying the key issues at stake in current controversies.

Clashing Views on Justice

The main problem with relying on claims of justice-as-equity to override or discount concerns about autonomy is that it fails to acknowledge the lack of agreement on a unified theory of justice in modern American society (Barry, 1989; Beauchamp and Childress, 2001; Sandel, 2010a). I think that the driving force behind the most contentious debates about the provision of public health and medical care services in America today turns on disputes between advocates of egalitarian theories of justice and proponents of meritocratic theories, or theories of moral desert. In theories of justice based on moral desert, people get what they deserve: good people are rewarded, and bad people punished (Kekes, 1995; Kekes, 2006; Sandel, 2010b). Based on this outlook, a wide swath of the American public believes that individuals should do what they can to stay healthy and should be held accountable for the decisions they make on such matters (Wikler, 2004). To them, it seems unfair to burden those who make healthy choices with higher taxes or higher health insurance premiums because of the imprudent decisions of morally irresponsible individuals (Buchanan, 2010; Wikler, 2004). To those who hold this outlook, public health injunctions regarding "the social determinants of health" are overstated and untenable (Lowe, 2010). The phrase seems to imply that people are compelled to overeat, smoke, and take drugs by latent forces rooted in their social conditions. It denies people the ability to make choices, which flies in the face of personal experience, commonsense intuitions, and bedrock notions of moral responsibility. If the vast majority of people who grow up in poverty do not, for example, take drugs, then a large cross-section of the lay public believes that those who do should bear personal responsibility for their decision. Supporters of this view want to preserve the notion of individual moral accountability and are troubled by rationalizations that appear to denigrate this core value. In this outlook, differences in health status due to choices people make may result in health inequalities, but they do not therefore oblige society to act. Rather, they are the result of choices made by different individuals, for which such persons should be held accountable. From the position of moral desert, if someone gets sick or injured because he chooses to engage in foolish, reckless, and imprudent activities, then he is getting what he deserves, which is not only not unjust but fair and right in this view.

In contrast, the idea that poor and minority people who are obese should be held accountable for their behaviors almost invariably provokes reflex charges of "blaming the victim" in progressive public health circles (Ryan, 1976; Crawford 1977; Lipscomb, Loomis, McDonald *et al.* 2006; O'Hara and Gregg 2006). In response to such accusations, it is important to examine key assumptions underlying this position. One major criticism of liberal egalitarian theories, in general, and of Rawls's theory, in particular, is that they fail to take into account the role of human agency in moral deliberations. As Scheffler (1992) points out,

> none of the most prominent contemporary versions of philosophical liberalism assigns a significant role to desert at the level of fundamental principle . . . according to the dominant philosophical defenses of liberalism that are current today, desert has no role whatsoever to play in the fundamental normative principles that apply to the basic social, political, and economic institutions of society. (301, 304)

Continuing, Scheffler traces this lacuna to an uncritical acceptance of

> a thoroughgoing naturalism [that] leaves no room for a conception of individual agency substantial enough to sustain such a notion. This problem, the problem of the relation between naturalism and individual agency, is of course a descendant of the problem of determinism and free will. (309)

In Scheffler's analysis, we can begin to see (1) the convergence of key mutually reinforcing assumptions across the scientific naturalistic foundations of public health, (2) the uncritical acceptance of the social determinants of health, and (3) the discounting of concerns about restricting human autonomy. Under the assumptions of naturalism, free will is an illusion, behavior is determined by antecedent causes (like any other empirical event), and the appropriate weight assigned to autonomy therefore morally negligible. Stemming from these assumptions, the field of public health frequently finds itself liable to charges of paternalism (Buchanan, 2008), a penchant that becomes more readily explicable in this light.

To recall, Dworkin (1999, 121) defines paternalism as: "interference with a person's liberty of action justified by reason referring exclusively to the welfare . . . of the person being coerced." With respect to the issues under discussion here, the most clear cut case of paternalistic policy proposals being put forward by public health advocates lies in efforts to regulate what poor people can or cannot buy with food stamps (now titled the Supplemental Nutrition Assistance Program [SNAP] in the United States). Although frequent comparisons are made between the fight against cigarette smoking and the current campaign against obesity, it is important to reiterate that one crucial moral difference between justifications to restrict smoking and justifications to restrict buying junk food is that exposure to second-hand smoke harms others, not just the self. Before the effects of second-hand smoke were scientifically substantiated, proposals to restrict smoking in public spaces did not gain much public traction, but public sentiment quickly changed when evidence of harm to others emerged. In the court of public opinion, the success of efforts to impose strict regulations on smoking turned on the harm principle, not on appeals to social justice and equality, precisely because such calls tend to gloss over concerns about respect for autonomy, as we now see in public reaction to proposed obesity regulations. In a kind of backhanded acknowledgement of the field's vulnerability to the charge of paternalism, one well-publicized research report claimed that obesity is "contagious" because exposure promotes acceptance of the empirical norm of being overweight (Cohen-Cole and Fletcher, 2008). While the merits of this study continue to be debated, there is a morally significant categorical distinction between the direct effects of ingesting a toxic substance and the indirect secondary influences of observing obese people, which may influence one to eat more, and thus cause obesity.

With respect to obesity, the question still stands: is the case for egalitarian justice sufficiently compelling to justify overriding respect for autonomy by the anticipated weight of benefits that will ensue from enacting such regulations? It is not, on both ethical and empirical grounds. In contrast to the promises to reduce or eliminate health disparities, the proposed restrictions at point of sale and regressive tax policy proposals on junk food mirror the public health policies enacted to reduce the prevalence of smoking over the roughly forty-year period after the publication of the US Surgeon General's *Report on Smoking and Health* in 1965, and prior to the second wave of regulations to ban smoking in public spaces to reduce exposure to second-hand smoke. In examining their impact on the distribution of smoking in the population, there is now ample evidence that health disparities with respect to smoking grew larger in the wake of their implementation (Nelson, *et al.* 1994; Pampel, 2007; Pierce, *et al.* 1989). Thus, by following the same prescription, there is good reason to expect that the obesity epidemic will follow in the footsteps of smoking epidemic, where virtually identical policies resulted in aggravating health disparities and further stigmatizing the targets of reform.

On ethical grounds, my concern is that supporters of bans and/or taxes on the sale of large sugary drinks appear to be largely insensitive to charges of paternalism and fail to give sufficient weight to autonomy as they draw on one particular theory of justice. As argued above, I believe that the grounds for taking this position are based on uncritical acceptance of a set of interlocking and mutually reinforcing assumptions that discount the idea that people exercise autonomy to a sufficient degree that merits moral concern and protection. As public health advocates rally to the cause of social justice, Rawls's theory resonates with the field's scientific/naturalistic assumptions and a strong stance on the social determinants of health, where the issues of choice, free will, and personal moral responsibility are given little weight, and hence, concerns about autonomy essentially rendered moot. In contrast, for those who think people can exercise self-control over the amount of food that they consume, they are not convinced that the level of obesity is a central indicator of the extent to which injustice prevails in society. (It must be noted that the extent to which the burden of obesity falls disproportionately on the poor can also be questioned, with reports published by the National Center on Health Statistics indicating a fairly random distribution across the total population at this time; see Ogden, Lamb, Carroll, and Flegal 2010.) Opponents perceive that the proposed regulations will mainly create petty inconveniences and impose additional costs felt largely by those who can afford it least, with little prospect of achieving significant health benefits. Appealing to different theories of justice, the crux of public debate about the proposed obesity regulations in this analysis is thus traced to the degree to which people believe that the propensity to become obese is significantly determined by one's position in the social structure, or whether it is reasonable and appropriate to assign a degree of personal responsibility for being overweight. As Wikler (2004, 115) puts it, "the locus of blame is key." Here, the issue becomes how much (if any) weight should be given to the principle of autonomy. Like the clashing views on justice, different conceptions of autonomy circulate in the modern American cultural milieu too. It is important for public health advocates not to allow the terms of the debate to be dictated by the facile equation of autonomy with negative liberty.

Freedom, Negative Liberty, and Autonomy

To clarify key issues at stake in debates about public policies to reduce obesity, it is also important to distinguish autonomy from liberty in arguments for and against such regulations (Gaylin and Jennings, 2003). Unfortunately, in popular public discourse, references to autonomy are casually used as a synonym for individual freedom, and public discussions of the issues in question here, consciously or unconsciously, reflect the views of John Stuart Mill's influential essay, *On Liberty,* published in 1859. In seeking to establish a principled basis for distinguishing the propriety or impropriety of government interference, Mill famously states:

> That principle is, that the sole end for which mankind are warranted [sic], individually or collectively, in interfering with liberty of action of any of their number, is self-protection. That the only purpose for which power can be rightfully exercised over any member of a civilized community, against his will, is to prevent harm to others.

In Mill's formulation, liberty is thus conceived as freedom *from* external constraint, freedom to do whatever one pleases as long as it does not harm others, what Berlin later described as negative liberty (Berlin, 1969; see also Taylor 1985). This view of liberty is now deeply entrenched in American culture and provides the seemingly impregnable foundation for claims that constraints on individual freedom are ethically unwarranted except when such actions may cause harm to others. Protests about respecting people's autonomy have then seeped indiscriminately into the populist forums that now dot the American social media landscape—typically in the juxtaposition of "freedom" and "autonomy," as in "every tax diminishes individual freedom and individual autonomy"–to buttress claims about the unacceptability of government interference with the individual's right to pursue whatever vision of life, liberty, and happiness that one pleases, as long as it does not harm others (see Appendix). Unfortunately, when the general public hears bioethicists raise concerns about potential violations of the principle of respect for individual autonomy, it is this view that comes first to mind.

In contrast, readers of this book may know that the concept of autonomy gained prominence in Western thought in the work of Kant. For Kant, autonomy is the source of all morality, such that freedom to choose and moral responsibility are inseparable. It is only rational agents who have autonomy, the capacity for moral choice based on reason. Because human beings have the unique ability to exercise autonomy, they can choose to regulate their behaviors, adopt constraints, and willingly submit to norms to which they have reason to give their assent. Etymologically, from the Greek for "self"-"rule," autonomy is defined in terms of positive freedom, self-mastery, being in charge of oneself. One can restrict one's behavior (e.g., not lie, not cheat, not take advantage, or more germane to the discussion here, not smoke, not eat dessert, not get drunk, not have unprotected sex, etc.), yet it is precisely in so doing that one demonstrates moral autonomy. It is this capacity–autonomy *per se*–that affords humankind its characteristic distinction of possessing dignity.

As we saw in the first chapter, Dworkin (1988) defines autonomy as the second order capacity of persons to reflect critically upon their desires, and to accept or to attempt to change them in light of higher order values. Exercising autonomy means consciously, deliberately, evaluating the many desires that humans feel and deciding whether or not to act upon them. Based on this distinction, freedom can then be defined as the absence of restrictions to act on *first-order* desires, i.e., whatever urges one happens to feel in the moment. In contrast, autonomy is the ability to formulate and act on second-order desires; it is the capacity to choose to act on felt first-order desires or not, based on values that give shape to the kind of person one strives to be and the life plans one seeks to achieve. Animals have desires, but it is only human beings who have the ability to evaluate a felt desire, not merely in terms of the feasibility of satisfying the urge, but especially and uniquely, in terms of whether its satisfaction is important and worthwhile. People know that not all their desires are good. Moral autonomy is realized by engaging in conscious reflection about the quality of one's preferences and choosing whether or not to act on felt desires in light of higher order values (see also Meyer, 1989 and 1995 for a largely consistent, less individualistic, more socialized account of autonomy). Making and maintaining the distinction between first- and second-order desires is essential to dispel the misunderstanding, confusion, and conflation of the terms liberty, freedom, and autonomy.

Frankfurt (1999) builds on the distinction to illuminate its importance in leading a meaningful life and finding direction in defining the kind of person one aims to become. In an essay titled "On Caring," Frankfurt (1999) distinguishes between caring and desiring, parallel to the division between second- and first-order desires noted above. Unlike merely wanting something, caring shapes human conduct because the person regards the object (e.g., person, project, pursuit) as something important to herself. People want things all the time, but that does not mean that they care about them. Satisfying an immediate desire does not necessarily lead to happiness or a sense of fulfillment, nor does failure to satisfy an immediate desire generally become a source of great distress. In contrast, the ability to do things that one cares about is essential to leading a meaningful life, and the thwarting or failing to realize projects that one cares about hurts. According to Frankfurt, people need to decide or to discover what they care about, what they regard as important to them, as an essential, intrinsic part of developing meaningful life plans.

Caring about something gives people direction; it enables them to choose between the things that they really want to do, to become the person that one really wants to be, and simply doing whatever whim bubbles to mind at the time. Acting on random urges is what people do when they do not have projects that they care about. It does not matter what one does now because there is nothing that is more important, nothing that would give one pause to reconsider whether all one wants to do is to act on the desire to sit around watching TV, eating potato chips and drinking beer all day. People need to have projects that they care about in order to put the urge for simple pleasures into some larger context, a rational framework that provides reasons to guide action, reasons for choosing one option over another. To make an autonomous choice takes having something better to do, having second-order desires to want to do something that matters, something that offers a sense of purpose and fulfillment. People are willing to set aside, to take a pass on easy indulgences, when they have something more worthwhile to do, for the pride of accomplishment, for what it tells them about themselves. People with genuine autonomy do it all the time. Based on the distinction delineated here, there is growing evidence that people who exercise the greatest degree of autonomy also experience the best health, and conversely, people with the least amount of autonomy have the poorest health (Wilkinson and Pickett, 2009). The distinguished epidemiologist, Len Syme, in fact, argues that having a sense of control over one's destiny is the most powerful factor in determining individual health status (Syme, 1998). The clear inference to be drawn from these data is that, to promote health, the field of public health should focus on expanding individual autonomy, not restricting it. Like the declining levels of smoking, we are now beginning to see the first signs that those who exercise the greatest degree of autonomy are responding to rational appeals to self-interest, to watch their weight in order to improve and extend their quality of life. With due appreciation of the moral significance of autonomy, it becomes more readily apparent that those segments of the population who exercise the greatest degree of autonomy choose not to smoke, to watch their weight, stay physically active, and so on, whether or not taxes on soda pop are raised and large sizes banned.

In this analysis, the problem is not that people have too much autonomy, it is that they do not have enough, or more precisely, that the capacity for exercising autonomy, in the ethically relevant meaning of the term, is unjustly distributed. For those interested in promoting the public's health and promoting justice, the main issue worth debating is not whether restricting access to soda pop will effect reductions in the BMIs of poor and minority people: the most important task before the field is to promote moral autonomy in light of the demands of the higher-order value of justice. People need to see that there are valuable and worthwhile things to do with their lives and that such socially valued pursuits are attainable, and not foreclosed due to social circumstances. It is the accidents of birth regarding the social position into which one is born that has the most decisive impact on people's ability to exercise moral autonomy, by creating conditions that nurture or stunt the development of human capabilities.

Justice Revisited

In recent years, there has been growing attention to a theory of justice called the capabilities approach. The capabilities approach is most closely associated with the work of Amartya Sen (1992, 1999a, 1999b, 2009) and Martha Nussbaum (1990, 1993, 2011). Powers and Faden (2006) and Ruger (2010) have extended this conceptual framework to issues in public health. In these various accounts, the central importance of autonomy in characterizing the just society can be found most directly in Nussbaum's description of "practical reasoning," and in Powers and Faden's discussion of "reasoning" in their recent texts.

In laying out this approach, Sen has mounted trenchant critiques of the Rawlsian principle of fair equality of opportunity, arguing that such opportunities are cruel fictions when many options are foreclosed or delimited by the effects of poverty, inferior education, racism, disproportionate exposure to environmental toxins (e.g., cockroaches as asthma triggers, lead paint in low-income housing, etc.), and other similar accidents of birth. Instead, Sen argues that the primary, principal concern of justice should be what people are *actually* able to achieve, a position Sen (2009) calls "substantive freedom." According to Sen (1992, 30), capabilities are defined as "a person's ability to do valuable acts and reach valuable states of being." If people's abilities are so stunted by existing social conditions that the range of opportunities that they can actually realize is severely restricted, then that society cannot be considered just, no matter how much people may believe that everyone has a fair and equal opportunity to assume any social position.

A familiar example of the application of the capabilities framework can be found in the justification for the Head Start program. There is widespread acknowledgement that students from vastly disparate social backgrounds cannot be said to have the same opportunity to succeed in school, and hence, society must compensate for evident deficiencies in order to enable everyone to succeed. More broadly, universal public education itself is an institutional structure set up to develop the capabilities of the general public to contribute to the common good. It is justified because illiteracy, innumeracy, ignorance of history, ignorance of geography, etc., are debilities that hold back human progress, individually and collectively, and therefore, should be remediated when and where possible to create a good and just society.

In the capabilities framework, the most serious concern for justice follows from the fact that the social position into which people are now born provides significantly different levels of support for developing one's capabilities to achieve a much broader, or much more restricted, range of socially valued projects, activities, and relationships. The most serious injustice is disregard for the deprivations that perpetuate deficits in people's capabilities. In this view, injustice can be assessed by the extent to which the current policies and practices of the major social institutions in modern society enable certain socially identifiable groups to develop the capabilities that make it possible for them to earn a decent living, to find work to support a family (or other living arrangements), and to engage in socially valuable activities, projects, and relationships, while others are left without the ability to make something of their lives, which diminishes their ability to garner the respect of their fellow citizens.

A long line of philosophical thought has held that the most distinguishing characteristic of humankind is the capacity to exercise moral autonomy. The analysis presented here suggests that the capacity to exercise moral autonomy is directly related to people's capabilities to do valuable acts and reach valuable states of being. It is having activities, pursuits, and relationships that one recognizes as worth the time and effort that enables one to make meaningful choices about what to do, by weighing the immediate decision at hand in light of a future that offers the prospect of greater fulfillment. In policy debates about topical health concerns, it is important to remember that there is a difference between freedom and autonomy. Public discussions and debates about potential violations of the principle of respect for moral autonomy need to be refocused on the issue of whether people can make meaningful choices about what they are able to do with their lives. People may have the freedom to choose between buying a 12- or 24-ounce bottle of soda pop, but we should not let ourselves get drawn into debating whether respect for autonomy turns on this distraction . . . nor in thinking that making it more difficult to purchase the extra-large option is an important step in improving people's lives and creating the just society.

Conclusion

Debates between the blame-the-victim versus nanny-state camps have grown rather stale by now. There are elements of truth in each position, and so, it may be time now to try to forge common ground. Dworkin's (2000, 2011) formulation of so-called luck egalitarianism is right to acknowledge the significance of individual responsibility, which then sets limits on the extent of social obligation. But this theory largely begs the question of distinguishing between freely chosen acts and acts that are determined by forces beyond the individual's control (Young, 2011). The capabilities approach is appealing because it highlights important considerations in analyzing the relationship between agency and structure. It calls attention to the ways in which extant social conditions may impair the individual's motivation to act reflectively, by interfering with people's capacity to envision a life worth living, leaving them instead to drift aimlessly, without projects that are worth their time and attention, where the lure of immediate sensual gratifications looms larger, because the amount of pleasure appears to be the only good that life has to offer.

In seeking a more coherent framework, the position outlined here has at least two distinct features that must be noted, although a full discussion will have to await another day. First, it is centrally premised on the tenet that "health" has an inextricable ethical dimension and hence can never be fully characterized by empirical measures alone. Achieving the goal of BMIs of 25 for everyone cannot be considered a success if it diminishes human dignity, and human dignity is defined by the exercise of moral autonomy (Rosen, 2012; Dworkin, 2011). The state can control what prisoners do or do not eat, but this is no one's idea of social conditions that foster human dignity, even if it could be highly effective in making sure everyone's weight stayed within well-defined bounds. To live a healthy life, people must be able to make choices about how they want to live their lives, including how much physical fitness matters to them, relative to other priorities they may have. There is more than sufficient evidence now that indicates that, if we can expand people's capacity to exercise moral autonomy, the obesity epidemic will for the most part take care of itself. As various policy proposals are floated to address the obesity epidemic, the litmus test must be whether the particular proposal at hand promotes or diminishes human dignity: does it enable people to pursue a broader or more restricted range of respect-worthy activities?

The field of public health does not now have a lot of experience in thinking along the lines of promoting autonomy, but there are a few noteworthy examples of a new framework for conceptualizing the relationship between justice and autonomy and strengthening the linkages between means and ends. For example, early childhood experiences have a powerful effect on the development of the capacity for impulse control, where living in chaotic social conditions damages the growth of this ability (Mischel, Ebbesen, and Zeiss, 1972; Mischel, Shoda, and Rodriguez, 1989; Kochanska, *et al.*, 1996; Eisenberg, Hofer, and Vaughan, 2007; Hammond, Potenza, and Mayes, 2011). Family support programs have been found to have a significant positive effect in filling this deficit, with lifelong implications for achieving greater success in school, staying out of trouble, and developing the perseverance to take on projects that require sustained time, attention, and effort to bring to fruition (Tangney, Baumeister, and Boone, 2004; Heckman, 2006; Heckman, 2013; Bowles, 2013). Likewise, there is growing evidence that a wide range of skills and competencies can be nurtured and developed during the period of late adolescence, including non-cognitive skills such as diligence and trustworthiness, which reduce high school dropout, increase high school graduation rates (or their equivalent), and increase employment prospects (Heckman and Rubinstein, 2001; Bloom and Haskins, 2010; Heinrich and Holzer, 2011). Based on the framework outlined here, public health professionals would stand on much stronger grounds, both ethically and empirically, in advocating for such policies and programs than in fighting for bans on large soda pop containers.

Although I think that such programs would ultimately prove to bring the greatest health and social benefits to their recipients, if these examples seem too far removed from the problem of obesity, it is not too difficult to think of capacity-building interventions more closely linked to the issue at hand. Such policies and programs would include support for community gardens in low-income neighborhoods, the expansion of recreational programs (e.g., basketball, soccer, swimming, dancing, weight-lifting, etc.) in local community centers, classes on meditation and open-mindedness, and classes to raise critical consciousness of the causes of chronic stress. An important clue is to look at what people who enjoy a robust sense of health do to maintain their cardiovascular fitness, and then, assure the conditions that would enable people of lesser means to pursue comparable activities. The potential health benefits of a tax on soda pop are purely speculative at this point, while there can be little question that the policy is both regressive and punitive.

The second distinct feature of the position put forward here is that it is distinctly teleological, raising complex questions about the nature of the good life for human beings and how we might decide what makes certain projects, activities, and relationships valuable and worthwhile, while others a frivolous waste of time. Rawls thought such questions intractable, and so, consistent with the modern temper, boldly constructed a theory of justice that gave priority to the right over the good. So, too, the field of public health would like to maintain a firm separation between facts and values, and proceed as if health and human well-being could be defined without reference to the values that define the nature of the good that we are seeking to realize. In contrast, Sen, Nussbaum, Powers and Faden, Ruger, and others must be applauded for putting forward explicit enumerations of the constituent qualities of good lives. Without a more fully fleshed out account of the goals we are seeking to achieve, efforts to improve the human condition are sure to miss their mark (see also Griffin, 1986 and Parfit, 1984 on such objective lists of human well-being). No doubt such specifications will continue to be controversial.

Setting ethical standards to guide policy development in response to the obesity epidemic should uphold key principles. It is imperative to be clear about the goals that the policies are intended to achieve, and only then, to identify the most appropriate means for achieving them. Current constrictions on people's capacity to exercise moral autonomy are more damaging to their health than overweight and obesity.

References

Baker, Elizabeth, Marilyn Metzler, and Sandro Galea. 2005. "Addressing Social Determinants of Health Inequities: Learning from Doing." *American Journal of Public Health* 95 (4): 553–57.

Barry, Brian. 1989. *Theories of Justice.* Berkeley, CA: University of California Press.

Beauchamp, Dan. 1976. "Public Health as Social Justice." *Inquiry* 13 (1): 3–14.

Beauchamp, Tom, and James Childress. 2001. *Principles of Biomedical Ethics*, 5th edition. New York: Oxford University Press.

Berlin, Isaiah. 1969. "Two Concepts of Liberty." In *Four Essays on Liberty.* London: Oxford University Press.

Bloom, Dan, and Ron Haskins. 2010. "Helping High School Dropouts Improve Their Prospects. Brief." The Future of Children, Princeton Brookings. Accessed July 20, 2014. http://futureofchildren.org/futureofchildren/publications/docs/20_01_PolicyBrief.pdf

Bowles, Samuel. 2013. "A (Science-Based) Poor Kids' Manifesto." *Science* 340: 1044–45.

Braveman, Paula, and Sylvia Gruskin. 2003. "Defining Equity in Health." *Journal of Epidemiology and Community Health* 57: 254–58.

Buchanan, David. 2008. "Autonomy, Paternalism and Justice: Ethical Priorities in Public Health." *American Journal of Public Health* 98: 15–21.

Buchanan, David. 2010. "Should People with Unhealthy Lifestyles Pay More for Health Insurance Premiums?" *Journal of Primary Prevention* 32 (1): 17–21.

Cohen-Cole, Ethan, and Jason M. Fletcher. 2008. "Is Obesity Contagious? Social Networks vs. Environmental Factors in the Obesity Epidemic." *Journal of Health Economics* 27: 1382–87.

Crawford, Robert. 1977. "You Are Dangerous to Your Health: The Ideology and Politics of Victim Blaming." *International Journal of Health Services* 7: 633–80.

Dworkin, Gerald. 1988. *The Theory and Practice of Autonomy*. Cambridge, England: Cambridge University Press.

Dworkin, Gerald. 1999. "Paternalism." In *New Ethics for the Public's Health,* edited by Dan Beauchamp and Bonnie Steinbock. New York, NY: Oxford University Press.

Dworkin, Ronald. 2000. *Sovereign Virtue: The Theory and Practice of Equality*. Cambridge, MA: Harvard University Press.

Dworkin, Ronald. 2011. *Justice for Hedgehogs*. Cambridge, MA: The Belknap Press of Harvard University Press.

Eisenberg, Nancy, Claire Hofer, and Julie Vaughan. 2007. "Effortful control and its socio-emotional consequences." In *Handbook of Emotional Regulation,* First Edition, edited by James J. Gross, 287–307. New York: Guildford Press.

Fields, Scott. 2004. "Fat of the Land: Do Agricultural Subsidies Foster Poor Health?" *Environmental Health Perspectives* 112 (4): A820–A823.

Finkelstein, Eric A., Justin G. Trogdon, Joel W. Cohen, and William Dietz. 2009. "Annual Medical Spending Attributable to Obesity: Payer- and Service-specific Estimates." *Health Affairs* 28 (5): w822–31.

Frankfurt, Harry G. 1971. "Freedom of the Will and the Concept of a Person." *Journal of Philosophy* 68 (1): 5–20.

Frankfurt, Harry. 1999. *Necessity, Volition and Love.* Cambridge: Cambridge University Press.

Gaylin, Willard, and Bruce Jennings. 2003. *The Perversion of Autonomy: Coercion and Constraint in a Liberal Society.* Washington, DC: Georgetown University Press.

Griffin, James. 1986. *Well-Being: Its Meaning, Measurement and Moral Importance*. Oxford: Clarendon Press.

Hales, Craig M., Carroll, Margaret D., Fryar, Cheryl D., and Ogden, Cynthia L. "Prevalence of Obesity and Severe Obesity Among Adults: United States, 2017–2018." 2020. *National Center for Health Statistics Data Brief*, No. 360, February 2020.

Hammond, Christopher J., Marc N. Potenza, and Linda C. Mayes. 2011. "Development of Impulse Control, Inhibition, and Self-Regulatory Behaviors in Normative Populations Across the Lifespan." In *The Oxford Handbook of Impulse Control Disorders,* edited by Jon E. Grant and Marc N. Potenza. New York: Oxford University Press.

Heckman, James. 2006. "Skill Formation and the Economics of Investing in Disadvantaged Children." *Science* 312 (5782): 1900–02.

Heckman, James. 2013. *Giving Kids a Fair Chance*. Boston: The MIT Press.

Heckman, James, and Rubinstein, Yona. 2001. "The Importance of Non-Cognitive Skills: Lessons from the GED Testing Program." *AEA Papers and Proceedings* 91(2): 145–49.

Heinrich, Carolyn J., and Harry J. Holzer. 2011. "Improving Education and Employment for Disadvantaged Young Men: Proven and Promising Strategies." *The Annals of the American Academy of Political and Social Science* 635: 163–91.

Hofrichter, Richard. 2003. "The Politics of Health Inequities: Contested Terrain." In *Health and Social Justice: Politics, Ideology and Inequity in the Distribution of Disease,* edited by Richard Hofrichter, 1-56. San Francisco: Jossey-Bass.

Jia, Haimiao, and Erica Lubetkin. 2010. "Trends in Quality-Adjusted Life-Years Lost Contributed by Smoking and Obesity." *American Journal of Preventive Medicine* 38 (22): 138-44.

Kekes, John. 1995. *Moral Wisdom and Good Lives.* Ithaca, NY: Cornell University Press.

Kekes, John. 2006. "Justice: A Conservative View." *Social Philosophy and Policy* 23: 88-108

Kochanska, Grazyna, Kathleen Murray, Tanya Y. Jacques, Amy L. Koenig, and Kimberly Vandegeest. 1996. "Inhibitory Control in Young Children and Its Role in Emerging Internalization." *Child Development* 67: 490-507.

Lipscomb, Hester J., Dana Loomis, Mary Anne McDonald, Robin A. Argue, and Steve Wing. 2006. "A Conceptual Model of Work and Health Disparities in the United States." *International Journal of Health Services* 36 (1): 25-50.

Lowe, Jane. 2010. "Why We Need a Better Way to Talk about the Social Determinants of Health." In *A New Way to Talk about the Social Determinants of Health.* Princeton, NJ: Robert Wood Johnson Foundation. Available at: https://www.rwjf.org/en/library/research/2010/01/a-new-way-to-talk-about-the-social-determinants-of-health.html

Meyer, Diana T. 1989. *Self, Society and Personal Choice*. New York: Columbia University Press.

Meyer, Diana T. 1995. "Self-Respect and Autonomy." In *Dignity, Character and Self-Respect,* edited by Robyn Dillon, 218–50. New York: Routledge.

Mill, John Stuart. 1859/1956. *On Liberty*. Indianapolis, IN: Bobbs-Merrill.

Mischel, Walter, Ebbe B. Ebbesen, and Antonette Raskoff Zeiss. 1972. "Cognitive and Attentional Mechanisms in Delay of Gratification." *Journal of Personality and Social Psychology* 21 (2): 204–18.

Mischel, Walter, Yuichi Shoda, and Monica L. Rodriguez. 1989. "Delay of Gratification in Children." *Science* 244: 933–38.

Moss, Michael. 2013. *Salt, Sugar, Fat: How the Food Giants Hooked Us.* New York: Random House.

National Center for Health Statistics. *Health, United States, 2012.* 2013. Hyattsville, MD:.US Department of Health and Human Services.

Nelson, David E., Seth L. Emont, Robert M. Brackbill, Lorraine L. Cameron, John Peddicord, and Michael C. Fiore. 1994. "Cigarette Smoking Prevalence by Occupation in the United States: A Comparison Between 1978 to 1980 and 1987 to 1990." *Journal of Occupational Medicine* 36 (5): 516–25.

Nussbaum, Martha. 1990. "Aristotelian Social Democracy." In *Liberalism and the Good,* edited by R. Bruce Douglass, Gerald Mara, and Henry Richardson, 203–52. New York, NY: Routledge.

Nussbaum, Martha. 1993. "Non-Relative Virtues: An Aristotelian Approach." In *The Quality of Life,* edited by Martha Nussbaum and Amartya Sen, 242–69. Oxford: Clarendon Press.

Nussbaum, Martha. 2011. *Creating Capabilities: The Human Development Approach*. Cambridge: Belknap Press.

O'Hara, Lily, and Jane Gregg. 2006. "The War on Obesity: A Social Determinant of Health." *Health Promotion Journal of Australia* 17 (3): 260–63.

Pampel, Fred C. 2007. "Persistence of Educational Differences in Smoking, United States 1976-2005." Working Paper, Institute of Behavioral Science, University of Colorado at Boulder. Available at: http://www.colorado.edu/ibs/pubs/pop/pop2007-0001.pdf

Parfit, Derek. 1984. *Reasons and Persons*. New York: Oxford University Press.

Pierce, John, Michael Fiore, Thomas Novotny, Evridiki Hatziandreu, and Ronald Davis. 1989. "Trends in Cigarette Smoking in the United States: Educational Differences Are Increasing." *JAMA* 261: 56–60

Powers, Madison, and Ruth Faden. 2006. *Social Justice: The Moral Foundations of Public Health and Health Policy.* New York: Oxford University Press.

Rosen, Michael. 2012. *Dignity: Its History and Meaning*. Cambridge, MA: Harvard University Press.

Ruger, Jennifer Prah. 2010. *Health and Social Justice*. New York: Oxford University Press.

Ryan, William. 1976. *Blaming the Victim*. New York: Vintage Book.

Sandel, Michael. 2010a. *Justice: What's the Right Thing to Do*. New York: Farrar, Straus and Giroux.

Sandel, Michael. 2010b. "Aristotle: Who Deserves What?" In Michael Sandel, *Justice: What's the Right Thing to* Do, 184-207. New York: Farrar, Straus and Giroux.

Scheffler, Samuel. 1992. "Responsibility, Reactive Attitudes and Liberalism in Philosophy and Politics." *Philosophy and Public Affairs* 21: 299–323.

Sen, Amartya. 1992. *Inequality Reexamined.* Cambridge, MA: Harvard University Press.

Sen, Amartya. 1999a. *Development as Freedom*. New York: Alfred Knopf.

Sen, Amartya. 1999b. *Capabilities and Commodities.* New York, NY: Oxford University Press.

Sen, Amartya. 2009. *The Idea of Justice*. Cambridge: Belknap Press.

Syme, Leonard. 1998. "Social and economic disparities in health: thoughts about intervention." *Milbank Quarterly* 76(3): 493–505

Tangney, June, Roy Baumeister, and Angie Boone. 2004. "High Self-Control Predicts Good Adjustment, Less Pathology, Better Grades, and Interpersonal Success." *Journal of Personality* 72 (2): 271–324.

Taylor, Charles. 1985. "What's Wrong with Negative Liberty?" In Charles Taylor, *Philosophy and the Human Sciences*, 211-229. Oxford: Oxford University Press.

Tillotson, James. 2004. "America's Obesity: Conflicting Public Policies, Industrial Economic Development, and Unintended Human Consequences." *Annual Review of Nutrition* 24: 617–43.

Wikler, Daniel. 2004. "Personal and Social Responsibility for Health." In *Public Health, Ethics, and Equity,* edited by Sudhir Anand, Fabienne

Peter and Amartya Sen, 109–34. Oxford, England: Oxford University Press.

Wilkinson, Richard and Kate Pickett. 2009. *The Spirit Level: Why Greater Equality Makes Societies Stronger.* New York: Bloomsbury Press.

Young, Iris Marion. *Responsibility for Justice.* Oxford University Press, New York, New York, 2011

Appendix A

1. The number of populist social media channels is voluminous. Among the more well-known are the Cato Institute, Human Events, the Democracy Institute, and the Volokh Conspiracy. (Wikipedia lists 84 libertarian think tanks alone, but cautions the number is constantly changing.) In addition to distributing white papers and policy briefs, many such think tanks also publish their own journals, and their affiliates publish articles in a wide range of journals and magazines, ranging from the *Economist* to *Regulation*. Drawing on lessons learned by the tobacco industry, the junk food industry has quickly set up fronts such as the Center for Consumer Freedom (www.consumerfreedom. com) and Americans against Food Taxes (www.nofoodtaxes.com) to wage the battle for public opinion. These outlets in turn feed not only into the editorials of conservative newspapers, such as the New York *Post*, Washington *Times* and Boston *Herald*, but also provide fodder for reporters striving to provide a balanced view in more respectable newspapers such as the New York *Times* and Washington *Post*. The popularity of these views can also be seen in the small genre of literature that has sprung up to feed these appetites (e.g., Sullum, 1998; Metzl and Kirkland, 2010). Examples to illustrate the "pro-freedom" rhetoric surrounding the soda pop tax clash can be found in the following:

Bandow, Doug. "Drop the Soda, or Else!" Commentary posted by the Cato Institute, May 14, 2009. http://www.cato.org/blog/drop-soda-or-else

Basham, Patrick, and John Luik. "Hard Truths about Soda Taxes." Commentary posted on Human Events, July 6, 2010. http://humanevents.com/2010/07/06/hard-truths-about-soda-taxes. Reprinted by Cato Institute, http://www.cato.org/publications/commentary/hard-truths-about-soda-taxes

Basham, Patrick, and John Luik. 2010. "The War on Working Class Culture: How Political Elites De-Normalize a Way of Life." Working paper, Democracy Institute. http://www.democracyinstitute.org/Default.aspx?SiteSearchID=50&ID=/SearchResults.htm

Burrus, Trevor. "The Dangers of a Soda Tax." The Cato Institute, November 29, 2013. http://www.cato.org/Blog/Dangers-Soda-Tax

Chabot, Hillary. Editorial. *Boston Herald*, January 28, 2009.

The Economist. 2012. "Civilizing thirst: Bloomberg's Paternalism." *The Economist*, Jun 4. http://www.economist.com/blogs/democracyinamerica/2012/06/bloombergs-paternalism

Glickman, Lawrence B. 2009. "What Is Consumer Freedom? Baseline Scenario" Oct 9, 2009. http://baselinescenario.com/2009/10/09/what-is-consumer-freedom/

Goldstein, Jeff. "Just a Reminder, For Those Who Are Interested in Individual Autonomy." November 5, 2012. Accessed July 20, 2014. http:// proteinwisdom.com/?p=45083

Hayward, John. "New York's Soda Ban: The Nanny State Goes Wild." Human Events, February 25, 2013. http://humanevents.com/2013/02/25/new-yorks-soda-ban-the-nanny-state-goes-wild/

Koch, Wendy. "Groups: Don't Tax Our Soft Drinks; Industry launches $2M ad campaign." *New York Times,* August 17, 2009.

Marlow, Michael L. and Sherzod Abdukadirov. 2012. "Can Behavioral Economics Combat Obesity?" *Regulation* 35(2): 14–18

Marlow, Michael L., and Alden F. Shiers. "Proposed Soda Ban Is a Bitter Pill." The Cato Institute, October 18, 2010. http://www.cato.org/publications/commentary/proposed-soda-ban-is-bitter-pill

Marlow, Michael L., and Alden F. Shiers. 2010. "Would Soda Taxes Really Yield Health Benefits?" *Regulation* 33(3): 34–38.

Metzl, Johnathan M., and Anna Kirkland, eds. 2010. *Against Health: How Health Became the New Morality*. New York: New York University Press.

Muth, M. "The War on Big Soda." *Human Events*, March 6, 2006. http:// humanevents.com/2006/03/06/the-war-on-big-soda/

Neuman, William. "Tempest in a Soda Bottle." *New York Times*. September 17, 2009.

Reynolds, Jeff. "Sin Taxes, The Nanny State and The Rejection of Personal Autonomy." Accessed on July 20, 2014. http://www.freedomworks.org/ content/sin-taxes-nanny-states-and-rejection-personal-autonomy.

Rizzo, Mario. "Threats to individual autonomy: Obamacare, Salt and Sugar." April 22, 2010. Accessed on July 20, 2014. http://thinkmarkets. wordpress.com/2010/04/22/threats-to-individual-autonomy-obamacare- salt-and-sugar/

Somin, Ilya. "Do Government Subsidies for Health Care Justify Paternalistic Soda Pop Regulations?" The Volokh Conspiracy, June 15, 2012. http:// www.volokh.com/2012/06/15/do-government-subsidies-for-health-care-justify-paternalistic-soda-pop-regulations/

Sullum, Jacob. 1998. *For Your Own Good: The Anti-Smoking Crusade and the Tyranny of Public Health.* New York: The Free Press.

Will, George F. "Uncle Sam Locks Up the Soda." *Washington Post*, August 23, 2012.

7. What Types of Public Health Proposals Should Agencies be Funding and What Types of Evidence Should Matter? Scientific and Ethical Considerations

David Buchanan and John Allegrante

The serial editions of the national *Healthy People* goal of eliminating health disparities have raised questions about the differences between individual medical interventions and community-wide public health interventions in terms of the best way to achieve this goal. When the focus of research shifts from investigating the efficacy of new experimental treatments on individuals to evaluating the effectiveness of community interventions in entire populations, however, at least two new major ethical considerations arise that deserve greater attention.

The first issue concerns the concept of and procedures for demonstrating respect for community autonomy. This topic is analogous to Beecher's (1966) original concept of individual informed consent and its primacy as an ethical component in research with human subjects. The second issue focuses on the demands of distributive justice and the ethical necessity of allocating scarce public resources fairly across different types of health research, in order to fulfill the National Institutes of Health (NIH) mission of uncovering "new knowledge that will lead to better health for everyone" (NIH, 2004). To address these concerns, this chapter delves into critical issues involved in finding an appropriate balance between scientific and ethical considerations in assessing the merits of community health intervention research, when the purpose of the research is to discover how health disparities can best be eliminated.

We begin this chapter with a description of the distinct characteristics of public health interventions, noting, in particular, how such interventions differ from clinical medical treatments. From there, we discuss the emerging challenges to the field posed by the call for "evidence-based" public health (Green, 2006). The main portion of the chapter addresses the need for achieving a sound balance across the demands for collecting the most rigorous scientific evidence possible, the intractable constraints faced in designing research on community interventions, and the rights of community members to be involved in the decisions about the goals and methods of community research, since such intervention research holds the potential to affect their lives in ways both intended and unintended. We then take up the question of ethical concerns regarding the fair allocation of public resources at NIH—a question of distributive justice. Based on the apparent disproportionate level of funding favoring clinical trials over community interventions, we argue that the skew toward individual interventions has resulted in an undue emphasis on individual behavior change as a common yet not necessarily warranted outcome measure in the hierarchy of funded research. In contrast, we present a proposal for broadening the types of evidence that should matter in assessing the potential value of community intervention studies. To address evident value conflicts between scientific promise and community responsiveness, the chapter concludes with a recommendation based on the work of Daniels and Sabin (1997) for using a fair procedure, called "accountability for reasonableness," for making decisions regarding the priority of different types of health research.

Public Health Interventions

In its landmark *The Future of Public Health* report, the Institute of Medicine defined public health as follows: "Public health is what we, as a society, do collectively, to assure the conditions for people to be healthy" (Institute of Medicine, 1998, p. 19). The definition is notable for its emphasis on a collective social responsibility for the health of the population, and for its focus on fostering the ecological conditions necessary to protect and to promote the health of people living in communities. Drawing on this definition and kindred reports (Institute of Medicine, 2002; Pew Health Commission, 1998), the two fundamental features generally considered to distinguish public health from medicine are: first, where medicine focuses on the individual patient, public health addresses the health of the population as a whole; and second, where medicine is mainly concerned with treating patients who are ill to restore health, public health focuses primarily on preventing disease to help people maintain and promote their health (Buchanan and Miller, 2006a). Based on these distinctions, public health interventions characteristically involve the endorsement and dissemination of new policies and programs that create changes in the physical and social environments; these changes are designed to protect people and to enable preventive actions that promote the health of entire population groups.

It may be helpful to consider a couple of examples to illustrate the differences between medicine and public health. One topical example is a syringe exchange programs and their effects on risk behavior and HIV prevention (Braine, Des Jarlais, Ahmad, Purchase, and Turner, 2004). Such programs create changes in both the physical and social environments that enable people at high risk to protect themselves from exposure to HIV. They are intended to prevent people from becoming infected with HIV, in contrast to medicine's principal obligation to treat people after they become infected. Another example is a program to reduce drunk-driving deaths developed by Holder and his colleagues (2000; 2002). This community-based intervention program had five major components: (1) community mobilization through media advocacy; (2) responsible beverage service training programs; (3) stepped up police roadblock sobriety checks; (4) crackdowns on alcohol sales to minors; and, (5) a reduction in the number of alcohol retail outlets. Clearly, this program involves a number of complex changes in the ecology of human behavior, changes that are intended to make drunk driving less likely. Illustrating the point, Hanson's chart of the "injury iceberg" (Figure 7.1) shows how public health programs characteristically seek to address a broad range of interpersonal, organizational, community, and societal level factors, whereas interventions that focus on the individual address only those biological, behavioral, and psychological causes of injury that are "above the waterline," while ignoring both physical and social environmental causes of injury that reside "below the waterline" (Hanson *et al.*, 2005). These examples lay the foundation for understanding the distinct challenges confronting efforts aimed at assessing the effectiveness of public health interventions in standard experimental research designs, demands that are increasingly being imposed on the field.

Figure 7.1: Injury Iceberg

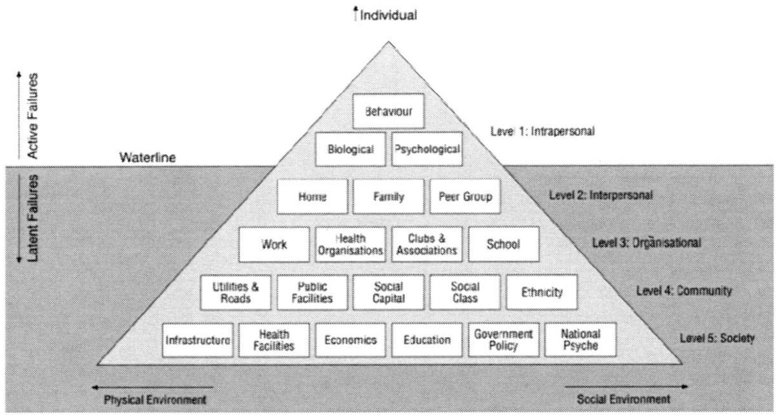

The "Injury Iceberg" ecological model, showing the relationship of the individual to the physical and social environment and levels of intervention. From "The Injury Iceberg: An Ecological Approach to Planning Sustainable Community Safety Interventions," by D. Hanson, J. Hanson, P. Vardon, K. McFarlane, J. Lloyd, R. Muller, *et al.*, 2005, *Health Promotion Journal of Australia, 16(1), 6.* Copyright © 2005 by the *Health Promotion Journal of Australia.* Reprinted by permission.

Challenges Facing Evidence-Based Public Health

In the wake of calls for "evidence-based" medicine (Evidence-Based Working Group, 1992; Brownson, Fielding, and Maylahn, 2009), the field of public health has faced mounting pressures to gather evidence that public health programs and policies do, in fact, achieve their stated goals of decreasing morbidity and mortality rates and reducing health disparities (Green, 2006). Based on certain scientific standards for assessing the quality of research evidence, a hierarchy of research designs has by now become well established. At the pinnacle of this hierarchy is the randomized controlled trial (RCT) (see Table 7.1), which is universally regarded as the "gold standard" of health research, because other research designs fail to control for various well-known threats to the validity of the research results (see Table 7.2). Unfortunately, due to their distinct goals and methods, public health interventions face a number of what we refer to as "structural impediments" that frequently make rigorous testing community interventions in RCTs virtually impossible. These structural impediments include practical, political, economic, and other constraints.

Table 7.1: Hierarchy of Knowledge		
C O N F I D E N C E	↑	▪ Randomized Controlled Trials ▪ Quasi-Experimental Research Designs ▪ Prospective Cohort Studies ▪ Cross-sectional Studies ▪ Retrospective Case-Control Studies ▪ Case Series and Registries ▪ Cases Studies - Evidence-Based Working Group. Evidenced-Based Medicine: A New Approach to Teaching the Practice of Medicine. *JAMA,* 268(17):2420-2425, 1992.

Table 7.2: Common Well-Known Threats to Internal Validity
• History • Maturation • Testing • Instrumentation • Statistical regression • Selection biases • Attrition • Hawthorne effect

Practical Constraints

The first major challenge to designing and executing studies of community interventions is that, in contrast to well-controlled laboratory studies, communities are open and dynamic systems, with a virtually unlimited number of factors that may influence health outcomes. To improve the quality of community interventions, Flay (1986) has recommended testing the interventions under consideration in phases, from pilot tests, to prototype studies, to efficacy trials, and so on. But, due to the many variables operating at the community level, single discrete interventions have often been found to yield a null or minimal effect. Because it is impossible to control for the innumerable factors influencing community dynamics, public health interventions generally require tests of the cumulative impact of multiple interventions simultaneously, in order to achieve a "critical mass" to produce a detectable effect at the population level. Significantly, since it is often not possible to demonstrate the efficacy of the individual components first, community health intervention research faces a much greater burden in providing compelling preliminary evidence to demonstrate the plausibility of achieving positive results in a full-scale trial. Responsible beverage service training programs, for example, seem like a good idea, but it is difficult to demonstrate their impact on alcohol-involved traffic fatality rates when tested independently of other complementary efforts. On the other side of this same coin, plans for data analysis in community intervention research are necessarily much more complicated than clinical studies, which involve fewer confounding or uncontrolled factors that need to be taken into account. This problem imposes unavoidable demands for even larger sample sizes in public health research.

The question of calculating adequate sample sizes for testing community interventions is controversial. Because such interventions are intended to produce effects at the community level (e.g., changes in a particular targeted morbidity or mortality rate for a geographic region), statisticians generally argue that the most appropriate unit of analysis is the community as a whole. Hence, the most rigorous research designs require randomly assigning communities, rather than individuals, to the different study conditions, in what are called group-randomized trials. When communities are the unit of analysis, however, studies of public health interventions are burdened with recruiting a large number of communities to participate in the research, a difficult, labor-intensive and time-consuming process (Luepker, *et al.*, 1994). Moreover, group-randomized trials are highly susceptible to selection biases, differential histories, and contamination due to the inherently small sample sizes (i.e., the number of communities) (Murray, 2001). That is, if the number of groups is less than 20, odds are that systematic differences between groups cannot be overcome by standard randomization procedures. In such situations, the recommended course is to use matched stratification procedures, but matching can be implemented only if the most significant variables influencing community dynamics are known in advance, and then, if known, subsequently identifying communities that can be so matched. Even with such matching procedures, due to the relatively small numbers, it takes only a few unanticipated events that differentially affect the target communities (e.g., teens killed in a drunk-driving accident) to undermine the validity of the research results. In short, in terms of concrete practical considerations, community-wide intervention studies face major hurdles.

Political Constraints

In addition to practical constraints, one of the most significant challenges confronting research on community interventions is that public health interventions often involve policy changes, and randomly assigning communities to comparison conditions is frequently unacceptable for patent political reasons. For instance, it is reasonable to hypothesize that limiting the amount of added sugar in food products will reduce obesity rates, but politically, it is simply not feasible to randomly assign counties or states to treatment and comparison conditions to test this hypothesis. Similarly, many public health professionals are concerned about the impact of junk-food advertising on children's television but demonstrating the positive impact of banning such ads in an RCT is politically impossible.

The feasibility of using RCTs becomes even more tenuous if there is speculation about potential unintended adverse effects. Syringe exchange programs, for example, have long been embroiled in arguments about whether their establishment condones drug use (Buchanan, *et al.*, 2003). Due to such moral and political compunctions, many public health interventions cannot be investigated in RCT research designs but frequently must yield to convenience samples for political reasons.

Economic Constraints

As noted above, the most robust research designs for testing the efficacy of public health interventions require large numbers of communities to be assigned to the intervention and comparison conditions. Such studies, however, are enormously expensive. A small number of group-randomized research designs have been conducted; the most well-known is the

COMMIT trial, in which 22 U.S. cities were randomly assigned to treatment and comparison conditions in an experiment designed to reduce smoking prevalence (Community Intervention Trial for Smoking Cessation [COMMIT], 1995a, 1995b). The cost of the COMMIT trial has been estimated at approximately $60 million, but unfortunately, as Murray (2001, p. 310) notes, "The disappointing results for several large trials have led some to question the value of group-randomized trials." Given their high cost and questionable track record, it appears unlikely that major group-randomized community intervention trials will be funded in the foreseeable future.

Other Constraints

On top of these challenges, a lively debate swirls around questions of external validity and the degree to which local contextual factors may influence outcomes (Green and Glasgow, 2006). Green (1977), for example, has argued that achieving a balance between high internal validity, or "true efficacy," and high external validity, or "true effectiveness," in broader applications is one of the key dilemmas facing public health researchers when designing evaluation studies. Suffice to say, because communities are open, dynamic, and complex systems, an unresolved question is whether there are limits on the generalizability of community interventions, or conversely, the degree to which factors unique to the specific context (e.g., the particular political actors, the historical background, community composition, etc.) largely determine the success or failure of different efforts. A key point of contention, with little resolution in sight, is how much interventions can be adapted to suit local conditions before they should be considered a "different" or "new" program.

There are other technical issues that we could list, but the thrust of these concerns has been to underscore questions about the feasibility of conducting RCTs to determine the effectiveness of community interventions. When the combined impact of various structural impediments poses virtually insurmountable barriers to conducting the most rigorous research possible on public health interventions, then it is critically important to ask what a fair and equitable resolution of this state of affairs might be. The question is: Should research on public health interventions simply be relegated to a lower status and lower priority in the allocation of limited research funding because such investigations will inevitably produce less rigorous, and more uncertain, questionable results? Beyond the rigor of the research, are there ethical considerations that merit further consideration in seeking a fair resolution of these tensions?

Ethical Considerations in Community Intervention Research

In addition to the problems caused by structural constraints, research on community interventions presents unique ethical challenges as well. In such public health research, one major concern is that the specification of an ethical process that is morally equivalent to the individual informed consent process used in clinical trials has not yet been formulated (Buchanan and Miller, 2007). In clinical research, the process of gaining informed consent is straightforward: the purpose of the research, its methods, risks, and benefits (if any) are explained and the individual decides whether she wants to participate. But how is this procedure supposed to be extended to an entire community? If community members have a right to autonomy and it is ethically unwarranted for researchers to conduct health research on them without their agreement, then the critical ethical challenge is to lay out how respect for community autonomy should be secured.

In past practice, despite the fact that Institutional Review Boards are required to have at least one community representative, respect for community autonomy has generally been neglected. Based on IRB deliberations about whether the risks are sufficiently minimal that individual informed consent can be waived, IRB approval alone has been considered adequate to authorize community health intervention research. When an experimental intervention has been determined to pose minimal risks, IRBs have waived the consent requirement and permitted community intervention trials to proceed.

While IRB review for community health intervention research may be adequate in certain limited circumstances, it restricts the scope of investigations to relatively innocuous interventions (e.g., mass media campaigns), and thus, is not sufficient for the majority of public health interventions. Consider the aforementioned public health research question regarding the effect of police roadblocks to screen for impaired drivers, with the goal of identifying effective strategies to reduce traffic fatalities. At the individual level, is it fair to assume that the average social drinker would consider participating in the roadblock experiment in one's interest? At the community level, do community members have a right to question why their community was selected, whether they wish to participate, or whether alternative strategies should be considered? Would an IRB be justified in designating such research as posing only minimal risk?

To test more powerful community interventions, IRB approval alone cannot suffice. There must be a process that serves the same ethical function as individual informed consent, where the community as a whole can decide whether it is in their interests to participate. The dual needs for avoiding exploitation and affirming the community's right to autonomy have led researchers to try to address these concerns by establishing Community Advisory Boards (CABs), based on the model of oversight at federally-funded community health centers.

Stipulating an ethical standard that requires establishing a CAB is an important first step in addressing the ethical challenges posed by conducting public health research, but it is not enough. It immediately raises questions about representation: Who should sit on these boards? Who can legitimately speak on behalf of community interests? How should they be selected? What is an appropriate number of CAB members? What is the scope of their responsibilities? What sorts of decisions (e.g., research methods, budget allocations, personnel, etc.) should they be authorized to make? (Buchanan, *et al.*, 2008).

Other researchers, particularly advocates of community-based participatory research, have recommended that additional processes should be required to ensure the legitimacy of the consent process and to respect the community's right to self-determination. Recommended procedures include interviews with stakeholders and key informants, focus groups, community surveys, community forums, and partnerships with existing community associations (Buchanan, *et al.*, 2007; Israel *et al.*, 2003). Likewise, Emanuel and his colleagues (2004) have recently articulated an ethical requirement for community collaboration in international health research; the requirement of community collaboration has been put forward as a necessary bulwark against the exploitation of vulnerable populations. They have identified seven indicators to gauge the degree to which this ethical requirement has been fulfilled. Moreover, the scope of researchers' duty to provide benefits to the community–in one form or another–has yet to be resolved, a debate that portends even greater demands on public health researchers (Belsky and Richardson, 2004).

To address this concern, we recommend the following standard as one possible model: the more powerful the intervention and the greater the possibility of exploitation, the more demanding the process of gaining community participation should be in ratifying the decision to allow the research to be conducted in their community. The most powerful interventions must implement processes that aim at maximum feasible participation. Strategies for responding to research proposals developed in Indian Country provide a model for broader community participation. Several tribes or tribal entities, most notably the Navajo Nation, have created their own separate Institutional Review Boards with stringent requirements of community support, evidence of community-wide benefit, and requirements to disseminate results to the appropriate tribal agencies and communities once the research is completed (American Indian Law Center, 1999).

For our purposes here, it is important to emphasize that (1) researchers have an obligation to respect the community's fundamental right to decide whether the goals of the research are valuable and the methods acceptable to them; and (2) such procedures entail exceptional efforts that make public health research more difficult than clinical trials. At a minimum, since the process of gaining community endorsement is much more complex and time-consuming than the process of gathering individual informed consent in clinical trials, there need necessarily be a much longer start-up phase in conducting public health research, and consequently, additional funding at a level appropriate to the scientific and ethical requirements entailed in conducting public health research.

Based on the preceding analysis of the unique scientific and ethical considerations that arise when the focus of the research shifts from clinical to public health contexts, we turn now to consider the implications for allocating federal health research funds.

Allocating Federal Health Research Funds Fairly

The question of allocating scarce public resources fairly is an issue of distributive justice. At the start of the third decade of the 21st century, the budget for the U.S. National Institutes of Health (NIH) was approximately $32 billion. Because funding comes from taxpayer dollars, fairness in the allocation of these funds is imperative. The mission of the NIH is "to uncover new knowledge that will lead to better health for everyone" (NIH, 2004). The critical issue is what kinds of new knowledge are most likely to lead to success in achieving the nation's goals for better health for everyone.

Based on a long history of scientific research, there can be little question that RCTs enable researchers to rule out the greatest number of threats to the validity of the research results, and hence, provide the most rigorous research results possible. However, if one acknowledges that many factors make community intervention trials less feasible than clinical studies, then it raises the issue of how the potential social and scientific value of public health research can be fairly assessed. The National Institutes of Health are steeped in a culture of clinical trials, but the way that the NIH sets its research priorities has not gone unquestioned (Agres, 2004; Buchanan and Miller, 2007; Dresser, 2001).

In response to a growing chorus of criticism, the NIH set out to make its decision-making processes more transparent in a report titled, *Setting Research Priorities at the National Institutes of Health* (Institute of Medicine, 1998). In this report, NIH officials identified five criteria that they said should guide fulfilling their fiduciary responsibilities to Congress and the American people: (1) public health needs, (2) scientific quality of the research, (3) potential for scientific progress, (4) portfolio diversification, and (5) adequate support of research infrastructure. The report asserted that all of these criteria are pertinent to setting priorities, and conversely, giving precedence to any one of them alone could potentially lead to squandering valuable resources. Allocating funding strictly according to the number of deaths, for instance, would neglect chronic diseases such as mental illness and arthritis that produce long-term disability and high costs to society. Still, a number of concerns have been raised about both the adequacy and the implementation of these standards. Critics start by pointing out that the criteria are so broad that, in effect, NIH officials have almost total freedom in exercising their discretion over the use of these monies.

With respect to public health needs, for example, an initial intuition might be that there should be a correlation between the distribution of disease burden and the allocation of research funds, with more funding going to those problems that cause a substantially greater burden of disease. But there are conflicting ways of measuring disease burden. Congressional representatives, for example, have complained that there appear to be widely disparate amounts of funding per afflicted person from one disease to the next, and they have pointedly asked why the NIH spends much more per death from HIV/AIDS than other causes of death, such as cancer, heart disease, or stroke, diseases whose prevalence rates are far greater than those for HIV/AIDS. In contrast, the prominent bioethicist Daniel Callahan (2000) has argued that far too much money is spent on research on the diseases of old age, such as cancer, and that priority should instead be given to diseases that cause premature death (before the age of 65).

In the face of on-going controversies about which health problems should have highest priority, an expedient resolution is simply to sidestep the question and fall back on the far less controversial standards of scientific promise in making funding decisions. Without explicit directives mandating that community intervention research receive higher priority, the peer review process is designed and intended to rank proposals according to the quality of the scientific design. As a result, critics charge that decisions at NIH are driven more by rigor than relevance, with an undue emphasis on basic science over practical application. Indeed, several commentators have lamented the overwhelming skew towards a biologically reductionistic emphasis on molecular and genetic determinants of health to the neglect and exclusion of research on social, behavioral, and environmental factors (McGinnis, Williams-Russo, and Knickman, 2002; Rees, 2004; Rogers, 2004; Kantor, 2008).

There is another important consequence of the bias towards clinical medical trials in NIH funding decisions. It produces an unwarranted–indeed we argue potentially counterproductive–emphasis on seeking ever more powerful methods for effecting individual behavior change. Two major factors have contributed to this state of affairs. Historically, Neubauer and Pratt (1981) have shown how the public health focus on creating healthy living conditions shifted toward a focus on isolating the agent of disease with the rise of the germ theory of disease around the turn of the last century. As infectious disease rates fell over time, the primary focus of research attention shifted again, to an emphasis on the host-individual behaviors–most especially, with then-Assistant Surgeon General Michael McGinnis's and former CDC Director William Foege's widely-cited report on the "actual causes of death" (McGinnis and Foege, 1993).

The second major factor relates to the relative ease or difficulty in conducting clinical trials with individuals versus public health interventions with whole population groups. If it is hard to conduct research on changing the social determinants of health, then conducting research on changing individual behaviors allows researchers to feel that they can still make worthwhile contributions to advancing public health goals. In combination, these two factors have created an atmosphere in which there is widespread acceptance of the idea that one of the most important outcomes of health research these days is demonstrating individual behavior change. To the extent that NIH funding priorities rise above the genetic and molecular level, there has been concerted scientific interest in determining whether researchers can control human behavior in precisely the same way that they have learned to control the virulence of micro-organisms. What is missing from this research agenda is an appreciation of how social position structures the choices that people can and do make (MacIntyre, 1986; Marmot and Wilkinson, 1999).

From an epidemiological perspective, there is now overwhelming and irrefutable evidence that socioeconomic status is powerfully associated with health status (Marmot, 2003, 2004). Conversely, people who have the least amount of control over their work conditions or other major life situations have the poorest health. The conclusion that we draw from these data is that, if researchers want to promote health, then they should focus on finding ways to promote autonomy, not restrict it. Public health research should focus on creating the conditions in which people can exercise the greatest degree of individual autonomy, and not trying to figure out how to develop new technologies for controlling their behavior (Buchanan, 2001, 2006a, 2006b).

As one further observation on this point, *Healthy People 2010* declared that one of the two principal goals for the nation is to improve quality of life (QOL) in this country. Little is actually said about what "quality of life" means in the document, but other scholars have illuminated the topic. The philosopher and bioethicist Dan Brock (1993, p. 105), for example, has defined quality of life as follows: "What is central to QOL is the capacity to exercise choice in forming and pursuing an integrated and coherent life plan." If the capacity for exercising choice is central to the meaning, and enjoyment, of quality of life, then research that aims to manipulate and control the choices people make is headed in the wrong direction, with potentially iatrogenic implications.

The thrust of these concerns has been to point out how demands for scientific rigor have resulted in shortchanging investment in community intervention research. The largely unquestioned mandate for upholding scientific standards serves to marginalize community intervention research, by relegating it to an inferior status not deserving priority in funding due to perceived deficiencies in scientific design. In light of the many structural impediments confronting community intervention studies, the invocation of "scientific promise" and the demand for "rigor in research" press towards individual clinical RCTs to the neglect of research on public health interventions. As a result, as the prospects for conducting research on the social determinants of health are diminished, so too is the likelihood of making a significant political commitment to eliminating health disparities.

Accountability for Reasonableness

The preceding section has shown how different value judgments are involved in assessing the relative merits of different types of health research. When faced with incompatible and seemingly irreconcilable value judgments, the demands of justice stipulate that groups ought to resort to fair procedures (e.g., democratic majority vote) to resolve their disagreements. Daniels and Sabin (1997) describe one such fair process for making controversial allocation decisions, a procedure they call "accountability for reasonableness." Daniels and Sabin developed their proposal to assist in setting priorities in medical care settings–specifically, insurers' decisions regarding coverage of particular medical interventions–but their recommendations are directly relevant to setting research priorities. They state that the decision-making process will be fair if the system has four features (see Table 7.3):

> One key feature is the provision of publicly accessible reasons, that is, a public rationale, for decisions. A second is that the rationale must constitute a reasonable construal of how to meet the [research] needs of a population under acceptable resource constraints. A third key feature is that there must be mechanisms for considering challenges to decisions that are made and for revisiting those decisions in light of counter-arguments . . . [Fourth], there is voluntary or public regulation of the process to ensure that conditions 1–3 are met. (p. 307)

Table 7.3: Accountability for Reasonableness
• Public rationale for decisions • Reasonable understanding of how to meet needs of affected population, given resource constraints • Mechanisms for challenging decisions and for revisiting decisions in light of counter-arguments • Voluntary or public regulation of the process

Regarding the fourth point, public regulation of the process, the NIH has acknowledged that its interactions with the public are "generally weak" and affirmed the need to more fully engage the public to redress concerns about the legitimacy and fairness of its distribution decisions (Institute of Medicine, 1998, p. 7). It is critically important at this time that community members and public health professionals vigorously advocate for oversight of the distribution of NIH funding by such public bodies. NIH officials and review groups are charged with evaluating proposals based on their prospects for uncovering new knowledge that will lead to better health for everyone. Their deliberations, however, must be reasonable with respect to the cogency of the rationales put forward regarding the prospects that the knowledge to be gained will result in improvements in population health. Justice demands that critical questions be posed and alternative criteria, beyond rigor in research, be judiciously considered.

What Types of Evidence Should Matter

If RCTs of community interventions are methodologically difficult and studies designed to influence individual behavior change possibly detrimental, then what types of evidence should matter in evaluating the merits of public health proposals? The future of public health research is largely dependent on the answer to this question.

First, public health needs to reclaim and honor its lineage. Historically, public health was founded on the science of epidemiology. Epidemiological research is based primarily on observational studies, retrospective case-control, and prospective cohort research designs. To certify the validity of these types of research, epidemiologists developed a set of "weight-of-evidence" standards, generally referred to as Hill's criteria, based on dimensions such as biological plausibility, consistency in association, and dose-response relationships (Hill, 1965; see Table 7.4). Despite the fact that many problems cannot be investigated in field experiments, public health researchers seem to have become almost apologetic about the quality of their research, rather passively seeming to accept the notion that epidemiology is a "second-rate" science relative to clinical trials (Parascandola, 1998; Parascandola and Weed, 2001).

Table 7.4: Hill's Criteria for Epidemiological Studies
• Temporal association • Strength • Dose-response relationship • Consistency • Biological plausibility • Alternative explanations • Specificity • Coherence

Fortunately, the Supreme Court ruling in *Daubert v. Merrell Dow Pharmaceuticals, Inc.* (in which the industry argued that claims, such as smoking causes cancer, that were not based on experimental research designs constituted "junk science") has served as a wake-up call for the field (Michaels and Monforton, 2005). A national organization and public health professionals across the country embarked on a major initiative, the Project on Scientific Knowledge and Public Policy (SKAPP), to advance understanding of different criteria for assessing scientific validity (National Research Council, 2012). Thus, to advance research on community health interventions, a more articulate justification of valid scientific standards is crucial.

Conclusion

In this chapter, we have argued that, for anyone interested in community intervention research, two key ethical concerns have yet to be resolved: (1) identifying an appropriate process for ensuring that the community members agree that the goals of the research are valuable and methods acceptable; and (2) deciding how to allocate scarce public resources designated for health research fairly. We have shown how there are evident tensions between scientific and ethical considerations and argued that a sound balance has yet to be achieved. As demonstrated here, RCTs may not be feasible in most community intervention research, and other standards are needed to assess the merits of proposed public health research. We have presented other types of evidence that should matter in trying to decide whether research on a proposed public health intervention is worthwhile. Due to the conflicting considerations between scientific promise and community responsiveness, we conclude that the NIH should establish fair procedures for resolving fundamental disagreements about the value of different types of research, a process embodied in the concept of "accountability for reasonableness."

References

Agres, Ted. 2004. "Questioning NIH priorities." *The Scientist* 5(1): 2.

American Indian Law Center. 1999. *Model tribal research code: With materials for tribal regulation for research and checklist for Indian health boards* (3rd ed.). Albuquerque, NM: American Indian Law Center, Inc.

Beecher, Henry K. 1966. "Ethics and Clinical Research." *New England Journal of Medicine* 274, 1354-1360.

Belsky, Leah and Henry Richardson. 2004. "Medical researchers' ancillary clinical care responsibilities." *British Medical Journal* 328(7454): 1494-1496.

Braine, Naomi, Don Des Jarlais, Seema Ahmad, Dave Purchase, and Charles Turner. 2004. "Long-term effects of syringe exchange on risk behavior and HIV prevention." *AIDS Education and Prevention* 16: 264-275.

Brock, Dan. 1993. "Quality of life measures in health care and medical ethics.: In *The Quality of Life*, edited by Martha Nussbaum and Amartya Sen, 95-132, Oxford: Clarendon Press.

Brownson, Ross C., Jonathan Fielding, and Christopher Maylahn. 2009. "Evidence-Based Public Health: A Fundamental Concept for Public Health Practice." *Annual Review of Public Health* 30:175-201.

Buchanan, David. 2001. *An Ethic for Health Promotion: Rethinking the sources of human well-being*. New York: Oxford University Press.

Buchanan, David. 2006a. "Moral reasoning as a model for health promotion." *Social Science and Medicine* 63: 2715-2726.

Buchanan, David. 2006b. "A new ethic for health promotion: Reflections on a philosophy of health education for the 21st century." *Health Education and Behavior* 33, 290-304.

Buchanan, David, and Franklin G. Miller. 2006. "A public health perspective on research ethics." *Journal of Medical Ethics* 32: 729-733.

Buchanan, David, and Franklin G. Miller. 2007. "Justice in research on human subjects." In *The Blackwell Guide to Medical Ethics,* edited by Rosamond Rhodes, Leslie Francis, and Anita Silvers, 373-392, New York: Blackwell.

Buchanan, David, Franklin G. Miller, and Nina Wallerstein. 2007. "Ethical issues in community-based participatory research: balancing rigorous research with community participation." *Progress in Community Health Partnerships* 2(1):153-160.

Buchanan, David, Priscilla Reddy, Sibu Sifunda, and Shegs James. 2008. "Assuring adequate protections in international health research: A principled justification and practical recommendations for the role of community oversight." *Public Health Ethics* 1(3):246-257.

Buchanan, David, Susan Shaw, Amy Ford, and Merrill Singer. 2003. "Empirical science meets moral panic: An analysis of the politics of needle exchange." *Journal of Public Health Policy*, 24(3–4): 427-444.

Callahan, Daniel. 2000. "Death and the research imperative." *New England Journal of Medicine*, 342(9): 654-656.

Community Intervention Trial for Smoking Cessation (COMMIT). 1995a. "I. Cohort results from a four-year community intervention." *American Journal of Public Health* 85(2): 183-192.

Community Intervention Trial for Smoking Cessation (COMMIT). 1995b. "II. Changes in adult cigarette smoking prevalence." *American Journal of Public Health* 85(2): 193-200.

Daniels, Norman, and James Sabin. 1997. "Limits to health care: Fair procedures, democratic deliberation, and the legitimacy problem for insurers." *Philosophy and Public Affairs* 26: 303-350.

Dresser, Rebecca. 2001. *When science offers salvation: Patient advocacy and research ethics*. New York: Oxford University Press.

Emanuel. Ezekiel, David Wendler, Jack Killen, and Christine Grady. 2004. "What makes clinical research in developing countries ethical? The benchmarks of ethical research." *Journal of Infectious Diseases* 189:930-7.

Evidence-Based Working Group. 1992. "Evidenced-based medicine: A new approach to teaching the practice of medicine." *Journal of the American Medical Association* 268(17): 2420-2425.

Flay, Brian. 1986. "Efficacy and effectiveness trials (and other phases of research) in the development of health promotion programs." *Preventive Medicine* 15: 451-474.

Green, Lawrence. 1977. "Evaluation and measurement: Some dilemmas for health education." *American Journal of Public Health* 67: 155-161.

Green, Lawrence. 2006. "Public health asks of systems science: To advance our evidence-based practice, can you help us get more practice-based evidence?" *American Journal of Public Health* 96: 406-409.

Green, Lawrence and Russell Glasgow. 2006. "Evaluating the relevance, generalization, and applicability of research: Issues in external validation and translation methodology." *Evaluation and the Health Professions* 29: 26-53.

Hanson, Dale, Jan Hanson, Paul Vardon, Kathryn McFarlane, Jacqui Lloyd, Reinhold Muller, and David Durrheim. 2005. "The injury iceberg: An ecological approach to planning sustainable community safety interventions." *Health Promotion Journal of Australia* 16(1): 5-10.

Hill, Austin B. 1965. "The environment and disease: Association or causation?" *Proceedings of the Royal Society of Medicine* 58: 295-300.

Holder, Hal. 2000. "Community prevention of alcohol problems." *Addictive Behaviors* 25: 843-859.

Holder, Hal. 2002. "Prevention of alcohol and drug 'abuse' problems at the community level: What research tells us." *Substance Use and Misuse* 37(8–10): 901-921.

Institute of Medicine. 1988. *The Future of Public Health*. Washington, DC: National Academies Press.

Institute of Medicine. 1998. *Scientific opportunities and public needs: Improving priority setting and public input at the National Institutes of Health*. Washington DC: National Academies Press.

Institute of Medicine. 2002. *Who will keep the public healthy? Educating public health professionals for the 21st century*. Washington, DC: National Academies Press.

Israel, Barbara, Amy Schulz, Edith Parker, Adam Becker, Alex Allen, Ricardo Guzman, and Richard Lichtenstein. 2003. "Critical issues in developing and following community based participatory research principles." In *Community-based Participatory Research for Health,* edited by Meredith Minkler and Nina Wallerstein, 31-44, San Francisco: Jossey-Bass.

Kantor, Lori. 2008. "NIH Roadmap for Medical Research." *Alcohol Research and Health* 31(1): 12-13.

Luepker, Russell, David Murray, David Jacobs, Maurice Mittelmark, Nell Bracht, Ray Carlaw, *et al.* 1994. "Community education for cardiovascular disease prevention: Risk factor changes in the Minnesota Heart Health Program." *American Journal of Public Health* 84: 1383-1393.

MacIntyre, Sally. 1986. "The patterning of health by social position in contemporary Britain: Directions for sociological research." *Social Science and Medicine* 23(4): 393-415.

Marmot, Michael. 2003. "Understanding social inequalities in health." *Perspectives in Biology and Medicine* 46(3): S9-23.

Marmot, Michael. 2004. "Social causes of social inequalities in health." In *Public health, ethics, and equity*, edited by Sudhir Anand, Fabienne Peter, and Amartya Sen, 37-62, Oxford: Oxford University Press.

Marmot, Michael, and Richard Wilkinson. 1999. *Social determinants of health*. New York: Oxford University Press.

McGinnis, J. Michael, and William Foege. 1993. "Actual causes of death in the United States." *Journal of the American Medical Association* 270: 2207-2212.

McGinnis, J. Michael, Pamela Williams-Russo, and James Knickman. 2002. "The case for more active policy attention to health promotion." *Health Affairs* 21: 78-93.

Michaels, David and Celeste Monforton. 2005. "Manufacturing uncertainty: Contested science and the protection of the public's health and environment." *American Journal of Public Health*, 95(Suppl 1), S39-48.

Murray, David. 2001. "Efficacy and effectiveness trials in health promotion and disease prevention: Design and analysis of group-randomized trials." In *Integrating behavioral and social sciences with public health*, edited by Neil Schneiderman, Marjorie Speers, Julia Silva, Henry Tomes, and Jacquelyn Gentry, 305-320. Washington, DC: American Psychological Association.

National Institutes of Health. 2005. *Policy on enhancing public access to archived publications resulting from NIH-funded research*. Bethesda, MD: Office of Extramural Research. Available at: https://grants.nih.gov/grants/guide/notice-files/NOT-OD-05-022.html

National Research Council. 2012. *Using Science as Evidence in Public Policy*. Washington, DC: The National Academies Press.

Neubauer, Deane, and Richard Pratt. 1981. "The Second Public Health Revolution: A critical appraisal." *Journal of Health Politics, Policy and Law* 6(2): 205-228.

Parascandola, Mark. 1998. "Epidemiology: Second-rate science?" *Public Health Reports* 113: 312-320.

Parascandola, Mark and Douglas Weed. 2001. "Causation in epidemiology." *Journal of Epidemiology and Community Health* 55: 905-912.

Pew Health Commission. 1998. *Recreating health professional practice for a new century*. Philadelphia: The Pew Charitable Trusts.

Project on Scientific Knowledge and Public Policy. 2007. *About us*. Retrieved January 26, 2007, from http://www.defendingscience.org/About-Us.cfm

Rees, Jonathon. 2004. "The fundamentals of clinical discovery." *Perspectives in Biology and Medicine* 47(4): 597-607.

Rogers, Wendy. 2004. "Evidence based medicine and justice: A framework for looking at the impact of EBM upon vulnerable or disadvantaged groups." *Journal of Medical Ethics* 30: 141-145.

PART II

8. Moral Reasoning as a Model for Health Promotion

Social scientific research is a peculiarly self-reflexive form of inquiry. It not only seeks to explain the behavior of other human beings, but also to provide self-understanding. By the same token, researchers can reflect on their own behavior in the effort to gain insight into the actions of others. This chapter proposes that health researchers can improve their understanding of how people make health choices by examining how they attempt to change their own behavior with respect to conducting research.

During the course of conducting health studies, investigators are often confronted with ethical dilemmas about what they should do, which course of action is most appropriate in the situation at hand. There are competing moral principles at stake and they are not sure which should take precedence or carry greater weight. To resolve these dilemmas, the various parties involved–researchers, IRBs, bioethicists, research participants, and the lay public–engage in a process that philosophers formally call "normative analysis," which aims to identify good reasons for choosing one option over another. The research community seeks to reach free and uncoerced agreement that the particular analysis under consideration is correct; that is, they draw conclusions about which action is right in that situation based on the cogency and coherence of the reasoning put forward. To illustrate, the research community once thought that women should be excluded from participation in health research due to a perceived greater vulnerability. Later, however, they came to see and agree that it was unfair to conduct research only on men, since the benefits of the research for women would remain uncertain and justice demands that the benefits be distributed fairly. Based on analyses of the relevant moral considerations, researchers decided to change their behavior and now systematically seek to achieve gender balance in health studies (unless there are particular circumstances that indicate why it is not necessary).

The purpose of this chapter is to describe a model of moral reasoning used by researchers to guide their own conduct and to suggest that this model could be applied to good advantage in health education, by re-shaping both research and practice in health promotion. The field of health education is now devoted to discovering and developing a scientific explanation of behavior. Interest in "evidence-based public health" has put an even greater premium on testing hypotheses to determine the most effective means of changing people's behavior. In contrast, this essay proposes that the field needs to pay greater attention to the ethical dimensions of human agency to advance its understanding of human action. The model of moral reasoning described here offers an expanded view of the human condition that will enable researchers to develop a more comprehensive body of knowledge to advance the field. The proposed model also provides a promising approach for demonstrating greater success in the field by identifying a broader range of worthwhile outcomes.

The chapter starts with an outline of two frameworks for describing the human condition–called the "scientific" and "humanistic" models–and identifies several characteristics on which they can be compared and contrasted. To demonstrate the application of humanistic research methods, the article presents a synopsis of two normative analyses from the author's own research, the Kennedy-Krieger lead abatement study and early stopping rules for reasons of efficacy in clinical trials. The purpose of introducing these case examples is: (1) to illustrate the process that the research community uses to decide what to do and whether they need to change their behavior; and (2) to indicate, by way of analogy, a model for thinking about processes of behavior change outside of the research context in the quotidian world of human health behaviors. Reflecting on the ways that researchers make decisions regarding their conduct offers a distinct, and potentially more fruitful, way of thinking about how the field could be re-oriented. In contrast to the standard scientific model that now dominates the field, the model of moral reasoning would reconfigure the relationship between research and practice. As proposed here, research and practice in health promotion would be redirected toward the goal of promoting autonomy and responsibility by means of enhancing people's capacity for moral reasoning.

Two Views of the Human Condition

Over the course of human history, two basic worldviews about the human condition–some might say competing, but perhaps they are better understood as complementary–have emerged. While this brief sketch obviously must grossly oversimplify complex matters, these worldviews can be succinctly cast as ideal types, in Weber's sense of the term.

In the first perspective, the scientific model views human behavior as the product of antecedent factors that cause people to act in predictable ways. Behavioral research in the scientific model is thus directed towards verifying cause-and-effect relationships. Researchers test hypotheses in experimental research designs, towards the goal of developing the capacity to interrupt the causal chain of events that results in unhealthy behaviors.

In contrast, the humanistic model sees human beings as endowed with a free will that allows them to choose between different courses of action. It is the ability to choose that provides the very foundation for ascribing moral responsibility. In this view, human action is guided by reasons, which enable people to act on felt desires–or to choose not to act–based on values and principles that they hold to be important (Frankfurt, 1971). Research in the humanistic model is thus directed towards clarifying human values, good reasons for pursuing one course of action over another and the moral considerations that should properly guide conduct.

These two models can be contrasted on several characteristics. While space constraints preclude a full discussion here, the respective frameworks highlight different aspects of the human condition and use different rules of evidence to draw conclusions about different types of questions. (See Table 1.4 in Chapter One for a summary discussion.) Significantly, the issue of whether one model has been proven to be true, while the other patently false, has not been definitively resolved. It is an open question whether human beings have free will, but the dismal lack of progress in the social sciences and the lived experience of feeling like one can choose suggest that human agency and moral responsibility remain viable possibilities (Kane, 2002). In general, the respective models serve as a set of background assumptions that researchers in different fields largely take for granted in conducting research.

One advantage of the scientific model, which may explain why it has become so popular in the social sciences, is that it provides more clear-cut rules for deciding whether the evidence yielded by an investigation enables one to draw certain conclusions. There can be little question that the scientific model provides a greater degree of certainty in answering certain types of questions. But it is important to acknowledge that the questions that it can answer–questions about the size and path of cause-and-effect relationships–do not exhaust the sphere of human concerns: for example, is certain research (e.g., a natural history of syphilis in black men) socially valuable, or is it wrong? Hypothesis-testing research is incapable of answering such normative questions.

It is an unfortunate fact of the limits of human knowledge that the model that seeks to address the ethical dimension of human agency simply does not provide the same level of confidence that can be found the hypothesis-testing, scientific method (Taylor, 1985). In conducting normative analyses, bioethicists are the first to admit that one of the most vexing problems in ethics centers on the nature and limits of justification (Daniels, 1996). One crucial issue in seeking valid answers to ethical questions is the epistemological foundation for justifying moral judgments: When is a reason a *good* reason for a moral judgment? What reasons count, and how much weight should they be given? In answer to these questions, bioethicists posit that the standards for certifying the validity of ethical claims are ultimately based on reaching reasoned agreement. There is a subtle point to emphasize here: positions are justified *not* by the fact that people agree with it, but because they find good reason to concur with the analysis.

Many health researchers might consider the methods of humanistic inquiry foreign and irrelevant, but such analyses invariably comprise the starting point for any research that involves human subjects, especially health research, since it frequently poses risks to the participants. Because there are significant social values at stake–the potential benefits of the research versus the potential harms to participants–researchers must rely on rigorous, sound analyses about the ethically most appropriate way to proceed. Researchers decide what to do based on their recognition and acknowledgement that there are good reasons for choosing one course of action over another. Two case examples are presented to illustrate this process; readers are referred to the original studies for complete discussions.

Kennedy Krieger Institute Lead Abatement Trial

The first research project concerns the controversial Kennedy-Krieger Institute (KKI) Lead Abatement Trial (Buchanan and Miller, 2006; Buchanan and Miller, 2007). The purpose of the KKI research was to determine if less expensive lead abatement procedures could prevent lead poisoning in children living in high-risk environments. In 2000-2001, CDC data showed that 2.2% of all children 1-5 years old in the US, and 9.6% of African-American children, had blood lead levels above the recommended 10 micrograms (µg) (Centers for Disease Control, 2003). According to the Alliance to End Childhood Lead Poisoning, an estimated 5 million preschool children in the US still live in houses with significant lead hazards. When the KKI study was being conceived, 95% of low-income housing in identified neighborhoods in Baltimore was contaminated by lead-based paint. Studies at the time showed that 40-50% of the predominantly African-American children living in these high risk neighborhoods had elevated blood lead levels over 20 µg, deemed "moderate" blood lead elevation by CDC standards. But because of the high costs of standard lead abatement

(~$20,000 per house), little was being done about the problem (Needleman, 1998; Baltrop, 1974).

To address these conditions, researchers at the Kennedy-Krieger Institute, a pediatric research facility affiliated with Johns Hopkins University, developed low-cost lead abatement procedures that effectively reduced ambient lead paint dust levels by 80% or more. The researchers then wanted to test whether these low-cost methods would effectively reduce blood lead levels in children living in houses that had been so abated.

The study included 108 houses in five comparison groups: three treatment groups that used the new lead abatement procedures, costing $1,650, $3,500, and $6,500, respectively; and, two comparison conditions, composed of housing abated by the city of Baltimore and housing built after 1978, which were presumably lead paint-free (Environmental Protection Agency, 1997; Farfel and Chilsom, 1991). By design, the researchers chose not to include a control comparison of existing housing that had received no abatement procedures, because they thought that it would be unethical to follow children being exposed to a known health hazard without remediation, despite the fact that this was the condition of the majority of children living in these neighborhoods. The study was designed to collect blood samples at baseline, 6 months and 24 months; children whose blood lead level exceeded 20 μg or whose blood level increased by 5 μg or more were referred for medical and environmental attention. The results showed significant reductions in lead dust in all five study conditions. Overall, the blood lead levels of children residing in the KKI-treated homes stayed constant or went down, although there were a few cases of increases.

Shortly after the trial was completed, two families sued KKI, stating that they were not fully informed of the trial purposes and that KKI had failed to inform them in a timely manner of the results of their children's blood tests. The case was thrown out by the lower courts, but the families appealed and in August 2001, in *Grimes vs. Kennedy Krieger Institute*, the Court of Appeals (Maryland's highest court) issued a scathing 96-page ruling comparing the research to the Tuskegee syphilis study and Nazi research on prisoners (Maryland Court of Appeals, 2001). The judges called it a "callous scientific experiment that put children in harm's way," saying the children were being used merely as "measuring tools."

The judges' decision made national headlines, and in the ensuing controversy, numerous articles analyzing the case have appeared in public health, legal, medical, and bioethics journals (Glantz, 2002; Mastroianni and Kahn, 2002; Hoffmann and Rothenberg, 2002; Ross, 2002; Spriggs, 2004). Critics have questioned the value of the research, and going even further, whether such research might undermine efforts to enforce just social policies. Moreover, they claim that the research is unfair, because it treats different population groups unequally, by providing participants with an intervention that is less effective than the best known treatment available. Finally, they contend that the research exploits the participants, by sacrificing their welfare to accomplishing the goals of the research.

In our analysis, the KKI case raises the broader question of whether research designed to test less costly interventions that might not be as effective as existing treatments can ever be ethically justified. In seeking to resolve whether such research should be allowed to proceed, we have determined that this type of research can be ethically justified only under carefully circumscribed conditions. To justify research aimed at developing less expensive yet less effective interventions, four conditions must be met: (1) a large population in need; (2) the existence of a treatment that is more effective yet substantially more expensive than a lower standard that would be cheaper but still significantly effective; (3) economic or political constraints that prohibit extensive provision of the higher standard; and, (4) a high likelihood that the less costly intervention will be implemented on a wide scale.

In response to arguments that such research should never be allowed, we identified the following reasons for permitting research on less expensive treatments to go forward, under the conditions enumerated above. The value of this research lies in developing an intervention that can provide relief to potentially millions of children in their lifetime. Indeed, the failure to conduct such research causes the greater harm, because it limits health interventions to the *status quo* of those who can afford currently available options and deprives disadvantaged populations of the benefits of imminent incremental improvements in health conditions. Such research represents a fair contract with the participants, where the risks to subjects are reasonable and proportionately balanced in relation to the prospective health benefits to them and the value of the knowledge to be gained. Contrary to the misplaced charges of exploitation, all of the participants in KKI study stood to benefit from reduced exposure to lead effected by the research intervention. Thus, the KKI study offered a favorable risk-benefit ratio both in terms of potential benefits to the participating children by living in safer housing, and in terms of the knowledge to be gained about cost-effective means of lead abatement.

Early Stopping Rules for Reasons of Efficacy

The second case example focuses on early stopping rules for clinical trials (Buchanan and Miller, 2005; Buchanan, Dunn, Slutsman and

Miller, 2004). Data and Safety Monitoring Boards (DSMBs) are responsible for reviewing emerging data from clinical trials and recommending that trials be stopped for reasons of toxicity, efficacy, or futility (Ellenberg, Fleming and DeMets, 2003; Food and Drug Administration, 2001). While it is obvious that trials should be stopped as soon as firm evidence emerges indicating that a new treatment is harmful, it is less clear when trials should be stopped when data indicate that a new drug appears to be beneficial. Given that valuable data will be lost, a critical question that researchers must answer is, when should clinical trials be stopped for reasons of efficacy?

The issue received considerable attention because three major national breast cancer treatment trials were stopped early for reasons of efficacy in the early 2000s (Goss, Ingle, Martino, Robert, Muss, Piccart, *et al.*, 2003; Coombes, *et al.*, 2004; Baum, *et al.*, 2002). The decision to stop these trials provoked heated controversies. While many researchers decried the loss of data, more surprisingly, the decisions were also criticized by the National Breast Cancer Coalition, the nation's largest breast cancer patient advocacy group, and the New York Times editorial board, who declared the decision to stop one trial an exercise in "ethical overkill" (Bryant and Wolmark, 2003; Cannistra, 2004; Twombly, 2003; New York Times Editors, 2003).

Currently, decisions about when to start and stop trials are founded on the concepts of equipoise and the therapeutic obligation. The therapeutic obligation derives from the Hippocratic Oath. In swearing allegiance to this Oath, physicians make a commitment to do everything in their power to benefit the patient. Once physicians assume this obligation, however, it creates a potential ethical dilemma in conducting research, as research participants will inevitably be exposed to a treatment found to be inferior to the other trial arm.

To resolve this dilemma, Fried (1974) developed the concept of "equipoise." Based on the concept of equipoise, it is ethical to start trials only when clinicians are in genuine doubt about the benefits of a new treatment. The reason that a clinician must be in a state of equipoise is that, if a physician knew that one therapy was worse than another, then it would be unethical for the physician to randomize patients to the inferior condition, because it would violate their therapeutic obligation to provide the best treatment possible to patients. Following this line of thinking, in landmark papers, Marquis (1983) claimed that, due to the therapeutic obligation, it is "ethically mandatory" to stop a trial as soon as it is "more probable" that one treatment regimen is better than another. Likewise, Freedman (1987) re-affirmed that trials should be stopped as soon as one discovers that one treatment is superior: "Should the investigator discover that one treatment is of superior therapeutic merit, he or she is ethically obliged to offer that treatment. This may occur well short of the original schedule for the termination of the trial."

In practice, the decision about when there is sufficient evidence to conclude that one treatment is superior is based on rejecting the null hypothesis (Freedman, Glass, and Weijer, 1996). As Figure 8.1 illustrates, there are various early stopping rules, such as the O'Brien-Fleming boundary, that define when this point has been reached (Jennison and Turnbull, 2000). It is important to note that these rules are all based on strict extrapolations of the p<.05 cut-off point for rejecting the null hypothesis, merely adjusted for taking serial peeks at the data. If the DSMB plans to look at the data every 6 months, then they need to adjust the p-value to take into account the repeated looks, such that the final p-value works out to the standard p<.05 convention for ruling out Type 1 errors. As soon as the data indicate that the magnitude of difference between the arms has crossed the designated boundary, the DSMB recommends the trial be stopped. In accordance with such rules, the letrozole trial, for example, was stopped after 2.4 years, instead of the original 5 years for which the trial was planned (Goss, *et al*, 2003).

There are many problems, however, associated with the loss of data that results from stopping early. Physicians and patients are left floundering with respect to the proper dose and length of treatment for the new drug. Other trials may be stopped, as the standard of care gets recalibrated, thus setting in motion a domino effect of toppling trials and losing even more information. Early stopping may lead to the need to conduct further trials to resolve unanswered questions, exposing even more subjects to research risks in the long run. Most importantly, stopping trials early may result in a therapy coming into practice that ultimately has an unfavorable risk-benefit ratio. As the results of the hormone replacement therapy and cox-2 inhibitor trials demonstrate, a new therapy may demonstrate immediate relief for hot flashes or pain but cause higher mortality rates with long-term administration (Rossouw, *et al.*, 2002; Horton, 2004).

In examining the basis for setting early stopping rules, we have proposed that the rules should be changed. In our analysis, the key question is, when should continuing a trial in the face of emerging evidence of benefit for the intervention group be considered morally equivalent to harming or exploiting participants in the control group due to the withholding of superior treatment? Based on the principle of non-exploitation (Wertheimer, 1996), we posit that the stringency of the stopping guideline should be proportional to the gravity of the harm incurred by withholding an efficacious treatment. In this framework, we delineate different types of primary outcomes, whether mortality, major morbidity, or minor symptom, and adjust the early stopping rules accordingly. The lesser the harm of the primary endpoint, the greater the amount of evidence it should take to stop a trial. (See Figure 8.2.)

Figure 8.1: Various Early Stopping Rules

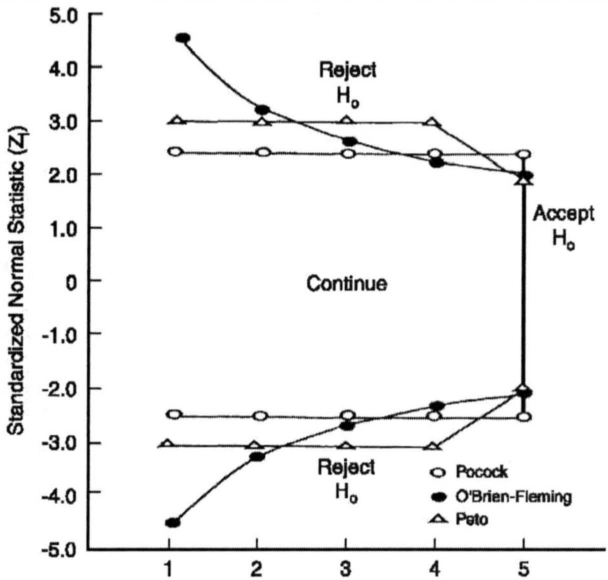

Figure 8.2: Proposed Schema for Stopping Trials Early

		Appropriate statistical cut-off point		
		Comparison of point estimates	Lower bound of 95% CI	Maximum acceptable difference
Primary endpoint	Mortality	Stop trial		
	Major morbidity		Stop trial	
	Minor Symptom			Stop trial

The alternative framework reflects the moral significance of the difference between practicing medicine and conducting research. In a medical setting, it may be morally acceptable for a physician to use any evidence (personal experience, rules of thumb, case studies, etc.) as the basis for trying a new treatment regimen with a particular patient. Sometimes, these "experiments" turn out to be ill-advised and the patient's condition aggravated, but the effects of individualized medical decisions have no ramifications beyond that single patient. However, in the context of randomized controlled trials, the decisions of DSMBs have implications for the whole of society. Since FDA approval and standards of practice often hang in the balance, the moral consequences of being wrong–of recommending a treatment that may turn out to increase the risk of serious morbidities or death–are more severe than individual clinical decisions. Therefore, it is appropriate to require a greater amount of evidence regarding the decision about when to stop a clinical trial than physicians in clinical practice may need to disturb equipoise. Under these more conservative rules, the decision to continue a trial is morally warranted because it is in both the participants' and the public's interest to establish greater certainty about the safety of the new drug, provided that this knowledge can be gained without exposing participants to undue risks.

Implications for Health Promotion

The purpose of presenting these case examples is to highlight the decision-making processes used by health researchers regarding their own behavior in conducting research. In contrast to this model, health researchers start from the assumption that the behavior of the people that they are studying is driven by antecedent factors that cause them to act in predictable ways, and thus, their behavior can be modified by manipulating these precursor social and psychological variables. If, however, health researchers act on the belief that their own behavior is guided by moral reasoning, then it may be worthwhile to consider the implications of normative analyses as a model for understanding the decision-making processes used by the lay public in deciding what they should do with respect to their health. In the situations described above, the researchers must decide what to do, and the way that they do that is to look for good reasons for proceeding in one direction versus another. I want to propose that the way that researchers decide about whether to go forward with their research or not is no different from the way that people in general decide how to conduct their lives: human beings look for good reasons for choosing one course of action over another.

Several characteristics of the action-guiding model described here are worth highlighting. First, contrary to the claims of some epistemologists, the conclusions drawn in these types of analyses are rational, defensible, and valid, even if no hypotheses have been tested. Perhaps the most striking aspect of the analyses presented above is that they immediately raise questions and invite a response. The reader seeks clarification of points before deciding whether she agrees. One wants to raise objections, hear rebuttals and strive to reach common ground that may, and often does, entail shifting one's original position in response to points that uncover flaws in one's initial reasoning.

Second, it appears that the researchers' decisions are based on free choice. While the possibility of free will remains an open question, it certainly seems like nothing causes or determines the outcome in advance; researchers must choose whether to continue the trial, or not. The grounds for justification and the validity of decisions are based on judgments about the strength of the arguments; researchers choose based on what they consider the more coherent case for one position over another. Third, as consumers of these analyses, researchers would consider it inappropriate if someone tried to manipulate their decision to adopt one pre-determined position over another; it is critically important to the ethical integrity of the researchers that they provide their free assent based on what they have determined is the right course of action.

Adopting an expanded view of the human condition that included the ethical dimensions of human agency would have major implications for both research and practice in health promotion. For researchers, it would mean opening important new vistas concerning both the means and ends of health promotion. In embracing a humanistic orientation, an important part of researchers' work would focus on conducting normative analyses to identify more compelling reasons why people should take up behaviors that promote physical fitness. It would also require researchers to think more deeply about the goals that the field seeks to achieve. For example, it would be important to address the question of the degree to which developing the technologies of behavior control is more important and should override the goal of promoting human autonomy and responsibility in seeking to realize human well-being (Buchanan, 2000).

Reflection on the ends of health promotion would open new avenues for empirical investigation. Rather than uncritically accepting pre-determined goals (largely set by bureaucratic imperatives for cost-effectiveness), researchers might consider the extent to which human beings achieve a sense of well-being through living lives of personal integrity and pursuing life projects that connect them to transcendent values that bring meaning to their lives. For example, many studies have shown that physical health does not bring happiness, while conversely, finding a sense of purpose leads to better physical health (Ostir, *et al*, 2000; Ostir, *et al*, 2001; Segerstrom, *et al*, 1998; Diener, 2000). Likewise, it appears that those people in our society who can now exercise the greatest degree of individual autonomy also enjoy the best health. If these findings hold up, then it would seem that promoting autonomy, rather than attempting to control and restrict choice, offers the more promising prospect of promoting physical health.

If health behavior research was re-directed towards identifying good reasons for choosing one course of action over another, it would open the field to the possibility that a broader range of outcomes for evaluating health promotion programs might be relevant and important. By ignoring the possibility of free choice, the field has set itself up for failure. Currently, researchers have declared that the success of health promotion efforts can best be measured – and to many researchers, *only* be measured – by the degree to which programs change people's behavior. Based on a research agenda restricted to identifying the causes of human behavior, the field has promised to deliver programs that are as effective in making people lose weight as physicians are in reducing blood pressure with prescription medications. Yet, it is difficult to make a convincing case that the field is making commensurate progress in controlling people's behavior. The reason that the field of health promotion has not been able to make greater progress is largely because it has overlooked the ethical dimensions of human agency. One major concern is that, in light of the field's evident lack of progress to date in developing effective behavior change programs, policymakers and funding agencies may conclude that health behavior research does not hold the same scientific promise as other avenues, and therefore, should be afforded lower priority in funding allocation decisions.

In contrast, the humanistic model provides a more realistic possibility for demonstrating the success of health education programs. Rather than narrowly focusing on behavior change, the field could consider the possibility of helping people to develop their own capacity for exercising autonomy and responsibility (Bellah, 1983). At an individual level, humanistic criteria of evaluating health promotion programs might focus on evidence of informed decision-making; for example, (1) awareness of alternative courses of action; (2) the ability to enumerate the advantages and disadvantages of the major alternatives; (3) greater self-understanding of one's reasons for choosing one course of action over another; (4) greater satisfaction with one's decision; and, (5) greater reassurance that one's decision better advances one's own life projects. At the community level, humanistic criteria could include: (1) the degree to which the community provides input and exercises control over research and community programs; (2) the degree to which community members feel their advice is respected; (3) the degree to which participants feel their concerns have been addressed; and finally, (4) the degree to which community members trust the researchers (Emanuel, Wendler, Killen and Grady, 2004).

In terms of practice, a humanistic orientation would require health educators to be open to the idea that, however they might think people should behave, they could be persuaded that community members have good reason for pursuing other courses of action and making choices that are valuable to them. For example, health promoters could be convinced that people are right in stating that they have more important things to do, like taking care of their children, developing their skills, or helping out in the community, than spending 45 minutes a day exercising at the gym, or that they would rather focus their attention on more worthwhile projects than losing 10 pounds. Similarly, while public health has declared smoking the number one public health problem, health promoters could better appreciate why certain communities might see drugs and violence as having higher priority. The field of health promotion could even be persuaded that it might be equally if not more important to recommend that community members devote 30 minutes a day to promote social justice, as a valued effort necessary to achieve the goal of reducing health disparities.

Emanuel and Emanuel (1992) provide an apt description of a humanistic orientation to health promotion, contrasting their "deliberative" model with the more traditional paternalistic process of seeking patient compliance:

> The aim of physician-patient interaction is to help the patient determine and choose the best health-related values that can be realized in the clinical situation. To this end, the physician must delineate information on the patient's clinical situation and then help elucidate the types of values embodied in the available options. The physician's objectives include suggesting why certain health-related values are more worthy and should be aspired to. The physician aims at no more than moral suasion; ultimately coercion is avoided and the patient must define his or her life and select the ordering of values to be espoused.

As these authors make clear, adopting a model of moral reasoning would in no way mean that health promoters would simply nod their heads in passive acquiescence to any nonsense that anyone put forward about why they plan to go living a self-destructive lifestyle. It is dialogical. It aims at reaching reasoned agreement about the good life for human beings (Bellah, 1983).

Discussion

Two possible objections to the proposed model might be that it is too rationalistic or too individualistic. Health education has found its *raison d'etre* in the fact that people frequently appear to act irrationally, take up self-destructive activities (such as smoking), and fail to change their behavior when informed of the dangers. Since giving people information is apparently insufficient to effect change, so the thinking goes, then the field must conduct research to uncover the "true," deeper, and presumed hidden and pathological causes of behavior. Based on the expert knowledge produced by such research, skilled professionals are supposed to design and implement programs that are effective in getting people to adopt pre-determined health behaviors, irrespective of whether such programs help people to gain insight into their own motivations.

In contrast to promoting physical fitness, the humanistic model described here seeks to achieve the goal of helping people to gain greater self-understanding and greater self-control–precisely, in that sense, of becoming more rational–even if it means that people decide they have more important things to do besides going to the gym 3-4 times per week. In the moral reasoning model outlined here, the purpose of both research and practice is to elucidate the reasons why people might consider the ("unhealthy") choices that they have made as acceptable and consistent with the kind of person that they want to be and life projects that they want to pursue at this point in their life. To the extent that health promoters are convinced that good physical health is important, then their practice would become directed towards articulating more compelling reasons for adopting certain health behaviors. Such programs, however, would be built around the notion of an argument. In this model, health promoters would (continue to) offer people various considerations about why they might want to change their behavior, reasons that most health promoters remain genuinely convinced are important (e.g., disease and disability restrict the range of opportunities open to individuals, and therefore, maintaining healthy functioning is helpful in pursuing valuable life projects), yet the measure of success would not necessarily be restricted to behavior change, but rather might include the degree to which people understand the implications of their decision and can explain why such a decision is right for them at this point in their lives. As Habermas (1984) reminds us, the goal of the enlightenment project is to realize the ideal of human rationality, not to develop ever more powerful technologies to force people to adopt regimens of physical fitness.

Second, a model of health promotion based on moral reasoning might appear to be too individualistic, directed at the decision-making processes of the individual, in contrast to the social determinants of health. This claim is a red herring. There is nothing inconsistent between the model outlined here and the goal of making changes in the social and physical environments to make them more conducive to healthy behaviors. On the contrary, the only way to gain support for public policies that would change environmental conditions is to convince people that proposed policies are more valuable than the current direction in which society is headed. For example, it appears that a broadly libertarian meritocratic conception of justice now prevails in the US. To achieve the goal of reducing health disparities, the field of public health must do a better job of convincing people that a more egalitarian conception of justice is the kind of society that all citizens would find more consistent with the values they wish to uphold. Making the case for revising public convictions about the justice of extant social conditions can only be accomplished by improving people's capacity for moral reasoning (while the field would need to remain open to the possibility that other theories of justice might prevail).

Finally, the moral reasoning model is more consistent with the goals of public health. One of the two overarching goals identified in *Healthy People 2010* is to improve the quality of life. To paraphrase Brock (1993), quality of life is defined by the capacity to deliberate and choose valued goals and activities for achieving them. Thus, if the field is truly interested in improving quality of life, then its primary mission must be to improve people's capacity for exercising autonomy and responsibility (Buchanan, 2000).

In his famous *Two Cultures* essay written more than 50 years ago, C. P. Snow (1964) lamented:

> I believe the intellectual life of the whole of western society is increasingly being split into two polar groups . . . Between the two, a gulf of mutual incomprehension–sometimes (particularly among the young) hostility and dislike, but most of all, a lack of understanding . . . It is all destructive. Much of it rests on misinterpretations, which are dangerous. The degree of incomprehension on both sides is a kind of joke which has gone sour . . . For the moment, I want to concentrate on the intellectual loss . . . When those two senses have grown apart, then no society is going to be able to think with wisdom.

Reflecting Snow's concerns, the field of health promotion currently seems obsessed with establishing its scientific credentials, to the neglect of the ethical dimensions of human agency. This position is perilously shortsighted.

To develop a more coherent body of knowledge, the field of health promotion must broaden its intellectual horizons, embrace a humanistic understanding of human motivation, and reject the destructive misinterpretations and intellectual loss that comes from too narrow a view of what constitutes valuable research and practice.

References

Barltrop, Donald. 1974. "Children and lead." *American Journal of Diseases of Children* 127(2): 165-166.

Baum, M., A. Buzdar, J. Cuzick, *et al.* 2003. "Anastrozole alone or in combination with tamoxifen versus tamoxifen alone for adjuvant treatment of postmenopausal women with early-stage breast cancer: results of the ATAC (Arimidex, Tamoxifen Alone or in Combination) trial efficacy and safety update analyses." *Cancer* 98(9):1802-1810.

Bellah, Robert. 1983. "Social Science as Practical Reason." In *Ethics, The Social Sciences, and Policy Analysis*, edited by Daniel Callahan and Bruce Jennings, 37-64, New York: Plenum Press.

Brock, Dan. 1993. "Quality of life measures in health care and medical ethics.: In *The Quality of Life,* edited by Martha Nussbaum and Amartya Sen, 95-132, Oxford: Clarendon Press.

Bryant, John and Norman Wolmark. 2003. "Letrozole after tamoxifen for breast cancer: what is the price of success?" *New England Journal of Medicine* 349(19): 1855-1857.

Buchanan, David. 2001. *An Ethic for Health Promotion: Rethinking the sources of human well-being*. New York: Oxford University Press.

Buchanan, David, Barbara Dunn, Julia Slutsman, and Franklin G. Miller. 2004. "Early Stopping for Efficacy: An Ethical Quandary and a New Proposal." Presentation at the annual meeting of the American Society for Bioethics and the Humanities, October 28-31, Philadelphia, PA.

Buchanan, David and Franklin G. Miller F.G. 2005. "Principles of Early Stopping of Randomized Trials for Efficacy: A critique of equipoise and an alternative ethical framework." *Kennedy Institute of Ethics Journal* 15(2):163-180.

Buchanan, David and Franklin G. Miller. 2006. "Justice and fairness in the Kennedy Krieger Institute Lead Paint Study: The ethical justification for public health research on less expensive yet less effective interventions." *American Journal of Public Health* 96(5):15-22.

Buchanan, David, and Franklin G. Miller. 2007. "Justice in research on human subjects." In *The Blackwell Guide to Medical Ethics,* edited by

Rosamond Rhodes, Leslie Francis, and Anita Silvers, 373-392, New York: Blackwell.

Cannistra, Stephen. 2004. "The ethics of early stopping rules: Who is protecting whom?" *Journal of Clinical Oncology* 22(9): 1542-1545.

Centers for Disease Control and Prevention. 2003. "Surveillance for elevated blood lead levels among children, United States, 1997-2001." *Morbidity and Mortality Weekly*. Sep 12; 52(10): 1-21. Washington DC: Government Printing Office.

Coombes, R. Charles, Emma Hall, Lorna J. Gibson, Robert Paridaens, Jacek Jassem, Thierry Delozier, *et al.* 2004. "A randomized trial of exemestane after two to three years of tamoxifen therapy in postmenopausal women with primary breast cancer." *New England Journal of Medicine* 350(11): 1081-1092.

Daniels, Norman. 1996. *Justice and justification: Reflective equilibrium in theory and practice*. New York: Cambridge University Press.

Diener, Ed. 2000. Subjective well-being. *American Psychologist* 55(1): 34-43.

Ellenberg, Susan, Thomas Fleming, and David DeMets. 2002. *Data monitoring committees in clinical trials: A practical perspective*. Hoboken, NJ: J. Wiley.

Emanuel, Ezekiel and Linda Emanuel. 1992. "Four models of the physician-patient relationship." *JAMA* 267(16): 2221-2226.

Emanuel, Ezekiel, David Wendler, Jack Killen, and Christine Grady. 2004. "What makes clinical research in developing countries ethical? The benchmarks of ethical research." *Journal of Infectious Diseases* 189:930-7.

Environmental Protection Agency. 1997. "Lead-based Paint Abatement and Repair and Maintenance Study in Baltimore: Findings Based on Two Years of Follow-up". December, EPA Report No. 747-R-97-005.

Farfel, Mark and J. Julian Chisolm. 1991. "An evaluation of experimental practices for abatement of residential lead-based paint: Report on a pilot project." *Environmental Research,* 55(2): 199-212.

Food and Drug Administration. 2001. *Guidance for Clinical Trail Sponsors: On the Establishment and Operation of Clinical Trial Data Monitoring Committees.* Rockville, MD: US Department of Health and Human Services, Food and Drug Administration; November.

Frankfurt, Harry G. 1971. "Freedom of the Will and the Concept of a Person." *Journal of Philosophy* 68 (1): 5–20.

Freedman, Benjamin. 1987. "Equipoise and the ethics of clinical research." *New England Journal of Medicine* 317(3): 141-145.

Freedman, Benjamin, Charles Weijer and Kathleen Glass. 1996. "Placebo orthodoxy in clinical research. I: Empirical and methodological myths." *Journal of Law, Medicine and Ethics* 24(3): 243-251.

Fried, Charles. 1974. *Medical experimentation: Personal integrity and social policy*. New York: American Elsevier.

Glantz, Leonard. 2002. "Non-therapeutic research with children: Grimes v Kennedy Krieger Institute." *American Journal of Public Health* 92(7): 1070-1073.

Goss, Paul E. James N. Ingle, Silvana Martino, Nicholas J. Robert, Hyman B. Muss, *et al*. 2003. "A randomized trial of letrozole in postmenopausal women after five years of tamoxifen therapy for early-stage breast cancer." *New England Journal of Medicine* 349(19): 1793-1802.

Habermas, Jürgen. 1984. *The Theory of Communicative Action*. Boston: Beacon Press.

Hoffmann, Diane and Karen Rothenberg. 2002. "Whose duty is it anyway? The Kennedy Krieger opinion and its implications for public health research." *Journal of Health Care Law and Policy* 6(1): 109-147.

Horton, Richard. 2004. "Vioxx, the implosion of Merck, and aftershocks at the FDA." *Lancet* 364(9450): 1995-1996.

Jennison, Christopher and Bruce Turnbull. 2000. *Group sequential methods with applications to clinical trials*. Boca Raton: Chapman and Hall/CRC.

Kane, Robert (Ed.) 2002. *Free Will*. Malden, MA: Blackwell.

Marquis, Don. 1983. "Leaving therapy to chance." *Hastings Center Report* 13(4): 40-47.

Maryland Court of Appeals. 2001. *Ericka Grimes v Kennedy Krieger Institute, Inc.* No. 128, September Term, 2000. Available at: http://www.courts.state.md.us/opinions/ coa/2001/128a00.

Mastroianni, Anna and Jeffrey Kahn. 2002. "Risk and responsibility: Ethics, Grimes v Kennedy Krieger, and public health research involving children." *American Journal of Public Health,* 92(7): 1073-1076.

Needleman, Herbert. 1998. "Childhood lead poisoning: The promise and abandonment of primary prevention." *American Journal of Public Health* 88(12): 1871-1877.

New York Times Editors. 2003. "Halting a Breast Cancer Trial." *New York Times* p. 10. October 12.

Ostir, Glenn, Kyriakos Markides, Sandra Black, and James Goodwin. 2000. "Emotional well-being predicts subsequent functional independence and survival." *Journal of the American Geriatrics Society* 48(5): 473-478.

Ostir, Glenn, Kyriakos Markides, M. Kristen Peek, and James Goodwin. 2001. "The association between emotional well-being and the incidence of stroke in older adults." *Psychosomatic Medicine* 63(2): 210-215.

Ross, Lainie. 2002. "In defense of the Hopkins lead abatement studies." *Journal of Law, Medicine and Ethics* 30(1): 50-57.

Rossouw, Jacques E., Garnet L Anderson, Ross L Prentice, Andrea Z LaCroix, Charles Kooperberg, *et al.* 2002. "Risks and benefits of estrogen plus progestin in healthy postmenopausal women: Principal results from the women's health initiative randomized controlled trial." *JAMA* 288(3): 321-333.

Segerstrom, Suzanne, Shelley Taylor, Margaret Kemeny and John Fahey. 1998. "Optimism is associated with mood, coping, and immune change in response to stress." *Journal of Personality and Social Psychology* 74(6): 1646-1655.

Snow, Charles Percy. 1964. *The Two Cultures: And a second look* (2nd Ed.). New York: The New American Library.

Spriggs, Merle. 2004. "Canaries in the mines: Children, risk, non-therapeutic research, and justice." *Journal of Medical Ethics* 30(2): 176-181.

Taylor, Charles. 1985. "Interpretation and the Sciences of Man." In Charles Taylor, *Philosophy and the Human Sciences*, 15-57. Cambridge: Cambridge University Press.

Twombly, Renee. 2003. "Critics question price of success in halted clinical trial of aromatase inhibitor letrozole." *Journal of the National Cancer Institute* 95(23): 1738-1739.

Wertheimer, Alan. 1996. *Exploitation.* Princeton, NJ: Princeton University Press.

9. Assuring Adequate Protections in International Health Research: A Principled Justification and Practical Recommendations for the Role of Community Oversight

By David Buchanan, Sibusiso Sifunda, Nasheen Naidoo, Shamagonam James, Priscilla Reddy

Since the conduct of the controversial HIV-perinatal transmission trials in the early 1990s, debates have raged about the ethics of international health studies. In that research, pregnant women in low-income countries were given low doses of AZT to determine whether a less expensive alternative could be developed to prevent mother-to-infant HIV transmission (Angell, 1997, 2000; Lurie and Wolfe, 1997). The research raised serious questions about the potential for exploitation and the adequacy of present protections for participants in international health research.

In response to these controversies, a number of bioethicists have recently issued calls to mandate community involvement in decision-making about the conduct of health research (Weijer and Emanuel, 2000; Emanuel *et al.*, 2004; Brody *et al.*, 2005). One major concern raised by these analyses is whether Research Ethics Committee (REC) reviews and individual informed consent provide sufficient ethical safeguards in all contexts (Macklin, 2004).

Key issues left unresolved by these calls are both the theoretical foundation that could provide the ethical justification for community monitoring and practical strategies for instituting an oversight process with legitimized authority. To advance the development of sound context-appropriate ethical standards, this chapter presents a principled justification for the ethical assessment of international health research protocols by community representatives. In addition, recommendations regarding a feasible process for achieving community oversight that demonstrates respect for community autonomy are provided.

From the outset, it is important to address potential concerns that requiring an additional layer of review might impede the timely conduct of research (Berkley, 2003; Dawson and Kass, 2005). A vastly disproportionate share of the world's research resources is now allocated to studies on diseases that affect only a minority of the global population (Global Forum, 2004). Additional review requirements on international health research would be unjust if the net result served only to decrease access to the benefits of research further for the majority of the world's population.

Our view is that, requiring another level of review is necessary, not only to ensure ethically appropriate oversight, but also to facilitate the conduct of research by building trust in its safety and importance. In Western industrialized nations, there has been a "paradigm shift" in public attitudes toward research participation, where the weight of concerns has shifted from apprehension about the risks of research participation to an appreciation of the potential benefits (Kahn *et al.*, 1998; Meslin and McCarthy, 1998; Powers, 1998; Buchanan and Miller, 2006a). With the onset of the AIDS epidemic, the urgent need for effective treatments led many people to view research participation not as a pernicious threat, but as an opportunity to obtain the most scientifically advanced therapies possible. Since community monitoring should reduce the threat of exploitation and thereby increase trust in its potential benefits, specifying clear policies with respect to the purpose and parameters of community review should bolster confidence among potential research volunteers, and thus facilitate the conduct of research in these settings.

The chapter starts with a synopsis of concerns that have been raised about the processes of individual informed consent and REC review. We then examine recent issues that have emerged from the field of public health ethics regarding the adequacy of currently accepted ethical review procedures, which were designed primarily to monitor clinical treatment trials, and growing recognition of the need to take into account population protections. Building on that framework, we present the ethical rationale for community involvement in assessing the ethical conduct of health research by upholding respect for community autonomy. Community oversight refers to a process of engaging community members equitably in monitoring health intervention research to ensure that ethical standards are upheld, and the interests of community members protected. We conclude with practical recommendations regarding issues of representation to ensure fair community participation in monitoring health research.

Problems with Individual Informed Consent

A number of concerns have been raised about the adequacy and appropriateness of the individual informed consent standard in the context of international health research. These concerns include: the definition of "informed" and criteria for assessing its attainment; the cultural appropriateness of individualistic decision-making processes; concerns about the priority of individual autonomy over other moral considerations; questions about the utility of individual informed consent *per se*; and, finally, reconsiderations of the overarching purpose of informed consent requirements.

Faden and Beauchamp (1986) make a distinction between "philosophical" and "policy-oriented" definitions of informed consent. A philosophical definition refers to a substantial understanding of the overall research process and its implications for human interests. A policy- oriented definition refers to the legal requirements enumerated in state law, such as the US Code of Federal Regulations (45 CFR 46.116(c) and 45 CFR 46.116(d)), which denotes eight elements that must be presented in written informed consent documents.

While some legal provisions are designed to foster the conditions in which the substantive philosophical ideal can be attained, there are currently no established standards or criteria for determining the degree to which individuals truly understand what their participation entails. Critically, there is a much greater distance between the philosophical ideal and the reality of individual comprehension in contexts where participants may lack formal education, be illiterate, live in poverty, be malnourished or face other stressful life conditions. Furthermore, researchers and others have noted that many languages do not have words or equivalent concepts for basic terminology such as "research" or "hypothesis," let alone more technical scientific language such as "placebo," "false positives," and "randomization" (Ekunwe and Kessel, 1984; Bayer, 1998; Moodley, 2002; MacQueen *et al.*, 2004; Molyneux *et al.*, 2004; Dawson and Kass, 2005). More broadly, many sociocultural conceptual frameworks regarding the etiology of disease are incongruent with Western scientific explanations. In such contexts, while the eight elements of informed consent can perhaps be satisfactorily explained to potential participants (thus fulfilling the policy-oriented definition of informed consent), it is difficult to maintain that they have a proficient understanding of the nature, goals and risks of the research, which is fundamental to providing one's permission for researchers to proceed with the experiment. The common requirement that informed consent documents be written in plain language fails to address this important ethical problem.

Issues have also been raised about the imposition of Western norms of individual decision-making in contexts where such practices are foreign (Moodley, 2002; Dawson and Kass, 2005; Woodsong and Karim, 2005). The (Western) concern that others may exert undue influence may be based on the questionable assumption that the interests of the individual and the community are inherently in conflict. In different cultural contexts, however, social relationships may be understood to be (at least partially) constitutive of one's identity; for example, the traditional African concept of "ubuntu" has been defined as "umuntu ngumuntu ngabantu" – "you are who you are because of other people" (Biko, 1978). In the West, Sandel (1982) has described this broader self-understanding as a shift from thinking in terms of "I" to "we," where one's sense of identity is bound up with the realization of a common way of life, the reproduction of valued social practices, and the sense of community in which one takes pride. In such contexts, not only are the interests of the individual and the community commonly perceived to be synonymous, but the notion that persons *should* make decisions independently, divorced from their social relationships, is a flagrant violation of accepted social norms. The current push for requiring individual informed consent in all contexts appears to be based on the tacit assumption that low-income countries are traditional societies that have not yet attained a modern, enlightened mindset, in the sense of the emancipation of the individual and valorization of individual rights (Mamdani, 1996). This trajectory is apparently presumed to be unilinear, universal and normal, rather than historically contingent or problematic, where the possibility of developing ethical norms along divergent lines might remain open. In light of these opposing considerations, the proposed standards presented here seek to achieve an appropriate balance between concerns about the potential for individual exploitation and the need for respecting beneficent cultural practices.

Critics have also questioned the near-absolute priority placed on the principle of respect for individual autonomy (from which the mandate for individual informed consent derives) over other moral considerations in the brief history of bioethics, as it developed in the US (Weijer, 1999; Rhodes, 2005). As Levine (1986) notes, the work of the 1978 US National Commission must be seen in context of its time and thus can be faulted now for its overemphasis on individual rights, to the neglect of obligations to the larger community. More strongly, Taylor (1985) has assailed the central tenet of liberalism, which he calls the "primacy of rights," referring to the moral view that individual rights have priority over all other moral considerations, such as obligations to contribute to the collective good. However, as the well-known 1905 US Supreme Court ruling in *Jacobsen v.*

Massachusetts made clear, the principle of individual freedom cannot take absolute precedence over other moral principles. On the contrary, since the potential benefits to society and future generations are significant, other ethicists have taken the position that citizens *should* be morally obligated to participate in research, in order to advance the common good, distribute risk equitably, and mitigate the free-rider problem (Caplan, 1984; Harris, 2005; Orentlicher, 2005; Rhodes, 2005).

Moreover, Truog and his colleagues (1999) have questioned the "blind insistence" on obtaining individual informed consent. As they state, "There is little evidence to support the claim that informed consent, as currently practiced, provides protection against the exploitation of patients in research. Studies have shown that patients rarely have an adequate understanding of consent forms and often do not understand the meaning or implications of randomization." In its stead, they propose the use of a "reasonable person standard," which could be achieved by "the involvement of the community through the representation of people without medical backgrounds" on ethical review boards.

Finally, while great emphasis has been placed on the need for demonstrating respect for individual autonomy, another key purpose of informed consent has centered on reducing inequalities of power and knowledge (President's Commission, 1982). As described below, when novel interventions hold the potential for affecting the community as a whole, there is a critical need for putting processes in place that reduce inequalities of power between research institutions and communities targeted as potential pools for participant recruitment and eventual dissemination. Current interest in the USA in Community-Based Participatory Research (CBPR) appears to be directly related to reducing power differentials and mitigating these ethical concerns (Wallerstein *et al.*, 2005; Buchanan *et al.*, 2007). In many types of research, it is the community as a whole that both bears the risks and stands to gain the most from newly developed interventions. New policies are thus imperative for redressing power imbalances and giving due consideration to the community's right to self-determination.

Problems with Research Ethics Committee Review

A number of concerns have also been raised about the adequacy of the research ethics review process, including the composition, training, scope of authority, accountability and allegiance of review boards (Emanuel, *et al.*, 2004). The following analysis focuses primarily on the US system of Institutional Review Boards (IRBs), and thus is limited to USA and other countries that have adopted similar systems of research ethics review.

In a policy formulation that has since been called into question, the US Congress passed regulations that created a decentralized system of ethical review boards and that enumerated only minimal requirements regarding the composition of local IRBs. According to these regulations, IRBs must have at least five members "with varying backgrounds to promote . . . sensitivity to such issues as community attitudes," "at least one member whose primary concerns are in non-scientific areas," and "at least one member who is not otherwise affiliated with the institution" (US 45 CFR 46.116). In practice, this has generally meant that institutions appoint one outside community member to sit on a board with 10–12 other members recruited from the ranks of experienced researchers employed by the university or research organization. As a result, Marshall (2007, p. 17) notes that "most are dominated by scientists who are responsible for reviewing the research protocols of colleagues and friends." US regulations do not provide any further guidance with respect to how members should be selected.

Until quite recently, there were no requirements in the US regarding the training or qualifications of IRB members. In the wake of widespread public outcry over the deaths of two research participants in the early 2000s, however, the US Office of Human Research Protections instituted regulations that now require all researchers to gain certification in research ethics; this training is generally provided by new, on-line certificate programs designed for researchers with doctorates, which take about 1 hour to complete. Otherwise, IRB membership is open to people with no specific knowledge, training or experience in conducting ethical reviews.

Regarding the scope of their authority, one major concern is that IRBs in the USA derive their regulatory power from the conditions attached to federal funding; hence, privately funded research does not fall under the purview of IRB review but falls only under FDA inspection as it pertains to applications for licenses to sell new drugs or devices (Berg, *et al.*, 2001). Currently in USA, the volume and investment of health research conducted by the pharmaceutical industry exceeds that of publicly funded research (Bodenheimer, 2000; Rettig, 2000). While many private corporations have voluntarily adopted the federal code of ethics regulating health research, they are not mandated by law. In one report, Levinson (2007) found that FDA regulators do not know how many clinical trials are being conducted, audit less than 1% of the testing sites, and have only 200 inspectors to police an estimated 350,000 testing sites. Oversight of drug trials funded by private pharmaceutical companies in international settings is even less well monitored.

Critics have also pointed out that IRBs are accountable to no one, except the courts in instances when the institution is sued by participant(s) to redress allegations of harm (Berg, *et al.*, 2001). Presently, if researchers, participants, community members, or other third parties disagree with the decision to approve or not to approve the research by the IRB, or with any stipulations that are attached or not attached for modifying the protocol, there are no provisions or standing body for appeal where they can plead their case and seek remediation.

Finally, largely as a result of the cumulative impact of the above factors, concerns have also been raised about the allegiance of IRBs. Faced with growing fears of litigation and liability, several commentators have noted that IRBs appear to have adopted a narrow "regulatory model", focusing on meeting the letter of the law (e.g., ensuring that all eight elements are spelled out in an approved consent form), which appears to be aimed primarily at providing legal protection for the institution (London, 2002; Dawson and Kass, 2005). Capturing these concerns, in ruling on a lawsuit pressed by two families against Johns Hopkins' Kennedy Krieger Institute in their controversial Lead Paint Abatement Trial, the Maryland Court of Appeals issued a blistering critique that referred to the Hopkins IRB as "in-house agents" who were not "as sufficiently concerned with the ethicality of the research as they were with the success of the experiment" (Maryland Court of Appeals, 2000).

In succinct summary, the Office of the Inspector General of the US HHS issued a report on IRBs that concluded: "IRBs are reviewing too much, too quickly, with too little expertise; conducting minimal continuing review of approved research; facing conflicts of interest that threaten their independence; and providing little training for clinical investigators and board members" (Brown, 1998).

A Public Health Ethics Perspective

Since in the early 2000s, there has been growing attention to ethics from a public health perspective (Kass, 2001; Childress, *et al.*, 2002; Buchanan and Miller, 2006b; Buchanan and Miller, 2006c). Where medicine focuses on individual health, public health is concerned with the health of the entire population. Thus, in contrast to a fiduciary duty to the individual patient, public health ethics is founded on societal responsibility to protect and promote the health of the population as a whole. The moral obligation to protect population health holds important implications for identifying appropriate ethical standards to guide research ethics, including that conducted in international settings.

The emerging public health ethics framework builds on a line of reasoning that has focused on the role of justice in evaluating the conduct of health research; in so doing, it gives greater weight to concerns for the collective good relative to the current emphasis on individual rights (Meslin and McCarthy, 1998; Kass, 2004). As mentioned, observers have noted a "paradigm shift" in the evolution of public concerns about health research in USA, moving from a preoccupation with protecting participants from harm to an interest in improving access to clinical trials (Powers, 1998). In the historical context of public outrage at the egregious misconduct of researchers at Tuskegee and other research scandals, the Belmont Report concentrated accordingly on justice considerations internal to the research process (National Commission, 1979). Although concerns about distributing the benefits of research fairly in society are presented, the report focused primarily on protecting research participants from harm and exploitation. Over time, however, the weight of public moral concerns has shifted, from worries about the risks of participating in research to greater recognition of the potential benefits. For example, the research community once thought that women should be excluded from health research due to a perceived greater vulnerability. Later, they recognized that it was unfair to conduct research only on men, since the benefits of the research for women would remain uncertain and justice demands that the benefits be distributed fairly (Dresser, 1992; Kahn *et al.*, 1998; Weijer and Crouch, 1999). Thus, the inclusion of various population groups is now seen to be obligatory. The demands of justice have expanded the range of parties that ought to be considered morally relevant beyond the participants alone in determining the acceptability of the research under consideration.

From a public health perspective, the range of risks and benefits that are considered ethically significant must be extended to take into account the social impact of the research (Buchanan and Miller, 2006b, 2006c). In ethical reviews, research is ultimately justified on the basis of its social value; research without any social or scientific value cannot be justified because it would place participants at risk for no reason, that is, without compensating social benefit (Emanuel *et al.*, 2000). To determine the social value of research, a comprehensive analysis should consider not only the risks and benefits to the research participants themselves, but also the benefits and risks to the population as a whole. Adopting a public health perspective thus entails the moral obligation of researchers to consider the interests of the community as a whole as well as the individual research participants.

A public health perspective on research ethics is based on due recognition of the inherently social purpose of health research. The evolution of ethical standards regulating health research (which has been dominated historically by clinical medical research) can be traced directly to the Hippocratic Oath and the decree that physicians have an unqualified duty of fidelity to each individual patient (Miller and Brody, 2003; Miller and Rosenstein, 2003). Due to its historical development within the context of clinical medical trials, the currently prevailing research ethics framework has focused virtually exclusively on protecting and benefiting individual participants, to the neglect of weighing the consequences of the research for the community as a whole. While this standard may be appropriate in the context of providing medical care, research results have implications for the whole of society. Unlike the clinical context of providing personalized doctor-patient care, in the context of conducting research, the moral consequences of inadvertently inflicting harm–of conducting a trial that turns out to increase risk of serious morbidities or death–extend beyond the individual to the community at large. The consequences of the conduct of the research include, for example, the perceived trustworthiness of health research, the perceived value of health science, and the likelihood of community-wide adoption of a new intervention (e.g., HIV vaccine) should one eventually become available. In contrast to basing standards on ethical norms appropriate to providing individual medical care, a public health perspective provides the theoretical foundation for incorporating due consideration of protecting community interests and respecting community autonomy in setting ethical standards for the conduct of health research.

The Ethical Justification for Community Oversight

As developed here, an ethical standard that requires community oversight of health research is justified on three principled grounds: respect for community autonomy and their right to self-determination; due consideration of the consequences of the research for the community as a whole; and, a more fully developed understanding of human autonomy. Respect for community autonomy entails the fundamental right of community members to exercise a meaningful role in determining the conduct of research that affects their lives (Buchanan *et al.*, 2007). Vaccines, for example, are designed not only to protect individuals but to protect the community as a whole, including unvaccinated individuals via herd immunity, but this can be achieved only if a large proportion of the population gets vaccinated. Requiring community review is warranted on the basis that communities are distinguishable entities with interests distinct from individual interests and that must be protected accordingly (Weijer, 1999; Brody *et al.*, 2005).

The principle of respect for community autonomy acknowledges that the community has a non-negligible stake in the decision to conduct research on its membership. The community, for example, has a collective right to participate in decisions regarding the use of limited fiscal or social resources (e.g., health clinic personnel and facilities). Since justice demands that resources be allocated fairly, the community must have a say in determining whether scarce resources are being diverted from more pressing priorities or result in other potentially important opportunities being lost (Brody *et al.*, 2005). This right encompasses protection against exploitation, where exploitation is defined as one party taking unfair advantage of another. As Wertheimer (1996) explains, for exploitation to occur, it is not necessary for one party to harm another–only that the benefit to one side be disproportionate compared to the benefit to the other. Given the enormous power of the pharmaceutical and academic health research enterprises, it is critically important to establish a body with sufficient standing to set fair terms of participation and protect against the potential for exploitation. For our purposes here, it is worth recalling that originally the word "autonomy" originally referred not to individuals but to relationships among city-states and communal independence from imperial domination (Hill, 2001).

In addition to problems of diverting scarce resources and exploiting community assets, the community bears other types of risks that cannot be reduced to the individual level. The success of many health interventions depends on their adoption by the population. To the extent that the conduct of the research reinforces negative attitudes (e.g., human beings as "guinea pigs"), it undermines trust in Western health science, which will impede the adoption of effective interventions. Likewise, the community as a whole must understand the implications of participation in certain types of research; sero-conversion due to participation in HIV/AIDS vaccine trials, for example, has high potential for family, workforce and community disruption if there is not a widespread understanding of its significance. The use of public resources also calls for public accountability, a standard that transcends individual consent and is not now part of REC review. If researchers claim that making referrals to a research project will not take an inordinate amount of staff time, a body is necessary to monitor whether it is interfering with the timely care of patients waiting for an appointment.

The community should also have the capacity to determine the fair terms of benefits in return for their participation. The so-called "ancillary duties" of researchers have received increasing attention in recent years, taking up questions about the extent of researcher obligations, for instance, to share the results with the community, to offer related health services (e.g., HIV testing and counseling), and to provide medical care for the participants (Belsky and Richardson, 2004; Macklin, 2004). The key point here is that the scope of fair, nonexploitative benefits can be decided and endorsed neither by individual participants nor by research institution-based RECs but only by the community itself.

Finally, the ethical justification for community oversight can be established on the basis of a more complete understanding of human autonomy, in particular, as it relates to conceptualizing human identity. In liberal Western societies, starting in the writings of Hobbes and Locke, conceptions of personhood have evolved in the direction of a radically individualistic, atomistic view of the human condition (Taylor, 1985). In this line of thinking, society and social cooperation come to exist only for the instrumental pursuit of individual interests, and social norms are perceived to be fundamentally antagonistic towards the unfettered quest for maximizing personal pleasure. This set of assumptions about human identity presses toward the position that the only right that warrants recognition is the right of individuals to choose not to participate.

In contrast, a number of other schools of thought, including communitarian, feminist and non-Western traditions of communalism, have underscored the incoherence of such assumptions, noting that an individual's sense of identity is inextricably bound up with social relationships and membership in groups (Weijer, 1999; Lindegger and Richter, 2000; Moodley, 2002). This broader view gains traction starting with the fact that any expression of self-understanding can be articulated only in terms provided by a situated linguistic community. It is only through participation in the life of a community that one gains access to and learns the linguistic practices that make possible perceptions of self and the value of certain activities and ways of life. The very language used for claiming that one wants to do something for some reason (e.g., choosing to participate in research or not) presupposes membership in a community in which those terms have meaning. But if one can perceive certain desires only within a given cultural context, then one must have an obligation to preserve the larger social grouping and ensure its continuing vitality, for otherwise the community that reproduces the concepts that enable one to make sense of one's decisions (e.g., by discerning value in select activities) would be lost. As Taylor (1985) and others have argued, we find here a duty to protect the community in which membership provides the capacity to find satisfaction and fulfillment in proffered ways of life.

On the other side of this same coin, individuals are systematically identified by their classification into social categories; thus, individual agreements to participate in research inevitably raise questions about stigmatizing identifiable social groups (Brody *et al.*, 2005). For example, the higher prevalence of HIV/AIDS found in Africans, which provides the primary justification for targeting Africans in AIDS prevention research, has been widely assumed to be attributable to promiscuous sexual practices, rather than other possible explanations (Epstein, 2007). In multiracial, multiethnic or otherwise diverse societies, the targeting of one group over another carries many meanings, about which the community identified for inclusion should be entitled to decide whether they find the implications of their participation acceptable. Hence, in direct parallel to the justification for respect for individual autonomy, the community has a right to protect itself against potential injuries to its self-understanding and self-respect (Taylor, 1992).

If one accepts that communities *per se* deserve protection and have a right to self-determination, then standards must be set to ensure community engagement in monitoring the conduct of health research. Based on the principle of community autonomy, we argue that the community is the best judge of its own interests; this position is analogous to the principle of individual autonomy, where respect is afforded the individual's right to determine his or her own best interests. Hence, a process must be put in place whereby the community can meaningfully deliberate about the implications of participating in a research project for its own interests. One process for achieving such community oversight is establishing Community Advisory Boards (CABs) (Buchanan *et al.*, 2007). Under the conditions specified below, CABs provide a sound mechanism for securing community ratification indicating that the research goals are valuable and methods acceptable to the community, before the research is allowed to proceed.

Practical Recommendations for Securing Legitimate Community Oversight

Currently, many CABs are set up for the express purpose of gaining access to groups targeted for recruitment purposes, and individual CAB members are identified and selected by the researchers for their "gate keeping" ability to open doors and provide entry to these populations (Cox *et al.*, 1998; Strauss *et al.*, 2001; Morin *et al.*, 2003; Reddy *et al.*, 2007). In contrast, once the ethical imperative for community oversight is acknowledged, then two key issues must be addressed. First, the body charged with responsibility for assuring community oversight must be vested with legitimate authority duly recognized by the community affected by the research to make decisions on their behalf. The second issue of concern here is specifying how community is defined.

While space constraints preclude a full discussion, in general, the two most common sources of legitimate civil authority are divine right and democratic procedures (Weber, 1915/1946; Friedman, 1990; Raz, 1990; Weijer and Emanuel, 2000; Richardson, 2002). To set up bodies with valid decision-making power, extant community norms and practices cannot be circumvented; unless decisions are made by a recognized source of legitimate authority, they will not be considered binding on community members. Thus, it is essential that researchers work within the existing system of power and authority at both the national and local levels.

The second major issue is the question of defining a community. A starting point for this discussion is the well-known distinction between geographic and sociological definitions of community (Clark, 1973; Plant, 1974). Health research projects have geographic locations,* the catchment area(s) for participant recruitment are defined in the research protocols. The research protocols will also specify the inclusion and exclusion criteria for participation, which provide the criteria for defining community sociologically (e.g., ethnic, cultural, linguistic, religious, gender, age, sexual orientation, racial, etc.).

Thus, we see two major sources of authority–leaders with inherited power and democratically elected representatives–and three major constituencies (existing authorities, residents, and potential participants) that must be acknowledged when vesting CABs with legitimate authority. Based on the preceding considerations, we make three recommendations with respect to instituting community oversight of health research.

The first is that national health ministries and national legislatures enact policies that require community review of health research. These national policies should specify the type of authority that will be recognized in constituting CABs, the level of geographic specificity, and the types of sociologically defined communities that merit protection against potential exploitation, and thus, representation on CABs. The national assembly should also establish an appeals process for groups not previously recognized to petition for inclusion.

---

* - The growing use of internet-based research belies this statement to some extent, suggesting a seemingly boundary-less domain. However, since the issue of concern here is specifying an identifiable community, questions raised by the use of the internet may be moot, as any meaningful sampling process capable of being generalized will require the same specification of geographic and sociological parameters (e.g., physicians practicing in the US).

The second recommendation is that the make-up of CABs should accord with existing social practices for making communally binding decisions.[†] In contexts where customary inherited authority is recognized, researchers must respect their executive agency and gain their approval and authorization to proceed. The ruling authority should be empowered to designate an agent or agents who will provide permission, approval and agreement on the terms and conditions of local participation. National legislation should stipulate whether any further community review is required at the local level. In other locales, there may be well-established practices of democratic decision-making and representation. There, we recommend that CAB members should be elected by both geographic and sociological community members (see third recommendation below).

Many countries have coexisting systems of rule by inherited power and democratic plebiscites. The South African Constitution, for example, provides one model for achieving an appropriate balance between political rights to vote for representatives to legislative bodies and recognition of the authority of traditional leaders on matters at the local level. In such contexts, we recommend that both sources of communal authority be consulted. The issue of whether the respective approval processes remain separate, or be combined, leads into our final recommendation.

Third, we recommend that one of the two following models of representation on CABs be adopted. In Model A, the CAB is composed of equal numbers of representatives of the traditional authorities, democratically elected residents, and participant representatives. The CAB will deliberate as a whole to determine whether the research should be approved, not approved, or how it should be modified to make it acceptable to each of the three respective constituencies. In Model B, there are two separate CABs, one composed of traditional authorities, and the other of equal numbers of geographically representative residents and targeted participants. Since many sociological communities may not be formally organized, we recommend soliciting volunteers. If more people volunteer than there are seats on the board, we recommend a process of random selection to ensure fairness.

[†] - The issue of conducting research in nations with despotic regimes and a history of human rights abuses is complicated. To the extent that CABs are permitted because they are perceived as politically neutral and non-threatening, they may foster the growth and vitality of civil society, which may prove to be beneficial for the country in time. Thus, we would not dismiss the possibility out of hand.

Discussion

The ethical foundations of health research are currently in a state of disequilibrium, both in international settings and in industrialized nations. Appeals to the established practices of Research Ethics Committee review and individual informed consent are inadequate, unquestionably in developing countries, but largely so in developed nations as well. A growing appreciation of the impact of health research on the community as a whole is precipitating a reassessment of the relative weight and understanding of the different ethical principles involved in protecting populations from exploitation. We have demonstrated here how new claims on justice oblige that the rights, harms and benefits to the community as a whole be taken into account in deliberations about the ethical propriety of research in international settings, but the analysis holds equally important implications for research in industrialized nations as well. To regain reflective equilibrium, an ethical framework based on a public health perspective yields a more satisfactory balance between the goals of gaining new knowledge and providing adequate protections in conducting health research for countries across the entire development spectrum.

An ethical standard requiring the establishment of CABs raises a host of issues, some of which cannot be decided *a priori* but will have to evolve pragmatically through experience and practice. One issue that needs to be addressed is the operational independence of CABs. Currently, CABs are largely set up and run by the individual research projects, which are responsible for providing trainings or other resources for their operations. This relationship of dependence is untenable. In consultation with community representatives, national governments and international sponsors need to begin discussions about sufficient set-asides to ensure the CABs' functional independence (Reddy *et al*, 2010). The level of resources necessary to make CABs operationally effective and the responsibility for its provision are issues that will likely vary from setting to setting but must be addressed as policies instituting their establishment are enacted.

The full scope of powers of CABs may also evolve in practice, most likely initially in relation to the setting and type of research proposed (e.g., experimental versus epidemiological). At a minimum, CABs should have the same scope of powers of Research Ethics Committees in conducting prior review of research protocols, and stipulating provisions to meet recognized ethical standards. But over time, we envisage that CABs might play an appropriately more active role in requiring greater community involvement, more consistent monitoring of the research in progress. For example, there are already evolving practices of CABs calling for more in-depth assessments of community perceptions of the acceptability of the goals and methods of research, through processes such as community forums, key informant interviews, focus groups, community surveys, and so on. The reliance on such practices is now seen as part and parcel of community empowerment, respect for human rights, support for self-determination and the promotion of civic responsibility for the justice of extant living conditions in the population. It is important that these practices be periodically reviewed, and the best practices codified into policy statements.

In contrast, one can readily imagine proposals to empower CABs to waive the right to individual informed consent (or assent), by appealing, for example, to new forms of proxy decision-making. Given the long track record of historical abuses, we cannot find support for this position at this time. In conclusion, the preceding analysis has shown how community oversight is ethically imperative to protect against exploitation, to minimize potential misunderstandings about the intent of the research, and to ensure fair terms of cooperation and standards of care.

References

Angell, Marcia. 1997. "The Ethics of Clinical Research in the Third World." *New England Journal of Medicine* 337: 847-849.

Angell, Marcia. 2000. "Investigators' Responsibilities for Human Subjects in Developing Countries." *New England Journal of Medicine* 342: 967-969.

Bayer, Ronald. 1998. "What is Informed Consent?" Durban, South Africa: Workshop on Ethical Issues in the Conduct of HIV Vaccine Trials.

Belsky, Leah and Henry Richardson. 2004. "Medical researchers' ancillary clinical care responsibilities." *British Medical Journal* 328(7454): 1494-1496.

Berg, Jessica, Paul Appelbaum, Lisa Parker, and Charles Lidz. 2001. *Informed Consent: Legal Theory and Clinical Practice*. 2nd edn. New York: Oxford University Press.

Berkley, Seth. 2003. "Thorny Issues in the Ethics of AIDS Vaccine Research." *Lancet* 362(9388): 992.

Biko, Steve. 1978. *I Write What I Like*. Johannesburg, South Africa: Heinemann.

Bodenheimer, Thomas. 2000. "Uneasy Alliance: Clinical Investigators and the Pharmaceutical Industry." *New England Journal of Medicine* 342: 1539-1544.

Brody, Baruch, Laurence McCullough, and Richard Sharp. 2005. "Consensus and Controversy in Clinical Research Ethics." *JAMA* 294: 1411-1414.

Brown, June. 1998. *Institutional Review Boards: The Emergence of Independent Boards*. Washington, DC: Office of Inspector General, Department of Health and Human Services, OEI-01-97-00192. Available at: http://oig.hhs.gov/oei/reports/oei-01-97-00192.pdf.

Buchanan, David and Franklin G. Miller. 2006. "Justice and fairness in the Kennedy Krieger Institute Lead Paint Study: The ethical justification for public health research on less expensive yet less effective interventions." *American Journal of Public Health* 96(5):15-22.

Buchanan, David, and Franklin G. Miller. 2007. "Justice in research on human subjects." In *The Blackwell Guide to Medical Ethics,* edited by Rosamond Rhodes, Leslie Francis, and Anita Silvers, 373-392, New York: Blackwell.

Buchanan, David, Franklin G. Miller, and Nina Wallerstein. 2007. "Ethical Issues in Community Based Participatory Research: Balancing Rigorous Research with Community Participation." *Progress in Community Health Partnerships* 2: 153-160.

Caplan, Arthur L. 1984. "Is there a Duty to Serve as a Subject in Biomedical Research?" *IRB* 6: 1-5.

Childress, James, Ruth Faden, Ruth Gaare, Lawrence Gostin, Jeffrey Kahn, Richard Bonnie, Nancy Kass, Anna Mastrioianni, Jonathon Moreno, and Phillip Nieburg. 2002. "Public Health Ethics: Mapping the Terrain." *Journal of Law, Medicine and Ethics* 30(2):170-8.

Clark, David. 1973. "The Concept of Community: A Re-Examination." *Sociological Review* 21(3): 397-416.

Cox, Lisa, Jack Rouff, Kenneth Svendsen, Madelyne Markowitz, and Donald Abrams. 1998. "Community Advisory Boards: Their Role in AIDS Clinical Trials." *Health and Social Work* 23(4): 290-297.

Dawson, Liza and Nancy Kass. 2005. "Views of US Researchers about Informed Consent in International Collaborative Research." *Social Science and Medicine* 61(6): 1211-1222.

Dresser, Rebecca. 1992. "Wanted: Single, White Male for Medical Research." *Hastings Center Report* 22: 24-29.

Ekunwe, Ebun and Ross Kessel. 1984. "Informed Consent in the Developing World." *Hastings Center Report* 14: 2224.

Emanuel, Ezekiel. 2002. "Institutional Review Board Reform." *New England Journal of Medicine* 347: 1285-1306.

Emanuel, Ezekiel, David Wendler, and Christine Grady. 2000. "What Makes Clinical Research Ethical?" *JAMA* 283: 2701- 2711.

Emanuel, Ezekiel, David Wendler, Jack Killen, and Christine Grady. 2004. "What makes clinical research in developing countries ethical? The benchmarks of ethical research." *Journal of Infectious Diseases* 189:930-7.

Emanuel, Ezekiel, Anne Wood, Alan Fleischman, Angela Bowen, Kenneth A Getz, *et al*. 2004. "Oversight of Human Participants Research: Identifying Problems to Evaluate Reform Proposals." *Annals of Internal Medicine* 141(4):282-91.

Epstein, Helen. 2007. *The Invisible Cure: Africa, the West, and the Fight against AIDS*. New York: Farrar Straus and Giroux.

Faden, Ruth and Thomas Beauchamp. 1986. *A History and Theory of Informed Consent*. New York: Oxford University Press.

Friedman, Richard B. 1990. "On the Concept of Authority in Political Philosophy." In *Authority*, edited by Joseph Raz, 56-91. New York: New York University Press.

Global Forum for Health Research. 2004. *The 10/90 Report on Health Research, 2003–2004*. Geneva: Global Forum for Health Research.

Harris, John. 2005. "Scientific Research is a Moral Duty." *Journal of Medical Ethics* 31(4): 242-248.

Hill, Thomas. 2001. "Autonomy of Moral Agents." In *Encyclopedia of Ethics,* edited by Lawrence Becker and Charlotte Becker, 112-115. New York: Routledge.

Jacobson v Massachusetts, 197 US 11. (1905). 2002. In *Public Health Law and Ethics: A Reader*, edited by Lawrence Gostin, Berkeley, CA: University of California Press.

Kahn, Jeffrey, Anna Mastroianni, and Jeremy Sugarman. 1998. "Changing Claims about Justice in Research: An Introduction and Overview." In Jeffrey Kahn, Anna Mastroianni and Jeremy Sugarman, *Beyond Consent: Seeking Justice in Research*, 1–10. New York: Oxford University Press.

Kass, Nancy. 2001. "An Ethics Framework for Public Health." *American Journal of Public Health* 91(11): 1776-1782.

Kass, Nancy. 2004. "Public Health Ethics: From Foundations and Frameworks to Justice and Global Public Health." *Journal of Law, Medicine, and Ethics* 32(2):232-42.

Levine, Robert J. 1986. *Ethics and Regulation of Clinical Research*, 2nd edn. New Haven, CT: Yale University Press.

Levinson, Daniel. 2007. *The Food and Drug Administration's Oversight of Clinical Trials*. Washington DC: Office of Inspector General, Department of Health and Human Services, OEI-01–06-00160.

Lindegger, G. and L. M. Richter. 2000. "HIV Vaccine Trials: Critical Issues in Informed Consent." *South African Journal of Science* 96, 313-317.

London, Leslie. 2002. "Ethical Oversight of Public Health Research: Can Rules and IRBs Make a Difference in Developing Countries?" *American Journal of Public Health* 92(7):1079-1084.

Lurie, Peter and Sidney Wolfe. 1997. "Unethical Trials of Interventions to Reduce Perinatal Transmission of the Human Immunodeficiency Virus in Developing Countries." *New England Journal of Medicine* 337(12): 853–856.

Macklin, Ruth. 2004. *Double Standards in Medical Research in Developing Countries*. New York: Cambridge University Press.

MacQueen, Kathleen, Katharine Shapiro, Quarraisha Karim, and Jeremy Sugarman. 2004. Ethical Challenges in International HIV Prevention Research. *Accountability in Research* 11(1): 49-61.

Mamdani, Mahmood. 1996. *Citizen and Subject: Contemporary Africa and the Legacy of Late Colonialism*. Princeton, NJ: Princeton University Press.

Maryland Court of Appeals. 2001. *Ericka Grimes v Kennedy Krieger Institute, Inc*. No. 128, September Term, 2000.

Marshall, Patricia. 2007. *Ethical Challenges in Study Design and Informed Consent for Research in Resource-poor Settings*. Geneva: World Health Organization on behalf of the Special Program for Research and Training in Tropical Diseases.

Meslin, Eric and Charles McCarthy. 1998. "The Evolving Story of Justice in Federal Research Policy." In *Beyond Consent: Seeking Justice in Research,* edited by Jeffrey Kahn, Anna Mastroianni and Jeremy Sugarman, 13-35. New York: Oxford University Press.

Miller, Franklin G. and Howard Brody. 2003. "A Critique of Clinical Equipoise: Therapeutic Misconception in the Ethics of Clinical Trials." *Hastings Center Report* 33: 19-28.

Miller, Franklin G. and Donald Rosenstein. 2003. "The Therapeutic Orientation to Clinical Trials." *New England Journal of Medicine* 348(14): 1383-1386.

Molyneux, Sassy, Norbert Peshua and Kevin Marsha. 2004. "Understanding of Informed Consent in a Low-income Setting: Three Case Studies from the Kenyan Coast." *Social Science and Medicine* 59(12): 2547-2559.

Morin, Stephen, Andre Maiorana, Kimberly A. Koester, Nicolas M. Sheon, and Anne Richards. 2003. "Community Consultation in HIV Prevention Research: A Study of Community Advisory Boards at 6 Research Sites." *Journal of Acquired Immune Deficiency Syndromes*, 33(4): 513-520.

Moodley, Keymanthri. 2002. "HIV Vaccine Trial Participation in South Africa – An Ethical Assessment." *Journal of Medicine and Philosophy* 27(2): 197-215.

National Commission for the Protection of Human Subjects of Biomedical and Behavioral Research. 1979. *The Belmont Report: ethical principles and guidelines for the protection of human subjects of research*. Federal Register Document 79–12065. Washington DC: Department of Health and Human Welfare, US Government Printing Office.

Orentlicher, David. 2005. "Making Research a Requirement of Treatment." *Hastings Center Report* 35: 20-28.

Plant, Raymond. 1974. *Community and Ideology*. London: Routledge.

Powers, Madison. 1998. "Theories of Justice in the Context of Research." In *Beyond Consent: Seeking Justice in Research,* edited by Jeffrey Kahn, Anna Mastroianni and Jeremy Sugarman, 147-165. New York: Oxford University Press.

President's Commission for the Study of Ethical Problems in Medicine and Biomedical Research. 1982. *Making Health Care Decisions*, Vol. 1. Washington, DC: US Government Printing Office.

Raz, Joseph. 1990. Authority and Justification. In *Authority*, edited by Joseph Raz, 115-141. New York: New York University Press.

Rettig, Richard. 2000. "The Industrialization of Clinical Research." *Health Affairs* 19(2):129-46.

Reddy, Priscilla, David Buchanan, Sibu Sifunda and Shegs James. 2010. "The Role of Community Advisory Boards in Health Research: Divergent Views in the SAAVI Experience." *Journal of Social Aspects of HIV/AIDS* 7(3):1-8.

Rhodes, Rosamond. 2005. "Rethinking Research Ethics." *American Journal of Bioethics* 5(1): 7-28.

Richardson, Henry. 2002. *Democratic Autonomy: Public Reasoning about the Ends of Policy*. New York: Oxford University Press.

Sandel, Michael. 1982. *Liberalism and the Limits of Justice*. Cambridge, UK: Cambridge University Press.

Strauss, Ronald, Sohini Sengupta, Sandra Crouse Quinn, Jean Goeppinger, Cora Spaulding, Susan M. Kegeles, and Greg Millett. 2001. "The Role of Community Advisory Boards: Involving Communities in the Informed Consent Process." *American Journal of Public Health*, 91(12): 1938-1943.

Taylor, Charles. 1985. "Atomism." In Charles Taylor, *Philosophy and the Human Sciences, Philosophical Papers*, Vol. 2, 187-210. Cambridge, UK: Cambridge University Press.

Taylor, Charles. 1992. *Multiculturalism and "The Politics of Recognition."* Princeton, NJ: Princeton University Press.

Truog, Robert, Walter Robinson, Adrienne Randolph and Alan Morris. 1999. "Is Informed Consent Always Necessary for Randomized Control Trials?" *New England Journal of Medicine* 340:804-807.

Wallerstein, Nina, Bonnie Duran, Meredith Minkler, and Kevin Foley. 2005. "Developing and Maintaining Partnerships with Communities." In *Methods for Community Based Participatory Research,* edited by Barbara A. Israel, Eugenia Eng, Amy J. Schulz, and Edith A. Parker, 43-68. San Francisco, CA: Jossey Bass.

Weber, Max. 1915/1946. "The Social Psychology of the World Religions." In *From Max Weber: Essays in Sociology,* edited by Hans H. Gerth and C. Wright Mills, 267-301. New York: Oxford University Press.

Weijer, Charles. 1999. "Protecting Communities in Research: Philosophical and Pragmatic Challenges." *Cambridge Quarterly of Healthcare Ethics* 8:501-513.

Weijer, Charles and Robert Crouch. 1999. "Why Should We Include Women and Minorities in Randomized Controlled Trials?" *Journal of Clinical Ethics* 10(2):100-6.

Weijer, Charles and Ezekiel Emanuel. 2000. "Ethics: Protecting Communities in Biomedical Research." *Science* 289(5482): 1142-1144.

Wendler, David, Ezekiel Emanuel, and Reidar Lie. 2004. "The Standard of Care Debate: Can Research in Developing Countries be both Ethical and Responsive to those Countries Health Needs?" *American Journal of Public Health* 94(6): 923-928.

Wertheimer, Alan. 1996. *Exploitation.* Princeton, NJ: Princeton University Press.

Woodsong, Cynthia and Quarraisha Karim. 2005. "A Model Designed to Enhance Informed Consent: Experiences from the HIV Prevention Trials Network." *American Journal of Public Health* 95(3): 412-419.

10. AUTONOMY, PATERNALISM, AND JUSTICE: ETHICAL PRIORITIES IN PUBLIC HEALTH

There has been a wave of interest in public health ethics over the past two decades and whether or how it might be different from clinical bioethics. Whereas medicine focuses on individual health, public health is concerned with the health of the entire population. Thus, in contrast to the primary fiduciary duty to the individual patient found in clinical medicine, public health ethics is founded on a societal responsibility to protect and promote the health of the population as a whole (Buchanan and Miller, 2006). On the basis of this distinction, many commentators have suggested that one major issue that distinguishes public health ethics from clinical ethics is identifying when paternalistic interventions that override individual autonomy are justified (Bayer and Fairchild, 2004; Harris and Martin, 2004; Gostin, 2005; Mariner, Annas, and Glantz, 2005; Colgrove and Bayer, 2005; Gostin and Javitt, 2001; Jones and Bayer, 2007).

The considerable attention paid to identifying plausible justifications for restricting individual autonomy to change unhealthy behaviors is largely misguided. This focus fails to give sufficient weight to the shift from infectious to chronic diseases as the leading causes of morbidity and mortality. In light of this shift, public health would be better served by seeking to expand autonomy through promoting justice. Although the call for social justice is frequently voiced in public health, it is critically important for the field to address major differences in definitions of justice found in the general public.

The issues of promoting autonomy and clarifying principles of justice are significant for several reasons. Undue attention to justifying interventions designed to limit and control unhealthy behaviors distracts attention from potentially more fruitful strategies. Currently, excessive time and energy are devoted to questions about whether "sin" taxes are inherently regressive, debating the efficacy of advertising bans, and the like (Bayer, 2003). A related concern is that seeking to shore up support for paternalistic interventions may result only in undermining trust of public health authorities (Bayer, 2003; Annas, 2002; Buchanan, 2001; Kass, 2001). More importantly, to achieve public health goals, greater consideration must be directed toward promoting a common understanding of a just society, about which there are gaping divisions in modern American society.

Undue Attention to Justifying Paternalism

Many authors have claimed that the central moral concern of public health ethics is articulating sound reasons for overriding individual freedom for the sake of promoting public health. In the landmark 1974 report on health promotion, Lalonde (1974, p. 36) laid the foundation for this focal concern:

> The ultimate philosophical issue . . . is whether and to what extent the government can get into the business of modifying human behavior, even if it does so to improve health.

In the many efforts since that time to justify this proposition, almost everyone points to the signal contribution of the 1905 Supreme Court ruling *Jacobson v Massachusetts*, which many consider the cornerstone of public health ethics. There, the court found that

> the liberty secured by the Constitution of the United States to every person within its jurisdiction does not impart an absolute right in each person to be, at all times and in all circumstances, wholly freed from restraint. There are manifold restraints to which every person is necessarily subject for the common good. (cited in Gostin, 2000, p. 207-208)

As we saw earlier (see Chapter 6), Dworkin (1988) defines paternalism as "interference with a person's liberty of action justified by reason referring exclusively to the welfare . . . of the person being coerced." Paternalism is the usurpation of decision-making power, by preventing people from doing what they have decided, interfering in how they arrive at their decisions, or attempting to substitute one's judgment for theirs, expressly for the purpose of promoting their welfare. The moral concern is that the presumption that one is right, and therefore justified in seeking to override other people's judgment, constitutes treating them as less than moral equals. It denies people the right to choose their own ends of action, because it would not be necessary to supplant their decision if they shared the public health professionals' goals (Dworkin, 1988).

In addressing this concern, Bayer (2003, p. 147) has reframed questions about the propriety of paternalistic interventions as follows:

> What are the appropriate limits of the state in a liberal society in regulating, restricting or prohibiting behaviors that lead to premature morbidity and mortality; [or] in shaping, molding or influencing the preferences and desires of its citizens?

Taking up the challenge, numerous researchers have sought to identify the conditions in which paternalistic public health interventions are justified.

For example, Childress *et al.* (2002) devoted the bulk of their oft-cited paper to specifying 5 "justificatory conditions" that indicate when public health interventions that infringe on individual autonomy are ethically warranted. The 5 criteria that they identified are (1) effectiveness, (2) proportionality, (3) necessity, (4) least infringement, and (5) public justification. Gostin *et al.* provided an illustrative example of the application of these criteria in discussing the proposed Model State Emergency Health Powers Act (MSEHPA) (Gostin, Sapsin, Teret, *et al*, 2002).

In the MSEHPA, to avert a significant threat to the public's health, public health authorities should be considered justified in exercising the police powers of the state over individuals for purposes including compulsory vaccinations, blood tests, physical examinations, treatment, isolation, and quarantine if the following conditions are met: (1) an occurrence or imminent threat of illness that (2) is caused by bioterrorism, infectious agent, or toxin and that (3) poses a high probability of substantial harm. Given the threat to civil liberties, Gostin *et al.* (2002) specified 4 principled limitations on exercising these powers. Such public health interventions must be (1) necessary to avert significant risk, first, in the judgment of health officials but, ultimately, to the satisfaction of a judge; (2) well-tailored to address the risk and not going beyond what is necessary in the situation; (3) authorized in a manner allowing public oversight; and (4) correctable in the event of a mistake. Conversely, they noted that such infringements would not be justified if (1) the problem was not as serious as initially believed, (2) the measure taken was unresponsive to the problem, or (3) the measure was more restrictive than necessary to abate the threat.

Although the MSEHPA demonstrates the prototypical process for specifying the conditions in which paternalism is warranted, the justification for restricting individual autonomy in this case rests on the relatively uncontroversial (albeit not entirely [Annas, 2002]) claim that failure to intervene would result in widespread harm to the public at large. There is, however, a critical distinction between communicable biological agents or dispersible chemical toxins and the causes of chronic diseases.

The Limits of Paternalism

Although public health proudly points to the *Jacobson* ruling as providing authoritative support for its right to restrict individual autonomy to protect and promote public health, there is a morally significant difference between controlling disease agents and controlling host behaviors, a difference reflected in the phrase "epidemiological transition." As countries develop economically, the field of public health has come to see a familiar shift in the leading causes of morbidity and mortality. This shift has important implications for thinking about public health interventions in both moral and scientific terms.

In their famous 1993 paper on the "actual causes of death," McGinnis and Foege (1993) explained that, although people may die from heart attacks or cancer, for example, the true "causes" of death were the lifestyle behaviors of smoking, ingesting fatty diets, lack of exercise, alcohol misuse, and so on. As these causes of morbidity and mortality have risen in prominence, public health professionals have grappled with providing a sound ethical justification for interventions intended to change unhealthy behaviors. Examples of these types of interventions include seat belt and motorcycle helmet laws; policies to restrict access to certain items (e.g., blue laws); excise taxes and advertising bans on "unhealthy" products; proposed tax breaks for people who maintain low blood pressure, body mass indexes under 25, etc.; prohibitions (e.g., of trans-fatty acids, marijuana); mandatory screenings; social marketing campaigns; drug testing; 2-tiered insurance premiums and long-term care plans; lower priority in treatment queues (i.e., people who have brought their health problems on themselves having lower priority in being treated than people who suffer ill health through no fault of their own); restrictive employment policies (i.e., discrimination through firing or not hiring people because of unhealthy lifestyle habits such as smoking or being overweight); and censorship.

The critical ethical concern here is that, although preventing harm to others for purposes of infectious disease control is ethically defensible, the justification for thwarting a person's choices for their own good in chronic disease prevention rests on morally tenuous grounds. The 3 most common lines of argument put forward to justify such paternalistic interventions are appeals to voluntary and informed consent, weak paternalism, and utilitarianism.

In the first line of defense, many public health professionals argue that behavioral interventions are ethically acceptable because individuals provide their voluntary and informed consent for treatment (e.g., a smoking cessation class) (Green and Kreuter, 2005). And at the individual level, there is no significant ethical concern; individuals may seek assistance in changing behaviors with which they are dissatisfied in the same way they might see a clinical therapist. It becomes problematic, however, when an intervention is targeted toward the whole population, where the process of gaining individual informed consent is infeasible and hence obviated (Buchanan, 2006; Buchanan, Miller and Wallerstein, 2007).

On another front, public health professionals have, in general, implicitly assumed a form of weak paternalism. Weak paternalists take the position that interventions to prevent people from harming themselves are justified when there is a defect in their decision-making that leads them to engage in self-harming activity (in contrast to strong paternalists, who maintain that interfering is justified even when the decision is fully voluntary and totally unimpaired) (Dworkin, 1999; Beauchamp and Childress, 2001). Hence, vast sums of federal research dollars are committed to developing more effective behavioral interventions based on the tacit assumption that unhealthy behaviors must be irrational and driven by pathological factors (peer pressure, dysfunctional family dynamics, internalized oppression, etc.) because they are self-evidently so contrary to one's self-interest. In response, critics point out that this assumption is questionable; people may simply place a higher value on the pursuit of goals other than physical fitness (Bayer, 2003; Wikler, 2004). If this is the case, which seems plausible, then it is mistaken to presume that there must be a defect in people's decision-making, and therefore that interventions to change their behaviors have ethical justification based on weak paternalist reasoning.

Finally, public health has long been associated with the utilitarian school of moral philosophy (Cole, 1995; Gostin, 2003). Utilitarianism is essentially consequentialist in analyzing issues, holding that the most ethically reasonable course of action is that which produces the greatest good for the greatest number. Thus, the most common criticism of utilitarianism is that the ends are used to justify the means. This school of thought frequently leads into protracted debates about the apparent costs and benefits of an intervention (e.g., does smoking cessation truly save the government money?) (Elixhauser, 1990).

Another prominent example of the resort to utilitarian arguments arises in debates about social marketing. As Bayer (2003, p. 151) puts it,

> Could not the manipulative capacity of advertising be mobilized for public health goals? Can the protection of individuals from the manipulative activity of commercial advertisers justify counter-manipulation in the name of public health?

Social marketing techniques are an integral part of political campaigns, seen for example, in the Swift Boat ad in Kerry-Bush presidential campaign and the "Harry and Louise" ads against Clinton's Health Care reform plan ads of the 1988 Bush-Dukakis race (Farhi, 2004; Milbank, 2004). Such ads are intentionally designed to provoke base emotional reactions such as fear and anger and bypass rational thought processes. Public health has supported similar campaigns, such as the Partnership for a Drug-Free America (PDFA), borrowing on utilitarian thinking to justify these efforts. In evaluations of the PDFA campaign, reviewers discount questions about whether any meaningful information is communicated and focus strictly on whether the desired ends are achieved by employing such marketing techniques (Buchanan, Hossain, and Reddy, 1994).

Whether or not these criticisms are valid and a satisfactory justification to support paternalistic interventions can eventually be worked out, my first point is that the interest in restricting individual autonomy to promote population health is largely misguided, both ethically and empirically. As noted earlier, on empirical grounds, there can be no question that people who exercise the greatest degree of individual autonomy also enjoy the best health (West, Heith and Goodwin, 1996; Macintyre, 1992). The clear inference is that, to promote health, public health should focus on finding ways to expand individual autonomy, not restrict it.

On ethical grounds, many different philosophical accounts identify autonomy as a defining constituent element in human well-being and, further, the fundamental precondition for moral agency (Dworkin, 1988; Wilkinson and Marmot, 2003; Griffin, 1986; Crisp and Hooker, 2000). Importantly for our purposes here, in the works of both Immanuel Kant and John Rawls, the state of autonomy provides the critical link between principles of justice and the idea of free and equal human beings. Autonomy is the *sine qua non* that enables moral agents to give free and rational assent to any proposed public principles of justice.

Given the drift in American culture today, it is important to distinguish autonomy from liberty (Brock, 1993). Most Americans view autonomy as synonymous with liberty, consciously or unconsciously reflecting the views of John Stuart Mill's influential work *On Liberty*, in which liberty is construed as negative freedom, freedom *from* restraint, freedom to do whatever one wants as long as it does not harm others. By contrast, the definition of autonomy of interest here, following Kant, is based on the integration of freedom and responsibility. Autonomous agents can adopt moral constraints, willingly submitting to norms to which they have given their consent. Autonomy here is equated with positive freedom, self-mastery, with being in charge of oneself. One can be restricted (e.g., celibate) yet still be autonomous. The critical point is being in the position of deciding, not being decided for, being able to choose to accept reasonable constraints on one's behaviors. As defined by Dworkin, autonomy is thus the capacity of a person to critically reflect upon and then attempt to accept or change one's desires, values, and ideals (Dworkin, 1988). This is the concept of autonomy that affords health benefits and needs to be promoted. Moreover, it is essential for securing agreement on those public principles of justice that should govern American society.

Clarifying Principles of Justice

Criticizing public health's focus on changing individual health behaviors may seem to many readers like beating a dead horse. Burgeoning attention to the "social determinants of health" in the field today leads many to conclude that such interventions merely blame the victim (Gaylin and Jennings, 2003). Thus, rather than seeking a warrant for paternalism, many instead invoke a call for social justice, to furnish the moral justification for efforts aimed at eliminating health disparities (Crawford, 1977; Krieger and Birn, 1998). Advocates' consistent recourse to qualifying "justice" with the modifier "social," however, points to an important public debate. Significant controversies swirl around the degree to which it is appropriate to assign personal or social responsibility for the prevalence of unhealthy behaviors (Wikler, 2004). My second major point is that efforts aimed at justifying paternalism should largely be redirected toward clarifying principles of justice.

As noted in Chapter 6, many Americans believe that individuals should do what they can to stay healthy and should be held accountable for the decisions they make (Wikler, 2004). They believe that it is unfair to burden those who make healthy choices with the costs of care in the form of higher taxes or insurance premiums for those who make irresponsible decisions (Wikler, 2004; Gostin and Powers, 2006). In this view, the phrase "social determinants" is too strong a term. It implies that people are compelled to start smoking, overeat, or take drugs by latent forces rooted in their social conditions. It denies people the ability to make choices, which flies in the face of personal experience, commonsense intuitions, and bedrock notions of moral responsibility. If the majority of people who grow up in poverty do not, for example, turn to drugs, then a large cross-section of the lay public believes that those who do should bear personal responsibility for their decision. They want to preserve the notion of individual moral accountability, and they are troubled by rationalizations that appear to denigrate this core value.

Opposed to this view, many public health professionals take the position that society as a whole bears responsibility for the pattern of distribution of unhealthy behaviors. Here, the field is deeply indebted to the work of Marmot and Wilkinson, who have repeatedly demonstrated the powerful association between social position and health status (Scheffler, 1992; Marmot, 2003; Marmot, 2004; Marmot and Wilkinson, 1999). As these data indicate, unhealthy living habits are strongly predicted by growing up and living in poverty. Significantly, Marmot *et al.* (1997) note that explaining the mechanisms underlying these associations is the major unsolved public health problem of the era.

On the basis of such findings, a prominent position in public health is founded on an egalitarian conception of justice, a stance signaled by appending "social" to the term justice. Given that one goal of the serial *Healthy People* reports is to eliminate health disparities (Marmot, Ryff, Bumpass, *et al*, 1997), this position holds that, because there is sufficiently plausible evidence linking health inequalities to social inequalities, to achieve equality in health, social inequalities must be eliminated. To paraphrase Hofrichter, social justice is defined by an opposition to inequality and thus demands an equitable distribution of collective goods, institutional resources, and life opportunities (Hofrichter, 2003, p. 12-13). As he continues,

> Achieving equality requires not merely redressing or ameliorating inequitable outcomes but creating a society that does not produce material inequality.

The problem with such statements is that they fail to acknowledge the lack of agreement about a unified theory of justice (Beauchamp and Childress, 2001; Barry, 1989; Buchanan, 1981). The social justice position, for example, runs directly counter to principles of justice based on the concept of moral desert (Taylor, 1994; Kekes, 1995). More broadly, principles of justice have been characterized as "patterned conceptions of distribution" with respect to rights and resources, in which different patterns (e.g., to each person an equal share, to each according to need, to each according to effort, etc.) have been derived from various social theories, including libertarian, communitarian, feminist, Marxist, and others (Powers, 1998; Buchanan and Miller, 2007). Thus, adopting the social justice position uncritically begs questions about the merits of alternative views; in particular, about whether any social inequalities could be considered fair and morally acceptable and about the degree to which individuals should be held accountable for making ill-advised choices, regardless of social circumstances. The field urgently needs to address these questions by shifting attention to clarifying principles of justice.

The Justice Project

Public health is in a unique position to open space in civil society for public deliberations about the extent to which justice prevails in modern American society. Nascent efforts along these lines are under way; they should be greatly expanded (Bloss, 2006; Hofrichter, 2002). To protect and promote the population's health, public health professionals need to engage the public in discussions and actions aimed at clarifying the role and character of justice in America today, an effort I call the "justice project."

To advance the discussion, one promising line of analysis regarding justice today, which holds high potential for finding common ground across the fault lines of America's culture wars, stems from the work of Sen (1992, 1999), Nussbaum (1990, 1993), and recently, Powers and Faden (2006). The starting point in this framework is the concept of capabilities, which, as we saw earlier, Sen (1992, p. 30) defines as "a person's ability to do valuable acts and reach valuable states of being."

The first topic for public deliberation is accordingly to identify a set of capabilities that citizens consider valuable. Community discussions might begin with questions like, "What do people need to be able to do or be in order to be successful in pursuing their life plans and lead a full and satisfying life?" drawing directly on the proposition that how well people are must be a matter of what they are succeeding in doing or being. These questions lead naturally to discussions about those capabilities that community members consider most valuable. To stimulate the conversation, examples of capabilities identified by Sen (1992, 1999), Nussbaum (1990, 1993), and recently, Powers and Faden (2006) are shown in the box below.

Table 10.1: Examples of Capabilities that Citizens Consider Valuable
From Sen (1992, 1999) 1. Adequate nourishment 2. Ability to achieve self-respect 3. Social integration 4. Adequate shelter 5. Ability to escape avoidable morbidity and premature mortality 6. Mobility, vacationing, and traveling 7. Happiness and enjoyment of life 8. A part in the life of the community

9. Ability to appear in public without shame
10. Ability to entertain friends and be close to people one would like to see
11. Ability to live life without being ashamed of one's clothing

From Nussbaum (1990)

1. Ability to live to the end of a complete human life, as far as possible; not dying prematurely, or before one's life is so reduced as to be not worth living
2. Ability to have good health, to be adequately nourished, to have adequate shelter, to have opportunities for sexual satisfaction, to move about from place to place
3. Ability to avoid unnecessary and non-useful pain and to have pleasurable experiences
4. Ability to use the 5 senses, to imagine, to think and reason
5. Ability to have attachments to things and persons outside ourselves, to love those who love and care for us, to grieve at their absence; in general, to love, to grieve, to feel longing and gratitude
6. Ability to form a conception of the good and to engage in critical reflection about the planning of our own lives
7. Ability to live for and to others, to recognize and show concern for other human beings, to engage in various forms of familial and social interaction
8. Ability to live with concern for and in relation to animals, plants, and the world of nature
9. Ability to laugh, to play, to enjoy recreational activities
10. Ability to live one's own life and nobody else's
10a. Ability to live one's own life in one's very own surroundings and context

From Powers and Faden (2006)

1. Health
2. Reasoning
3. Self-determination
4. Attachment
5. Personal security
6. Respect

After the identification of capabilities that community members consider valuable, the next step is to assess the degree to which existing social inequalities impair or deprive people of the opportunity to achieve them. Daniels has advanced a strong case that social inequalities are unacceptable to the extent that they produce health impairments that impede people's capacity to pursue the life plans that it would be reasonable for them to pursue if they were not so impaired (Daniels, 1985; Daniels, 2001). In this framework, the most serious injustice is thus the lack of opportunity to achieve one's full capabilities because of corrigible social conditions, the extent to which the current practices of various social institutions inflict unnecessary and intolerable disadvantages on fellow citizens.

Following Daniels's lead, it is critical to raise the level of public discourse to look beyond brute physical impairments to examine possible psychological and social impairments, such as the loss of hope for the future, or the sense of failure and the ridicule that derives from exclusion from material prosperity. A part of this effort is to continue conducting research aimed at explaining causal relationships between social inequalities and health impairments. Important work on chronic stress and stress hormones has already made valuable contributions toward building the case and needs to continue to illuminate the underlying social, psychological, and physiological processes (Geronimus, Hicken, Keene and Bound, 2006; McEwen, 2004; McEwen, 2003; Lynch, Smith, Kaplan and House, 2000). Although solid scientific research is essential for calling attention to significant underlying influences, I suspect that age-old questions about free will and the dialectics of agency and structure will not ultimately be resolved empirically. The majority of the public might find certain social inequalities to be either fair, because they are consistent with other socially desirable goals (e.g., rewarding those who make outstanding contributions to the common good), or irredeemable acts of fate beyond human control (e.g., genetic differences in susceptibilities).

Identifying socially important capabilities is an inescapably evaluative exercise, and people will attach different values to different items (Sen 1999). The public health community may have their preferred set, but one measure of the validity of moral norms is the degree to which reasoned public consensus can be achieved (Daniels, 1996; Habermas, 1984). Thus, the project recommended here is a "public reasons" approach (Rawls, 1971). It is based on the cooperative search for moral agreement, established on the basis of good reasons, in which nothing but the force of better argument should prevail. To aid in these discussions, Brock has identified a set of criteria that may serve as checks for avoiding potential distortions in public moral discourse (Brock, 1996; see Chapter 1). The goal of this project is to identify those capabilities that people consider essential for living a decent life. If consensus cannot be reached and seemingly irresolvable value judgments persist, modern democracies must often look to fair procedures to resolve their disagreements (Daniels and Sabin, 1997).

In the end, the field of public health needs to engage the public directly in building consensus on what we owe each other in creating a society in which all citizens feel supported in living decent lives characterized by dignity, integrity, and mutual responsibility (Institute of Medicine, 1988; Young, 2011)).

For public health professionals, the goal is to ensure that people have adequate opportunities to achieve good health, but not to insist that they must take up the offer (recognizing, for example, the difference between childhood lead poisoning and a personal decision not to worry about health). To be human is to have the ability to make decisions.

Other things being equal, a society in which people choose to behave responsibly, rather than being forced against their will–a maxim that applies as well to paying taxes as to smoking–is inherently more desirable. The goal of the justice project is to reach broader agreement about those institutional practices ("what we as a society do collectively") that foster responsible individuals who choose to take care of themselves and those around them. To improve quality of life and eliminate health disparities, public health would therefore be well served by recommending that community members devote 30 to 45 minutes a day 4 to 5 times a week to building consensus on the just society.

References

Annas, George. 2002. "Bioterrorism, public health, and civil liberties." *New England Journal of Medicine* 346:1337-1342.

Barry, Brian. 1989. *Theories of Justice.* Berkeley, CA: University of California Press.

Bayer, Ronald and Amy Fairchild. 2004. "The genesis of public health ethics." *Bioethics* 18:473-492.

Bayer, Ronald. 2003. "Ethics of health promotion and disease prevention." In *Ethics and Public Health: Model Curriculum,* edited by Bruce Jennings, Jeff Kahn, Anna Mastroianni and Lisa Parker, 147-158. Washington, DC: Association of Schools of Public Health.

Beauchamp, Thomas and James Childress. 2001. *Principles of Biomedical Ethics.* 5th edn. New York, NY: Oxford University Press.

Bloss, Doak. 2006. "Initiating social justice action through dialogue in a local health department: the Ingham County experience." In *Tackling Health Inequalities through Public Health Practice: A Handbook for Action,* edited by Richard Hofrichter, 33-58. National Association of City and County Health Officers. Available at: https://www.canr.msu.edu/outreach/uploads/files/Health%20and%20Nutrition/naccho_handbook_hyperlinks_000.pdf#page=115.

Brock, Dan. 1993. "Quality of life measures in health care and medical ethics. In *The Quality of Life,* edited by Martha Nussbaum and Amartya Sen, 95-132, Oxford: Clarendon Press.

Brock, Dan. 1995. "Public Moral Discourse." In *Society's Choices: Social and Ethical Decision Making in Biomedicine*, edited by Ruth Bulger, Elizabeth Bobby, and Harvey Fineberg, 215-240. Washington DC: National Academy Press.

Buchanan, Allen. 1981. "Justice: a philosophical review." In *Justice and Health Care*, edited by Earl Shelp, 3-21. Boston, MA: D. Reidel Publishing Co.

Buchanan, David. 2000. *An Ethic for Health Promotion: Rethinking the Sources of Human Well Being.* New York, NY: Oxford University Press.

Buchanan, David. 2006. "A new ethic for health promotion: reflections on a philosophy of health education for a new millennium." *Health Education and Behavior* 33:290-304

Buchanan, David, Sasiragha Reddy, and Zafar Hossain. 1994. "Social marketing: a critical appraisal." *Health Promotion International* 9(1): 49-57.

Buchanan, David, and Franklin G. Miller. 2006. "A public health perspective on research ethics." *Journal of Medical Ethics* 32: 729-733.

Buchanan, David, and Franklin G. Miller. 2007. "Justice in research on human subjects." In *The Blackwell Guide to Medical Ethics*, edited by Rosamond Rhodes, Leslie Francis, and Anita Silvers, 373-392, New York: Blackwell.

Buchanan, David, Franklin G. Miller and Nina Wallerstein. 2007. "Ethical issues in community based participatory research: balancing rigorous research with community participation." *Progress in Community Health Partnerships* 2(1):153-160.

Childress, James, Ruth Faden, Ruth Gaare, Lawrence Gostin, Jeffrey Kahn, Richard Bonnie, Nancy Kass, Anna Mastrioianni, Jonathon Moreno, and Phillip Nieburg. 2002. "Public Health Ethics: Mapping the Terrain." *Journal of Law, Medicine and Ethics* 30(2):170-8.

Cole, Philip. 1995. "The moral bases for public health interventions." *Epidemiology* 6(1):78-83.

Colgrove, James and Ronald Bayer. 2005. "Manifold restraints: liberty, public health, and the legacy of *Jacobson v Massachusetts.*" *American Journal of Public Health* 95(4):571-576.

Crawford, Robert. 1977. "You are dangerous to your health: the ideology and politics of victim blaming." *International Journal of Health Services* 7(4):633-680.

Crisp, Roger and Brad Hooker (Eds.). 2000. *Well-Being and Morality.* Oxford, England: Clarendon Press.

Daniels, Norman. 1985. *Just Health Care.* New York, NY: Cambridge University Press.

Daniels, Norman. 1996. *Justice and Justification.* Cambridge, England: Cambridge University Press.

Daniels, Norman. 2001. "Justice, health, and health care." *American Journal of Bioethics* 1:2-16.

Daniels, Norman and James Sabin. 1997. "Limits to health care: Fair procedures, democratic deliberation, and the legitimacy problem for insurers." *Philosophy and Public Affairs* 26: 303-350.

Dworkin, Gerald. 1988. *The Theory and Practice of Autonomy*. Cambridge, UK: Cambridge University Press.

Dworkin, Gerald. 1999. "Paternalism." In *New Ethics for the Public's Health*, edited by Dan Beauchamp and Bonnie Steinbock, 115-130. New York, NY: Oxford University Press.

Elixhauser, Anne. 1990. "The costs of smoking and the cost effectiveness of smoking-cessation programs." *Journal of Public Health Policy* 11:218-237.

Farhi, Paul. 2004. "Two political ads share more than fame and controversy." *Washington Post.* September 7, 2004, A02.

Gaylin, Willard and Bruce Jennings. 2003. *The Perversion of Autonomy: Coercion and Constraint in a Liberal Society.* Washington, DC: Georgetown University Press.

Geronimus, Arline, Margaret Hicken, Danya Keene and John Bound. 2006. " 'Weathering' and age patterns of allostatic load scores among Blacks and Whites in the United States." *American Journal of Public Health* 96(5):826-833.

Gostin, Lawrence. 2003. "Public health ethics: tradition, profession, values." *Acta Bioethica* 9:177-188.

Gostin, Lawrence. 2005. "*Jacobson v Massachusetts* at 100 years: police power and civil liberties in tension." *American Journal of Public Health* 95:576-581.

Gostin, Lawrence. 2007. " 'Police' powers and public health paternalism: HIV and diabetes surveillance." *Hastings Center Report* 37:9-10.

Gostin, Lawrence and Gail Javitt. 2001. "Health promotion and the First Amendment: government control of the informational environment." *Milbank Quarterly* 79(4): 547-578, iv.

Gostin, Lawrence and Madison Powers. 2006. "What does social justice require for the public's health? Public health ethics and policy imperatives." *Health Affairs* 25: 1053-1060.

Gostin, Lawrence, Jason Sapsin, Stephen Teret, Scott Burris, Julie Samia Mair, James G. Hodge and Jon Vernick. 2002. "The Model State Emergency Health Powers Act: planning for and response to bioterrorism and naturally occurring infectious diseases." *JAMA* 288: 622-628.

Green, Lawrence and Marshall Kreuter. 2005. *Health Promotion Planning: An Educational and Ecological Approach.* 4th edn. New York, NY: McGraw-Hill.

Griffin, James. 1986. *Well-Being: Its Meaning, Measurement and Moral Importance.* Oxford, England: Clarendon Press.

Habermas, Jürgen. 1984. *The theory of communicative action.* Boston, MA: Beacon Press.

Harris, Andrew and Robyn Martin. 2004. "The exercise of public health powers in an era of human rights: the particular problems of tuberculosis." *Public Health* 118(5):313-322.

Healthy People 2010: Understanding and Improving Health. 2000. Washington, DC: US Department of Health and Human Services.

Hofrichter, Richard. 2003. "The politics of health inequities: contested terrain." In *Health and Social Justice: Politics, Ideology and Inequity in the Distribution of Disease*, edited by Richard Hofrichter, 1-56. San Francisco, Calif: Jossey-Bass.

Hofrichter, Richard. 2002. "Creating health equity though social justice." Washington DC: National Association of City and County Health Officers. Draft working paper.

Institute of Medicine. 1988. *The Future of Public Health.* Washington, DC: National Academy Press.

Jones, Marian and Ronald Bayer. 2007. "Paternalism and its discontents: motorcycle helmet laws, libertarian values, and public health." *American Journal of Public Health* 97(2): 208-217.

Kekes, John. 1995. *Moral Wisdom and Good Lives.* Ithaca, NY: Cornell University Press.

Krieger, Nancy and Anne-Emnanuelle Birn. 1998. "A vision of social justice as the foundation of public health: commemorating 150 years of the spirit of 1848." *American Journal of Public Health* 88(11):1603-1606.

Lynch, John, George Smith, George Kaplan and James House. 2000. "Income inequality and mortality: importance to health of individual income, psychosocial environment, or material conditions." *BMJ* 320(7243): 1200-1204.

Macintyre, Sally. 1992. "The effects of family position and status on health." *Social Science and Medicine* 35(4):453-464.

Mariner, Wendy, George Annas and Leonard Glantz. 2005. "*Jacobson v Massachusetts*: it's not your great-great-grandfather's public health law." *American Journal of Public Health* 95(4): 581-590.

Marmot, Michael. 2003. "Understanding social inequalities in health." *Perspectives in Biology and Medicine* 46(3): S9-S23.

Marmot, Michael. 2004. "Social causes of social inequalities in health." In *Public Health, Ethics, and Equity*, edited by Sudhir Anand, Fabienne Peter and Amartya Sen, 37-62. Oxford, England: Oxford University Press.

Marmot, Michael, Carol Ryff, Larry Bumpass, Martin Shipley and Nadine Marks N. 1997. "Social inequalities in health: next questions and converging evidence." *Social Science and Medicine* 44(6): 901-910.

Marmot, Michael and Richard Wilkinson. 1999. *Social Determinants of Health.* New York, NY: Oxford University Press.

McEwen, Bruce. 2003. "Early life influences on life-long patterns of behavior and health." *Mental Retardation and Developmental Disabilities Research Reviews* 9(3):149-154.

McEwen, Bruce. 2004. "Protection and damage from acute and chronic stress: allostasis and allostatic overload and relevance to the pathophysiology of psychiatric disorders." *Annals of New York Academy of Science* 1032:1-7.

McGinnis, J. Michael and William Foege. 1993. "Actual causes of death in the United States." *JAMA* 270:2207-2212.

Milbank, Dana. 2004. "Bush campaign drops Swift Boat ad figure; Democrat's team says veteran's role in drive to discredit Kerry shows a link." *Washington Post.* August 22, 2004: A13.

Nussbaum, Martha. 1993. "Non-relative virtues: an Aristotelian approach." In *The Quality of Life*, edited by Martha Nussbaum and Amartya Sen, 242–269. Oxford, England: Clarendon Press.

Nussbaum, Martha. 1990. "Aristotelian social democracy." In *Liberalism and the Good*, edited by Gerald Mara, Henry Richardson and Bruce Douglass, 203–252. New York, NY: Routledge.

Powers, Madison. 1998. "Theories of Justice in the Context of Research." In *Beyond Consent: Seeking Justice in Research*, edited by Jeffrey Kahn, Anna Mastroianni and Jeremy Sugarman, 147-165. New York: Oxford University Press.

Powers, Madison and Ruth Faden. 2006. *Social Justice: The Moral Foundations of Public Health and Health Policy.* New York, NY: Oxford University Press.

Scheffler, Samuel. 1992. "Responsibility, Reactive Attitudes and Liberalism in Philosophy and Politics." *Philosophy and Public Affairs* 21: 299–323.

Rawls, John. 1971. *A Theory of Justice.* Cambridge, MA: Harvard University Press.

Sen, Amartya. 1992. *Inequality Reexamined.* Cambridge, MA: Harvard University Press.

Sen, Amartya. 1999. *Capabilities and Commodities.* New York, NY: Oxford University Press.

Supreme Court of the United States, *Jacobson v Massachusetts*, decided February 20, 1905. 2000. In *Public Health Law and Ethics: A Reader,* edited by Lawrence Gostin. Berkeley: University of California Press.

Taylor, Charles. 1994. "Justice after virtue." In *After MacIntyre: Critical Perspectives on the Work of Alisdair MacIntyre*, edited by John Horton and Susan Mendus, 16–43. Notre Dame, IN: University of Notre Dame Press.

West, Darrell, Diane Heith and Chris Goodwin. 1996. "Harry and Louise go to Washington: political advertising and health care reform." *Journal of Health Politics, Policy, and Law* 21(1):35-68.

Wikler, Dan. 2004. "Personal and social responsibility for health." In *Public Health, Ethics, and Equity,* edited by Sudhir Anand, Fabienne Peter, and Amartya Sen, 109–134. Oxford, England: Oxford University Press.

Wilkinson, Richard and Michael Marmot. 2003. *Social Determinants of Health: The Solid Facts.* 2nd edn. Copenhagen, Denmark: World Health Organization Publications.

Wilkinson, Richard. 2005.*The Impact of Inequality: How to Make Sick Societies Healthier.* New York, NY: W. W. Norton.

Young, Iris Marion. 2011. *Responsibility for Justice.* New York: Oxford University Press.

11. A NEW ETHIC FOR HEALTH PROMOTION: REFLECTIONS ON A PHILOSOPHY OF HEALTH PROMOTION FOR THE NEW MILLENNIUM

What is the purpose of health promotion? What are we trying to accomplish? The promise of a new millennium beckons us with new possibilities. This chapter offers reflections on the ends that we now seek and the ends that we should seek, with the aim of continuing a healthy debate.

To get into these questions, I want to explore a potential tension inherent in the juxtaposition of the terms, health and education. I want to describe two different models for thinking about what we are doing, a medical model and an education model, at once familiar yet with some interesting contrasting characteristics. I want to suggest that the dominant metaphor for thinking about what we are doing in health education is now a kind of medical model, in the sense that the overarching goal of health education seems to be to develop more effective interventions, just like effective medical treatments. The vast bulk of HE research is directed towards developing more powerful programs that will successfully prevent people from adopting behaviors that are harmful to their health: smoking, obesity, lack of exercise, unsafe sexual behaviors, violence, illicit drug use, teen pregnancy, alcohol abuse, low screening rates, drinking and driving, sunburn, low fruit and vegetable consumption, and so on. Just as physicians can prescribe medications that effectively control patients' blood pressure, so too health promoters want to run programs that will effectively control people's weight.

The prod for taking up this topic stems from my uneasiness with the direction that we are headed. My worry is this. Because there is such tremendous institutional inertia and intellectual and financial investment in the current program of behavioral and social scientific research, we have largely lost sight of the fact that telling people how we think they ought to live is a moral and political process, not a scientific problem to be solved. We need a new ethic. As an alternative, I want to describe a philosophy of education that might be more well-suited for engaging the public in examining the way we live and how we, individually and collectively, might choose to change it. Instead of the medical model, I propose the model of higher education as a more ideal philosophy for thinking about the purposes of health promotion.

To set the stage for the discussion that follows, I want to start by describing briefly several strands of thought that lay out some major differences for thinking about what we are doing, as hinted by the shorthand labels, medical model and philosophy of education. My thinking on these issues is deeply indebted to the work of Jürgen Habermas, and Charles Taylor. The principal theme running through these works is that there are fundamental differences between scientific reasoning and ethical reasoning, which, in turn, have major implications for thinking about the goals and methods of health education.

Scientific versus Ethical Analysis

In his early work, *Knowledge and Human Interests*, the German philosopher, Jürgen Habermas, recalls Aristotle's distinction between different types of human experiences–*theoria* and *praxis*–and the different types of knowledge corresponding to each (Habermas, 1971; Aristotle, 1962; McCarthy, 1982). As discussed in Chapters One and Two, according to Aristotle, *theoria* refers to the experience or observation of order in the unchanging realities of the natural world, events that appear constant, universal, and eternal. The knowledge that grows out of these experiences corresponds to what we now call the natural sciences. In contrast, *praxis* refers to the experience of initiating action in the flux of ever-changing, non-recurrent social situations. In Aristotle's analysis, the experience of *praxis* requires a categorically distinct kind of knowledge because human action, at its most fundamental level, is distinguished by choice, in circumstances that require sensitivity, perceptiveness and attentiveness to the unique morally salient features of the situation at hand. It is the kind of knowledge that we need when we must decide what we should do right here and now. As Aristotle put it, "The decision lies in the perception . . . For where it is in our power to act, it is also in our power not to act, and where we can say 'no,' we can also say 'yes' " (Aristotle, 1962, p. 65). It is this capacity for making choices that provides human beings with the unique capability for moral reasoning–for choosing on the basis of what we think is right, what we think we *ought* to do, and hence, our distinctive notions of moral responsibility. Because human beings can choose, Aristotle thought that human behavior could never be captured in the kinds of general laws that are found to govern cause-and-effect relationships in the natural world, the proper realm of *theoria*. In contrast, the kind of knowledge that emerges from the experience of *praxis* corresponds to what we would now call moral judgment, or wisdom.

Building on Aristotle's original distinctions, in his *Theory of Communicative Action*, Habermas traces how these different kinds of knowledge come down to us today in terms of what he calls communicative (moral-practical) versus instrumental (scientific-technical) reasoning (Habermas, 1987; Habermas, 1993; White, 1995; Passerin d'Entreves and Benhabib, 1997). Communicative rationality is consent-oriented, i.e., it is oriented towards gaining mutual understanding and agreement about the validity (moral rightness) of norms of behavior. In his analysis, communicative rationality is characteristic of the world of everyday human existence, a sphere he refers to as (following Husserl and Schutz) "lifeworld," which is described as that implicit "taken-for-granted" background of shared understandings, values, and routine ways of life in which one's social identity develops.* In contrast, instrumental rationality is goal- or success-oriented. The logic of this type of reasoning is organized around determining the most effective means to achieve identified goals, goals which are themselves determined by the structure of impersonal economic and administrative systems that are geared to profit maximization and bureaucratic efficiency. (For example, to maximize the most efficient use of its resources, the public health service has identified the leading causes of morbidity and mortality [heart disease, cancer] and their primary causes [smoking, obesity], and hence, the elimination of smoking and obesity are now its highest, most important goals.) Based on these distinctions, Habermas is deeply troubled by what he sees as the inappropriate imposition of instrumental thinking on the sphere of lifeworld affairs.

The process of "rationalization" is the extension of instrumental reasoning to ever more arenas of social life. In Habermas's analysis, the distinct logic of instrumental rationality is gradually displacing communicatively-oriented modes of socialization and social integration. Instrumental patterns of communication are strategic and manifest in the attempt to get others to conform to goals given by the economic system or administrative state; instrumental communication stands in contrast to communicative rationality, which is expressed in a mutually-open, reciprocal, two-way process of seeking consensus on appropriate norms of living in society. In response to pressures generated by economic and bureaucratic systems, consent-oriented patterns of communication and interaction are being progressively squeezed out and replaced by the instrumental modes of reasoning. As this process of rationalization is extended into new domains, consensus is subordinated to efficiency. Ultimately, Habermas traces the origins of various social pathologies evident in modern society to these systematically distorted patterns of communication, a process Habermas dramatically refers to as the "colonization of the lifeworld."* According to Habermas, social ailments such as anomie, hedonism, drug use, cynicism, apathy, violence, the withdrawal from responsible citizenship into a private world of pleasure-seeking and the maximization of self-interests, and so on, result from the erosion of social consensus about the norms and conditions of a just society. In tandem, our unique human capacity for autonomous moral reasoning is being increasingly threatened and impoverished by the increasingly predominant recourse to instrumental rationality, which is steadily encroaching upon the way we think about issues that are more appropriately resolved through the consent-oriented moral reasoning processes of the lifeworld domain.

Based on a related yet independent line of analysis, the Canadian philosopher, Charles Taylor, sees the growing recourse to "instrumental reason" as a "massively important phenomenon" underlying the perplexing sense of loss, malaise, and disintegration widely felt in modern culture (Taylor, 1992; Weber, 1978; Buchanan, 2000). Succinctly stated, instrumental reason is the intellectual tendency to give precedence to thinking about means, rather than ends. Coined by the great German sociologist, Max Weber, the term "instrumental reason" refers to a pattern of thinking dedicated to the methodical expansion of human control and domination "by means of an increasingly precise calculation of adequate means." Weber used the term to characterize the modern preoccupation with determining the most effective means to a given end, to the neglect of the evaluation of the ends themselves. As the sociologist Philip Selznick (1992) states, "Reason is instrumental when it abdicates responsibility for determining ends and restricts itself to ways and means."

In contrast to instrumental reasoning, Weber described another type of reasoning process that he called "value rationality" or "practical reason." Building on Weber's work, Taylor sees a compelling need for reviving the exercise of "practical reason" to counter-balance the growing prominence and hegemony of instrumental reason (Taylor, 1995). Practical reason addresses questions about the good for human beings. It is reflection on the goals, values, and purposes of human action. It is the thinking process involved in evaluating the quality of the ideals that we seek to realize in this life. Practical reason is the exercise of one's faculty of judgment in making qualitative distinctions of worth among different goals and choosing one course of action over another in light of the highest good people hope to realize.

With that as background, let us now take a closer look at two models for thinking about the purposes of health education.

The Medical Model

The metaphor of the medical model is quite familiar to those of us in health education, commonly encountered, for example, in the notion of making an "educational diagnosis" using the popular PRECEDE model (Green and Kreuter, 1991). It is worth remembering, however, that this is not the only way that we have thought about our work. One of the founders of the field, Godfrey Hochbaum (1976), noted a historical shift in the field dating to a time around 1950. Following in the wake of huge increases in funding for social scientific research after World War II, he observes that the field began to move away from its earlier goal of providing factual information towards "the need to influence these [social-psychological] factors if behavior is to be effectively modified." By 1960, another giant in the field, Mayhew Derryberry (1960), makes perhaps the earliest reference to the metaphor of the medical model: "the processes [of health education] are almost completely analogous to those used by physicians in the practice of medicine" and "the steps that the two groups go through in applying their respective sciences are almost identical." Following this train of thinking, Lawrence Green (1978), the developer of the PRECEDE model, thus could write in 1978: "Health education is found to be highly interwoven with the complementary and overlapping technologies of motivational and behavioral control such as mass communication and behavior modification." These days, with major funding from the National Institutes of Health, a research agenda that emulates the medical model is rarely questioned.

The reason that health education bought into the medical model (as outlined here) has everything to do with the awesome success of modern medical science, in particular, and the natural sciences, in general. Because of their undeniable success, many, if not most, researchers argue today that the best–or even more strongly, the *only*–way to gain valid knowledge about human behavior is to use the exact same research methods that researchers in the natural and medical sciences use, namely, an experimental, hypothesis-testing model. Researchers have opted for the scientific, hypothesis-testing model, by and large, because it provides clear and powerful criteria for determining the validity of claims about how the world works. But these very same criteria for assessing the validity of truth claims have a built-in bias: the power to effect change is inherent in the use of hypothesis-testing methods. One significant and inextricable by-product of the use of the criteria of prediction and control is that the confirmation of hypotheses can be demonstrated only by wielding instrumental power over the events being investigated: the dependent variable changes, as predicted, as a result of the experimentally-induced changes in the hypothesized independent variable(s). Based on this singular understanding of how one establishes the truth of propositions (what positivists call the verification principle), the scientific method has proven remarkably successful in extending man's power to control the course of events occurring in the natural world. Caught up in the larger cultural veneration of scientific success, the historical shift in orientation in the field of health education was set in motion by this particular understanding of what makes research valid, which over time has resulted in a reformulation of the goals and methods of the field. As the experimental, hypothesis-testing model of behavioral research has become dominant, the practice of health promotion has consequently come to be identified with developing effective interventions.

The medical model is based on the assumption that it is only by conducting experiments that one can verify claims about the nature and direction of relationships among observed events. Or more accurately, the medical model has developed a codified set of standards regarding levels of evidence that has established that prospective tests of hypotheses in experimental research designs provide the highest level of certainty and confidence about the truth of a given claim (Elwood, 1988; Ferreira, Ferreira, Maher, *et al*, 2002). Thus, while there are many other types of social scientific research, such as descriptive or correlational studies, the strength of evidence in these types of research is considered inferior and less trustworthy, and hence, these types of studies are generally regarded as preliminary steps along the way to the most robust test of science, experimental research designs. Researchers conduct experiments to test hypotheses about the nature and magnitude of conjectured cause-and-effect relationships between identified independent and dependent variables, called randomized controlled trials (RCTs). While there are many other types of non-experimental health studies, RCTs are the gold standard towards which all lines of research are directed. As anyone who has ever submitted a grant application to NIH knows, RCTs are the research design that all other types of research are ideally expected to culminate in order to meet the highest standards of credibility, proof, and validity. RCTs enable researchers to determine whether a change in an independent variable will or will not effect a change, as predicted, in the dependent variable of interest.

Whether it is in testing new drugs to treat AIDS or cancer, or new behavioral interventions to prevent overeating or promote exercise, it is the ability to effect change as predicted in testing hypotheses that is considered the most critical test for establishing valid knowledge in the medical/scientific model. By testing hypotheses, social scientists assume that they can identify the causes of people's behaviors (for instance, interest these days focuses on what causes people to eat too much). Drawing on the well-known canon of health behavior theories, theories such as social learning theory, the health belief model, the theory of reasoned action, and so forth, behavioral scientists formulate hypotheses about the relationship between various independent variables (e.g., self-efficacy, perceived susceptibility, attitudes, etc.) and the dependent variable of interest (e.g., overeating), which they then test by conducting experiments.

When the criteria used to assess the validity of claims are defined and set by an experimental, hypothesis-testing paradigm, then the goals and methods of the practice of health education follow directly. After researchers have tested and verified the relationships among the different variables in their theory, practitioners are expected to use the exact same methods to achieve the exact same results as the researchers. Just as lab scientists know precisely how to control electro-magnetic currents, or split atoms to make nuclear energy, or mix up a batch of pure unadulterated aspirin, or medical doctors know how to treat and cure bacterial infections, health educators are supposed to design programs to effect changes in a set of specified independent variables, which will then cause changes in the dependent variable, health behaviors. So, in response to the current epidemic of obesity, we plan to increase the target population's sense of susceptibility to the ill effects of being overweight, or their perception of the severity of diabetes, and so on. This point needs to be emphasized: in the medical model, intervening to change theoretically-specified independent variables to bring about targeted changes in the dependent variable is the ideal and expected relationship between research and practice, a link referred to in the scientific literature as "fidelity in implementation."

To sum up, in the medical model, the goals are identified by a bureaucratic system set up to maximize the most efficient use of resources by ranking the leading causes of morbidity and mortality (heart disease, cancer) and their causes (smoking, obesity), and then, the methods to achieve these goals are determined by discovering through scientific research the most effective way to interrupt the causal chain of events that causes people to eat too much or to start smoking. Health promotion practitioners are expected to replicate the methods identified by researchers to be the most effective in achieving the goals set by the administrative apparatus of the state. An "effective" program is one that consistently and reliably results in people behaving in accordance with these given goals.

There are significant and worthwhile questions about whether this model works on its own terms (that is, I think it is an open question about whether we are making *any* progress in identifying more effective weight control programs or smoking prevention programs), but setting aside the epistemological question about why this model has not been more successful in identifying the causes of human behavior, the question that I want to pursue here is the ethical one: is this the only way to think about what we are doing? Or are there other ways of thinking about the purposes of health education that we might find more worthwhile, more commendable in terms of pursuing higher goals beyond physical fitness (like, say, human wellbeing) through means that are ethically less problematic than behavioral control/modification? I am going to come back to some of the limitations of the medical model in the concluding section, and some of the worthwhile parts that might be salvaged in light of a different interpretation. But if this is a fair representation of how the field presently operates, then we can turn now to consider another way of thinking about our purposes, one that should be very familiar to readers of this journal, the model of higher education.

The Education Model

There are, of course, many different ideas about the purposes of education, so let me start by saying that the model that I have in mind is neither simple information transmission nor vocational skills training (such as auto mechanic school). It is, instead, the model of a broad liberal arts education, where the goal is to develop a cultivated "well-educated" mind. Five common purposes of a liberal education cited in the literature are: (1) to enhance one's faculty of critical judgment, (2) to gain deeper self-understanding, (3) to liberate, or free people from narrow, parochial, or prejudiced views of the world, (4) to refine moral sensibilities, by challenging and strengthening one's convictions and sense of obligation to advance justice in this world, and (5) to build respect and appreciation for the diversity of understandings of the good life for human beings and a commitment to reaching reasoned agreement about how we can best share a more decent and humane world (Oakeshott, 1989; Frankena, 1965; de Nicolas, 1989; Anderson, 1993). These purposes, I think, provide a better analogy for thinking about aims of health promotion. It is exactly what we do, in our best moments, as faculty members and graduate students.

Critical Judgment

In *The Republic*, Plato argues that the purpose of education is to develop one's capacity to distinguish the good life from the bad life and to form those habits of mind always to choose the better alternative from among all that are possible. It is a process of becoming more self-conscious about how one lives, to reflect at length about what one had previously just taken for granted, and to develop one's ability to justify and defend which courses of action and ways of life that, as individuals and as a society, one considers most worthwhile and fulfilling. It is a matter of developing one's aptitude in determining when information must be acted on, and when it is irrelevant. Education seeks to expand one's horizons in order to enrich and improve the process of making well-reasoned choices from among a wider range of envisioned alternatives. It is sustained inquiry into the good life for human beings. It aims to hone one's skills at discerning about what is best, a reasoning process that can never be fully captured by or reduced to algorithms or explicit computer-like rules for rank-ordering decisions.

Self-understanding

Oakeshott (1989, p. 3) defines education as "an encounter with self-understanding." Etymologically, "e-duc-ation" signifies a leading out, from darkness into light. Education is a process of immersion and comprehensive engagement in which we come to know ourselves and our place in the world more clearly. As Anderson (1993) writes,

> To be fully human is to be acutely conscious of purpose. Only when we think through our aims and objectives–when we ask probing questions about the "good" we seek, about the *telos* of our acts–do we act as humans are capable of acting (p. 5).

It is gaining greater insight into and awareness of areas of one's life that were formally opaque, obscured, and poorly understood. We study good literature in order to be better able to articulate and discriminate among feelings that were previously garbled and confused; or, as DeBotton (1997) writes,

> The value of a novel is not limited to its depiction of emotions and people akin to those in our own life; it stretches to an ability to describe these *far better* than we would have been able, to put a finger on perceptions that we recognize *as our own*, but could not have formulated *on our own* (p. 28, emphasis in original).

Greater self-understanding makes it possible to live a life that one can call "one's own." It is finding a way to be at home in the world and face it with more or less grace. Education begins with the idea, in Socrates's most famous words, "The unexamined life is not worth living."

Liberation

The ideal of a liberal education is the realization of a certain sort of freedom, to develop the capacity to think for oneself. Its opposite is acquiescence or acceptance of parochialism, bigotry and dogmatism. The goal of education emerges out of the recognition that ignorance is a form of slavery and dependence, of being blind to new possibilities. It is opening one's mind to see different paths and imagine what might be otherwise. It is becoming better able to formulate one's life plan and foresee the steps to pursue it. It is expanding one's ability to respond to situations with new and fresh interpretations, in lieu of thoughtless knee-jerk reactions.

Justice

The value of education lies in its capacity to make us better people; we trust that educated people will be better able to recognize and point out injustices, identify what must be done to correct them, and know how to make a more convincing case for taking action. A good education seeks to deepen one's commitment to advancing justice, "which means, above all, unflagging concern for those who have gained least from modern prosperity, education and democracy. A concern for justice takes seriously the rightful claims of all persons to life, health, dignity, and hope," a point Selznick (2002, p. 12) drives home. One purpose of education is to create more intelligent, more learned, wiser people who are committed to making our political and economic systems more responsive to the needs of all people.

Civility

Finally, the goal of a liberal education is to foster greater mutual respect and more civilized discourse about how we can best share this space on earth. It aims to promote the value and possibility of reaching reasoned agreement about the core constituent elements that define the common good of community life, the full extent of areas of cooperation, and the boundaries of private space where people are free to pursue their own vision of the good life. A well-educated person invites and is invested in dialogue. Through a good education, we become more open to the possibility that we may be persuaded by other points of view and change our minds about what is valuable and worth realizing.

To wrap up, one critical difference between the medical model and a philosophy of education is their respective constructions of the relationship between means and ends. In the medical model, the goals are seen to be independent of the means, both in how they are determined and in how they are achieved. In the medical model, goals are prioritized based on concerns for efficiency and effectiveness; smoking is the number one preventable public health problem not because people in the community are clamoring for smoking cessation programs but because statistical calculations have determined that it is the largest contributor to the leading cause of death, heart disease. Likewise, the methods for reducing smoking are seen to be unrelated to the process of goal determination. After a goal has been independently determined, the methods of achieving a given goal are considered largely interchangeable (e.g., counseling, prescription drug medications [e.g., buproprion], aversive conditioning, hypnosis, acupuncture, etc.) and to be selected on the basis of which is shown to be most effective.

In contrast, the model of higher education has always had difficulty in settling on precise operational definitions of what it means to be educated and appropriate ways to measure the outcomes of an education. We would find it awkward to speak of, let alone assess, an "effective" education. It takes a good education to appreciate the value of a good education (despite increasing pressures to define "learning objectives" these days). And the methods of education are inextricably linked to the outcomes; it is only through engaging in the process of education (encounters with the thinking of others, self-reflection, and dialogue) that one becomes educated. In an ironic commentary on differences described here, written early in the evolution of the field, Mendelsohn 1968, cited in Faden and Faden, 1978) describes the difference between education and persuasion:

> Education seeks to expand the intellectual horizons to facilitate rational choice from among alternatives; it does not seek to change behavior *per se*. Persuasion, on the other hand, is concerned with limiting choices and controlling perceptions to facilitate adoption of those behaviors promoted by communicator.

Based on these distinctions, he therefore concludes, "We must drop the euphemistic 'education' mantle. Educators do not make for effective persuasive communicators" (p. 10).

Fortunately, there is a long proud tradition in health education that has not treated people as a means to the field's ends. This philosophy of health promotion has worked to strengthen individual autonomy and social solidarity through practices centered on caring and fulfilling our collective responsibility for creating more humane living conditions for all people (Minkler, 1989; Nyswander, 1967). Change and growth are possible when community members connect with one another as human beings in caring relationships characterized by trust and mutual support. It is a type of health education practice that is fully accountable yet not dependent on exercising instrumental power to accomplish predetermined outcome objectives. It is based on the knowledge that, with a modicum of trust and institutional support, many good things can happen–many we may never have even considered before listening to, learning from, and engaging with fellow community members (Minkler and Wallerstein, 2003; Wallerstein and Bernstein, 1994).

Discussion and Conclusion

In a famous debate that appeared in *Science* in 1956 titled "Some Issues Concerning the Control of Human Behavior," B. F. Skinner and Carl Rogers agreed that the science of behavior control was both imminent and inevitable and the only question worth debating was who would have control over determining the goals to which the new technology would be put to use (Rogers and Skinner 1956). The stock response of those committed to the medical model of health education is that any qualms about manipulation will be absolved by securing voluntary and informed consent. Just as surgeons obtain the patient's informed consent before removing a tumor, so too the practice of health education can be ethically redeemed by gaining voluntary and informed consent before subjecting clients to the procedures that will effectively alter their behavior. And if we stick strictly to the question of whether such procedures would meet current ethical standards for clinical care, there can be little question that such a program would not only pass ethical scrutiny but would probably be warmly welcomed by all of us who have ever struggled with losing weight or freeing ourselves from our favorite addiction.[§]

If these technologies were ever developed, however, we would have to confront the profound and radical implications for our understanding of the meaning of the human condition, letting go of any pretensions to human autonomy, integrity, dignity, and moral responsibility. While we might lose weight, we would not gain the dignity and integrity that comes from becoming a self-disciplined agent capable of self-control. More concretely, if the medical model of health education ever were successful, we would need to address serious questions about who would control these program interventions, especially in a public health context when they are intended to be applied on a population basis. (Case in point, in the COMMIT trial, did every single citizen in all 22 cities sign an informed consent form volunteering to participate in the experiment?) As Huxley's nightmarish *Brave New World* vividly illustrates, we might all be made happy (with

BMIs of 25!), but we would no longer be living lives of our own choosing. Let me conclude with some final comments on the implications of a new ethic for research and practice.

First, the choice of models is driven largely by what we think makes research valid. Most social scientific researchers have opted for the hypothesis-testing model because it provides such clear-cut criteria for assessing the validity of factual claims. If our choice of models turns on this concern, then it may be time to consider whether there are other grounds for gaining confidence in the validity of claims besides testing hypotheses. One way of approaching the question of what makes research valid is to ask ourselves whether we have any grounds for claiming that statements about values are true, or not. How do we know if some way of living is good, or not? Or if some course of action that we are considering is the right thing to do? To the extent that one thinks that value claims can be reasonably debated and one can arrive at rational conclusions about their validity, then an alternative research framework to be considered is ethical or normative analysis. It is research aimed at the clarification of basic human values. Research in ethics seeks to articulate more clearly and comprehensively the reasons and justifications that support one course of action over another.

Although space constraints preclude a full discussion, the standards or criteria for establishing the validity of value claims are ultimately based on reaching reasoned agreement (Habermas, 1987). We gain confidence in the validity of propositions to the extent that others exercise their considered judgment and find good reasons to concur with the analysis. Based on this standard, it is clear that the validity of value claims will never attain the same level of certainty as factual claims verified by the scientific method. But here is where I part company with colleagues invested in the medical model: the certainty granted by the power to predict and control outcomes is not the only measure of the value of research. In the alternative model outlined here, the goal of the research–the good to be achieved–is to gain clarity, not to claim certainty.

In getting back to our roots in education, the field would return to its role as disseminators of factual information: what is known about the causes of death and disability. People have a right to this information, whether or not they choose to act on it. But rather than expecting people to change their behavior based on this information (or feeling frustrated when they do not), the more interesting challenge for the field would be to help people make critical value judgments about their priorities, the steps they want to take in pursuing their life plans, and the place of "good" health habits in their vision of the kind of person they want to be. In this model, the quality of a health educator's work would be evaluated not by its effectiveness in changing people's behavior, but by whether audiences find the dialogue valuable in helping them think about how they want to live their lives and the impact of their behaviors on the pursuit of their life goals.

For example, there is growing interest in the field of health promotion in advancing public policy initiatives designed to change the environment to support healthier living habits. In the education model outlined here, one critical role for health educators would be to stimulate discussions in public forums about whether community members think any changes need to be made in the organization of society, for example, regarding the role of large corporations in manipulating the content, cost, and availability of foods that are bad for people's health. Schlosser (2001), for example, provides a thought-provoking analysis of the impact of the food industry in shaping our eating habits that could be used as a stepping-off point for dialogue and deliberation. Building public support for policy initiatives aimed at redressing the vast inequities in the distribution of power in our society through educational forums are critical to the successful passage of such policy proposals. With democratic support from the majority of society, it becomes morally acceptable and politically feasible to use the instrumental power of the state to change the physical and social environment (e.g., passing more progressive tax policies to reduce inequalities in wealth, which have been associated with inequalities in health) in line with more people's vision of the good society.

The project recommended here is a "public reasons" approach, similar to the framework put forward by John Rawls (Rawls, 1971; Daniels, 1996; Brock, 1996). It is based on the cooperative search for moral rightness, which is determined solely on the basis of good reasons, in which nothing but the force of better argument prevails. As Habermas (1987) argues, we have a right not to be bound to norms other than those to which we give our uncoerced rational consent, and it is only by engaging in dialogue with others that one can become convinced of the validity of any proposed norm. The participants themselves are ultimately the only ones competent to judge the merit of various articulated justifications for a particular course of action (e.g., raising taxes on soda pop to deter consumption), for it is the consequences to their needs and interests that constitute the relevant reasons in terms of which the issue of normative validity must be decided. In Habermas's view, justice consists in permitting all persons to participate freely and equally in conversations aimed at reaching consensus on norms regulating their conduct.

This new direction would thus entail building health education programs around the notion of an argument, that is, a particular form of conversation in which something is at stake. Why should people spend 45 minutes a day exercising? Why is this more valuable than the other ways that they now choose to spend their time? In answer to these questions, I think that we as a field have been largely mute, mumbling something about living longer, saving the government money on Medicare, and making corporations more profitable by reducing absenteeism and paying less for insurance. Let me point out, however, that, when viewed in a more positive light, what many health education theories seem to do is to provide reasons for particular courses of action, except that they have become mixed up with incongruent expectations tied to the overlay of a scientific cause-and-effect framework. Telling people how serious diabetes is, how susceptible they are, and discussing the values that they might attach to different outcomes (a la Ajzen's [1988] breakdown of the component parts of "attitudes") is unintentionally offering reasons why they might want to change their behavior, ones that most of us remain genuinely convinced are important. One crucial difference in the approach recommended here, though, is that we would remain open to the possibility–indeed we could become convinced–that there may be more important issues in people's lives on which they are focusing their attention.

In conclusion, instead of devoting all of our time and energy to creating the technologies of behavior control, I think that we should be moving in precisely the opposite direction: we should be doing everything in our power to increase human autonomy. Instead of seeking to develop programs that are ever more effective in altering people's behavior, we should focus on aiding people to make their own choices about how they want to live in light of their best understanding of the good life for themselves (Haan and Bellah, 1983). To the extent that autonomy is associated with good health, then we should shift the emphasis in the field from the rather narrow focus on producing perfect specimens of physical fitness, to a broader concern for human well-being, here understood in terms enhancing autonomy, promoting greater self-understanding, liberating people from scientistic assumptions perpetuating the belief that human behavior is determined by antecedent causes that only highly trained scientists can divine, advancing the cause of social justice, and promoting respect and appreciation for the diversity of understandings of the good life for human beings.

At bottom, it is the dominance of this instrumental mindset that concerns me most. The medical model frames how we think about our relationship to others, dictating the development of more effective behavior change programs and the unquestioned pursuit of the power to make others behave the way we think they should behave as the overriding purpose of health education. We seem to have placed higher priority on the pursuit of scientific, technical expertise over the advancement of moral propriety. If the medical model is a fair characterization of the current direction and purposes of the field, then we have banked on the power of science and technology over democratic processes of engaging fellow citizens in forging a just society. But at the end of the day, figuring out how we should live, individually and collectively, is a moral and political process, not a scientific problem to be solved.

Notes

* - Lifeworld is "the intuitively present, in this sense familiar and transparent, and at the same time vast and incalculable web of presuppositions that have to be satisfied if an actual utterance is to be at all meaningful."

§ - I am not quite sure what such a program would look like, but probably some combination of a) genetic testing to determine genotypic predispositions and responsiveness to alternative therapies, b) psychotropic medications to regulate targeted reward pathways, c) cognitive therapy to reprogram those internal tapes with positive messages, and d) environmental contingency management (e.g., restrictions on what one can buy with food stamps).

References

Ajzen, Icek. 1988. *Attitudes, personality, and behavior*. Chicago: Dorsey Press.

Anderson, Charles. 1993. *Prescribing the Life of the Mind: An essay on the purpose of the university, the aims of liberal education, the competence of citizens and the cultivation of practical reason*. Madison: University of Wisconsin Press.

Aristotle. *Nichomachean Ethics*. 1962. Translated by Martin Ostwald. Indianapolis, IN: Bobbs-Merrill Educational Publishing.

Beauchamp, Thomas. 1980. "The Foundations of Ethics and the Foundations of Science." In *Knowing and Valuing*, edited by H. Tristam Engelhardt and Daniel Callahan, 260-68. Hastings-on-Hudson NY: The Hastings Center.

Brock, Dan. 1995. "Public Moral Discourse." In *Society's Choices: Social and Ethical Decision Making in Biomedicine*, edited by Ruth Bulger, Elizabeth Bobby, and Harvey Fineberg, 215-240. Washington DC: National Academy Press.

Buchanan, David. 2000. *An Ethic for Health Promotion: Re-thinking the sources of human well-being*. New York: Oxford University Press.

Daniels, Norman. 1996. *Justice and Justification*. Cambridge: Cambridge University Press.

DeBotton, Alain. 1997. *How Proust Can Change Your Life.* New York: Pantheon Books.

deNicolas, Antonio. 1989. *Habits of Mind: An Introduction to the Philosophy of Education.* New York: Paragon House.

Derryberry, Mayhew. 1960. "Health Education–Its Objective and Methods." *Health Education Monographs* 8:5-11.

Elwood, J. Mark. 1988. *Causal Relationships in Medicine: A Practical System for Critical Appraisal.* New York: Oxford University Press.

Ferreira, Paola, Manuela Ferreira, Christopher Maher, Kathryn Refshauge and Herbert R, Latimer J. 2002. "Effect of applying different 'levels of evidence' criteria on conclusions of Cochrane reviews of interventions for low back pain." *Journal of Clinical Epidemiology*; 55(11):1126-9.

Frankena, William. 1965. *Philosophy of Education.* New York: MacMillan.

Green, Lawrence. 1978. "Determining the Impact and Effectiveness of Health Education as it relates to Federal Policy." *Health Education Monographs* 6(1): 48-89.

Green, Lawrence and Kreuter, Marshall. *Health Promotion Planning: An Educational and Environmental Approach.* 2nd edn.on. Mountain View, California: Mayfield Publishing Company, 1991.

Haan, Norma and Robert Bellah. 1983. *Social Science as Moral Inquiry.* New York: Columbia University Press.

Habermas, Jürgen. 1971. *Knowledge and Human Interests*. Boston: Beacon Press.

Habermas, Jürgen. 1987. *Theory of Communicative Action*. Translated by Thomas McCarthy. Boston: Beacon Press.

Habermas, Jürgen. 1993. *Justification and Application: Remarks on Discourse Ethics.* Translated by Ciaran Cronon. Cambridge: MIT Press.

Hochbaum, Godfrey. 1976. "At the threshold of a new era." *Health Education* 7(4):2-4.

McCarthy, Thomas. 1982. *The Critical Theory of Jürgen Habermas*. Cambridge MA: MIT Press.

Mendelsohn, Harold. 1968. "Which shall it be: Mass education or mass persuasion for health." *American Journal of Public Health* 58:131-7. Cited in Ruth Faden and Alan Faden, 1978. "The Ethics of Health Education as Public Health Policy." *Health Education Monographs* 6(2):5-23.

Minkler, Meredith. 1989. "Health education, health promotion, and the open society: An historical perspective." *Health Education Quarterly* 16(1): 17-30.

Minkler, Meredith and Nina Wallerstein (Eds.). 2003. *Community-based participatory research for health.* San Francisco: Jossey-Bass.

Nyswander, Dorothy. 1967. "The open society: Its implications for health educators." *Health Education Monographs* 1: 3-13.

Oakeshott, Michael. 1989. *The Voice of Liberal Learning*. New Haven, CT: Yale University Press.

Passerin d'Entreves, Maurizio and Seyla Benhabib (Eds.). 1997. *Habermas and the Unfinished Project of Modernity: Critical essays on the Philosophical Discourse of Modernity*. Cambridge, MA: MIT Press.

Rawls, John. 1971. *A Theory of Justice*. Cambridge, MA: Harvard University Press.

Rogers, Carl and BF Skinner. 1956. "Some Issues Concerning the Control of Human Behavior." *Science* 124(3231): 1057-66.

Schlosser, Eric. 2001. *Fast food nation: The dark side of the all-American meal*. Boston: Houghton Mifflin.

Selznick, Phillip. 1992. *The Moral Commonwealth: Social Theory and the Promise of Community*. Berkeley: University of California Press.

Selznick, Phillip. 2002. *The Communitarian Persuasion*. Washington DC: Woodrow Wilson Press.

Taylor, Charles. 1985. "Interpretation and the Sciences of Man." In Charles Taylor, *Philosophy and the Human Sciences, Philosophical Papers, Volume 2,* 15-57. Cambridge: Cambridge University Press.

Taylor, Charles. 1992. *The Malaise of Modernity*. Cambridge MA: Harvard University Press.

Taylor, Charles. 1995. "Explanation and Practical Reason." In Charles Taylor, *Philosophical Arguments*, 34-60. Cambridge: Harvard University Press.

Wallerstein, Nina and Edward Bernstein. 1994. "Introduction to community empowerment, participatory education, and health." *Health Education Quarterly* 21(2): 141-148.

Weber, Max. 1978. *Economy and Society: An Outline of Interpretive Sociology*. Berkeley: University of California Press.

White, Stephen. (Ed.) 1995. *The Cambridge Companion to Habermas*. New York: Cambridge University Press.

12. Ethical Issues in Community-Based Participatory Research: Balancing Rigorous Research with Community Participation in Community Intervention Studies

By David R. Buchanan, Franklin G. Miller, Nina Wallerstein

A convergence of interests has raised questions about a potential tension between scientific rigor and community participation in health research. In this paper, we show how this tension can be traced to two major underlying ethical concerns: (1) demonstrating respect for community autonomy (including procedures analogous to obtaining individual informed consent); and (2) determining fair procedures for allocating scarce federal health research resources across different research designs. The paper examines how these two issues may have become conflated in controversies surrounding the increasing attention to community-based participatory research (CBPR). CBPR advocates are advised to attend to these underlying ethical concerns in responding to potential criticisms of this new research methodology.

From the outset, it is important to distinguish CBPR from community participation and from community health research. First, although a standardized definition of CBPR has not yet been formulated, proponents point out that community participation *per se* does not necessarily qualify a project as meeting nascent standards of excellence in CBPR. If community participation is seen on a continuum, then CBPR can be understood as an orientation to research that aims at maximum feasible community participation in all phases of the research. Thus, in principle, CBPR can be used with any research design, from epidemiologic studies to clinical trials. In this paper, we focus on randomized controlled trials (RCTs) to test community health interventions, because there are increasing calls for "evidence-based" public health and RCTs are considered the most rigorous research design. Second, in contrast to individual health, community health research seeks to discover new knowledge to improve population health. As such, community health intervention research does not necessarily have to use a CBPR approach, and traditionally, it has not. With these distinctions in mind, this paper examines the ethical issues raised by the use of CBPR to test community health interventions.

The chapter opens with an analysis of two new ethical issues raised by public health interventions. Unlike previous case studies (Minkler, 2004; Malone, Yerger, McGruder and Froelicher, 2006; Green, George, Daniel, Frankish *et al*, 1995; Chen, Jones and Gelberg, 2006) that have examined ethical dilemmas internal to the conduct of particular CBPR projects, this analysis addresses issues that are generic to the conduct of community health intervention research. We start with a discussion of the ethical challenges encountered when the locus of research shifts from the individual to the community level, specifically with regard to the issue of demonstrating respect for the community's right to self-determination. Next, we identify several "structural impediments" that make assessing the effectiveness of public health interventions in standard RCTs virtually impossible. This analysis raises the question of how research proposals aimed at the community level can be evaluated fairly, when it is infeasible to use research designs widely acknowledged as the most robust.

The paper then shows how these two concerns have converged in discussions about the merits of CBPR. We argue that these discussions have become bogged down because CBPR proponents and critics have failed to distinguish the distinct purposes of CBPR. These three distinct purposes are (1) an ethical function of demonstrating respect for community autonomy; (2) a research method for eliciting ideas for interventions to improve population health; and (3) as an intervention itself, seeking to enhance community capacities.

Based on this analysis, the paper concludes with two recommendations for achieving a sound balance between scientific promise and community responsiveness in public health research. First, we propose a model standard for respecting the community right to autonomy, and second, we present a process for allocating the limited public resources designated for health research fairly. In light of the recent federal investment in CBPR initiatives, it is critical to achieve a common understanding of appropriate ethical and scientific standards for evaluating community health intervention research in the 21st century.

New Ethical Considerations in Conducting Community Health Intervention Research

Since the promulgation of the Nuremberg Code, voluntary, informed consent has been recognized as a fundamental norm of health research.‡ Based on the principle of respect for autonomy, individuals have the right to decide if they want to participate after being informed about all relevant aspects of the research. In clinical trials, one important way that respect for autonomy is demonstrated is by obtaining written informed consent.

In clinical research, the process of gaining informed consent is straightforward. The purpose of the research, methods, and risks and benefits (if any) are explained and the individual decides whether she or he wants to participate. But how is this procedure supposed to be extended to a community? If community members have a right to autonomy and it is ethically unwarranted for researchers to conduct health research without their approval, then the major ethical challenge is to specify how respect for community autonomy should be secured. We see three progressively more inclusive possibilities.

In past practice, Institutional Review Boards (IRBs) have generally ignored the issue of respect for community autonomy. IRB approval has been considered sufficient to authorize community health intervention research, based on judgments about whether the risks are sufficiently minimal that individual informed consent can be waived. When an experimental intervention has been deemed to pose minimal risks, IRBs have waived the consent requirement and permitted community intervention trials to proceed.

Although IRB review of community health intervention research may be adequate in certain circumstances, it restricts the scope of investigations to relatively innocuous interventions (e.g., mass media campaigns), and hence is not sufficient in many cases. Consider the following: the effect of police roadblocks to test for impaired drivers, with the goal of identifying effective strategies to reduce traffic fatalities. At the individual level, is it fair to assume that the average social drinker would consider participating in the roadblock experiment in one's interest? At the community level, do community members have a right to question why their

‡ The analysis presented here is based on the ethical framework of principlism. The reader is referred to Beauchamp and Childress, 2001; Emanuel *et al.*, 2000; and Kass, 2001 for definitions of key principles of respect for autonomy and justice discussed in this report.

community was selected, whether they want to participate or not, or whether alternative strategies should be considered? Would an IRB be justified in designating such research as minimal risk?

To test more powerful community interventions, IRB approval alone cannot suffice. There must be a process that serves the same ethical function as individual informed consent, where the community as a whole can decide whether they want to participate. The dual needs for avoiding exploitation and affirming the community's right to self-determination lead into questions of representation: Who can legitimately speak on behalf of community interests? Drawing on the model of oversight in community health centers, one common procedure for addressing these concerns is to establish a Community Advisory Board (CAB).

Stipulating an ethical standard requiring oversight by a CAB is an important first step, but it is not enough. Further issues include the composition of CABs and the scope of their responsibilities: Who and how many should sit on these boards? How should they be selected? What should they be authorized to decide? Significantly, beyond CABs, CBPR proponents recommend other procedures to establish community approval of the research, including interviews with stakeholders and key informants, focus groups, community surveys, community forums, and partnerships with community associations (Wallerstein, Duran, Minkler and Foley, 2005).

Structural Impediments confronting Community Intervention Research

Like the rise of evidence-based medicine, public health interventions face mounting pressures to demonstrate that programs are effective in decreasing morbidity and mortality rates and reducing health disparities. Over time, certain scientific standards for assessing the quality of research evidence have become well established; the gold standard for conducting health research is the RCT (Evidence-Based Working Group, 1992; Rosen, Manor, Engelhard and Zucker, 2006). Like the challenges in identifying appropriate ethical requirements when one shifts from the individual to the community level, it is also complicated to specify appropriate scientific standards for assessing community interventions. For public health interventions, the most rigorous research design requires randomly assigning communities to the different study conditions, in what are called *group-randomized trials* (Murray, 2001). Conducting such research, however, is frequently not feasible, due to various structural impediments.

The most significant complicating factor is that public health interventions often involve policy changes, and randomly assigning communities to comparison conditions is generally not possible for pragmatic political reasons. For example, it is reasonable to hypothesize that limiting the amount of added sugar in food products will reduce obesity rates, but politically it is not feasible to randomly assign counties or states to treatment and comparison conditions to test this hypothesis. The feasibility of using RCTs becomes even more tenuous if unintended adverse effects are conjectured. Needle exchange programs, for instance, have been embroiled in arguments about whether their establishment condones drug use (Buchanan, Shaw, Ford and Singer, 2003). Because of such moral and political compunctions, many public health interventions cannot be investigated in RCTs.

Another major problem is that, in contrast with well-controlled laboratory studies, communities are open and dynamic systems, with a virtually unlimited number of factors influencing health behaviors. As discussed earlier (see Chapter 7), to produce an effect at the community level, public health interventions thus often require tests of the cumulative impact of multiple interventions simultaneously, to achieve a critical mass with detectable effects. Standard protocols for improving the quality of community interventions recommend testing interventions in phases, from pilot tests, to efficacy trials, and so on (Flay, 1986), but testing single discrete interventions have generally been found to yield a null or minimal effect because of the many influences operating at the community level. To recall, Holder (2000, 2002) implemented a study designed to reduce alcohol-involved traffic fatalities that involved five distinct components: (1) community mobilization through media advocacy, (2) responsible beverage service training programs, (3) stepped up police roadblock sobriety checks, (4) crackdowns on alcohol sales to minors, and (5) reductions in the number of alcohol retail outlets. Significantly, because it is frequently not possible to demonstrate the efficacy of individual components first, community health interventions face a much greater burden in providing convincing preliminary evidence to demonstrate the plausibility of achieving positive results in a full-scale trial. Moreover, because of small sample sizes (i.e., number of communities), group-randomized trials are particularly susceptible to selection biases, differential histories, significant challenges in matching communities, unanticipated events (e.g., teens killed in a drunk driving accident) that differentially impact different communities, and contamination (Murray, 2001).

There are additional technical issues that we could present (e.g., questions of external validity; Glasgow, Green, Klesges, *et al*, 2006; Green and Glasgow, 2006), but the point is that there are many intractable barriers to conducting RCTs of community interventions. A small number of group-randomized research designs have been conducted; the most well-known is the COMMIT trial, in which 22 cities were randomly assigned to treatment and comparison conditions in an experiment designed to reduce smoking prevalence (Community Intervention Trial for Smoking Cessation, 1995a, 1995b). Such studies, however, require an enormous investment of public resources and the disappointing results of such large trials to date have led many to question the value of group-randomized trials (Murray, 2001, p. 310) Based on their expense and intrinsic threats to their validity, it appears unlikely that major group-randomized community intervention trials will be undertaken in the foreseeable future.

Given the many factors that make group-randomized trials less feasible than clinical studies, one might then ask how the value of community health intervention research can be demonstrated and limited federal research resources allocated fairly. We return to this point in the final section.

Three Purposes of CBPR

In their 2003 text, Minkler and Wallerstein define CBPR as follows: "Although often and erroneously referred to as a research method, CBPR and other participatory approaches are not methods at all but *orientations to research*" (Minkler and Wallerstein, 2003, p. 4, emphasis in original). They state that fundamental characteristics of CBPR include that it (1) is cooperative, engaging community members and researchers in a joint process in which both contribute equally; (2) achieves a balance between research and action; (3) involves systems development and local community capacity building; and (4) is an empowering process through which participants can increase control over their lives.

In reviewing the literature (Green, George, Daniel *et al*, 1995; Minkler and Wallerstein, 2003; Israel, Eng, Schulz and Parker, 2005; Viswanathan, Ammerman, Eng *et al*, 2004; Green 2003; Israel, Schulz, Parker *et al*, 2003), three major purposes of CBPR stand out. CBPR is used to (1) demonstrate respect for community autonomy; (2) elicit ideas from community members for potential health interventions; and (3) strengthen the capacities of participants to gain control over the conditions that affect health. CBPR is thus a means to fulfill an ethical obligation, a method for identifying new interventions, and an intervention itself, a social process that is expected to change the participants positively as a result of their participation. These purposes are seen to operate simultaneously in a mutually reinforcing process. The multiple purposes, however, may foster potential confusions with regards to how CBPR initiatives should be evaluated. To ensure a fair process of evaluation, it is critically important to distinguish these three purposes and to identify appropriate criteria to evaluate the merits of each.

CBPR as Ethical Obligation

When proponents declare that CBPR is not a method but an orientation to research, it is fair to suggest that they mean the researchers' ethical orientation; that is, it is essential for researchers to demonstrate respect for community members. On this point, there should be no argument: all community health projects must fulfill this fundamental ethical obligation. We see CBPR as the most viable attempt to resolve the problem of respecting community autonomy in public health research today. However, problems may arise when the imperative to demonstrate respect is equated with blurring the respective roles of the different parties involved.

It bears repeating that the goal of health research is to discover new knowledge, with the aim of improving health. Federal agencies have a fiduciary responsibility to invest limited public resources to achieve this goal. Unfortunately, because federal grants are capped, there are direct trade-offs between the amount of money allocated to the intervention and the amount devoted to the research. In typical subcontracting arrangements, the percentage of funds going to the academic and community partners, respectively, may be perceived to reflect the relative value and respect due each partner, and hence, can cause serious frictions in these partnerships when funding appears imbalanced. Thus, it is imperative for CBPR consortia to acknowledge these constraints and determine a fair process for decision making about budgetary issues, where simple democratic "majority rules" procedures may not be appropriate. Based on a shared responsibility to use taxpayer dollars prudently, it is essential for all parties involved to uphold the highest scientific standards possible in conducting the research.

CBPR as Research Method

To the extent that CBPR is understood as a method for eliciting or adapting ideas for promising health interventions, then, in principle, these suggestions should be subjected to testing in the most rigorous research design possible. One primary justification for using CBPR is that efforts to develop effective interventions or translate them into more diverse settings have not been consistently successful. If identifying more effective interventions is the goal, then CBPR consortia must strive to achieve agreement about how evidence of effectiveness can best be produced.

As a method for eliciting ideas for interventions, the different steps in the research process need to be recognized and distinct responsibilities of the respective partners acknowledged. Just as it would be inappropriate for researchers to insist on implementing an intervention that community members found objectionable, so community members need to respect the knowledge that researchers bring regarding research design, validated measures, and statistical analysis. Questions about which methods are best suited to the situation need to be kept distinct from questions about whose opinions deserve more respect. The major pitfall is to accept compromises that would permit less than the highest quality research feasible.

CBPR as Social Intervention

Finally, to the extent that CBPR is seen as a process for enhancing community capacities, then it should be evaluated as a social intervention in itself. CBPR advocates refer to the "added value" of CBPR and criteria are evolving for assessing the impact of participation. Many see the benefits in terms of community empowerment, and so look to measures of the capacities of community members to engage in research, develop effective interventions, push for policy changes, and so on.

It is not difficult to pose the question of added value as a hypothesis, and one can imagine a group-randomized trial to test it, at least in theory. One problem is that consensus about the hypothetical added value has not yet been achieved, with ideas ranging from eliciting new ideas; to improving recruitment and retention rates; to enhancing adaptation and implementation of interventions in diverse settings; to those who suggest that the process of participation itself may have an even greater impact than the intervention under investigation. The challenge of capturing this broad range of outcomes is further compounded by unresolved questions about the primary beneficiary of community participation: all community members, all targeted community members, advisory board members, or only those who most actively involved?

To assess the "CBPR effect," the ideal research design would be a group-randomized trial that compared communities randomized to the CBPR process to communities assigned to the comparison condition of a traditional researcher-driven investigation. Such an investigation, however, would be tremendously complicated and practically impossible.

Recommendations to Achieve a Sound Balance Between Scientific and Ethical Considerations

In the preceding analysis, two underlying ethical issues emerged regarding perceived tensions between demands for scientific rigor and calls for community participation. First, CBPR proponents are concerned that the scientific community has paid insufficient attention to the ethical requirement of respect for community autonomy. Second, supporters are troubled that demands for scientific rigor have shortchanged the need for greater investment in community intervention research.

One problem that fosters continuing controversies is that these two issues often get fused, where calls for greater community participation are used almost interchangeably with calls for greater support for community health intervention research. In this line of thought, if community participation is more moral than traditional paternalistic approaches, then it deserves greater support in the National Institutes of Health (NIH) funding priorities. Conversely, anyone who questions the priority of community research must not respect community members and their right to participate in making decisions that affect their lives. It is critically important, however, to keep these two issues distinct and evaluate each on its own merits.

Respecting Right to Community Autonomy

As shown herein, there is an urgent need to develop new ethical guidelines that specify standards for obtaining community endorsement of the goals and methods of public health research. Therefore, we recommend a major revision of IRB review procedures. To ensure that the goal and methods are acceptable to community members, we propose that IRBs require researchers to use a progressively more inclusive process proportionately geared to the potential risks and threat of exploitation. The more powerful the intervention and the greater the possibility of exploitation, the more extensive the level of community participation, both in outreach to the community and in their involvement in all phases of the research. Models for community participation are now being put into practice, notably in the work of the Navajo Nation IRB (American Indian Law Center, 1999). As these models attest, the consent process must establish widespread community support, where residents agree that the proposed intervention is relevant and the methods of evaluation appropriate. There is growing debate about the ancillary duties of researchers these days (Belsky and Richardson, 2004), but in general, evolving model standards also include provision for community benefit and dissemination of the results to the community.

Fair Allocation of Federal Research Dollars

The second major ethical concern identified here entails allocating scarce public resources designated for health research fairly, a matter of distributive justice. The process for determining how federal research dollars should be allocated is a relatively neglected area of ethical analysis. The mission of the NIH is "to uncover new knowledge that will lead to better health for everyone." The key question is what kinds of knowledge are most likely to succeed in achieving better health for everyone.

In the 1997 report, *Setting Research Priorities at the National Institutes of Health*, NIH officials identified five criteria to guide distribution decisions: (1) public health needs, (2) scientific quality, (3) potential for scientific progress, (4) portfolio diversification, and (5) support for research infrastructure (Institute of Medicine, 1998). Clearly, different value judgments are involved in assigning different weights to the different criteria (Dresser, 2001; Buchanan and Miller, 2006). The issue that CBPR proponents raise is whether "scientific promise" has taken undue precedence over community responsiveness.

In light of these conflicting value judgments, we recommend that NIH establish fair procedures for resolving such disagreements. Daniels and Sabin (1997) have developed a procedure, called "accountability for reasonableness," to assist in setting priorities in medical care settings–specifically, decisions to cover particular medical interventions in insurance policies–but their procedure is directly applicable to setting research priorities. (See Table 7.3 for list of criteria.) Regarding the need for public regulation, NIH officials have acknowledged that their interactions with the public are "generally weak" and affirmed the need to more fully engage the public to redress concerns about the fairness of its distribution decisions (Institute of Medicine, 1998, p. 7). Thus, it is critically important that community members and public health professionals vigorously advocate for the just distribution of public resources held in trust at NIH. NIH officials and review groups are charged with evaluating proposals based on their prospects for uncovering new knowledge that will lead to better health for everyone. Their deliberations, however, must be reasonable with respect to the cogency of the rationales put forward about the prospects that the research results will lead to improvements in population health. Because of the feasibility constraints enumerated, we recommend that reviewer guidelines unequivocally affirm that methods other than experimental research designs are acceptable in assessing the merits of CBPR proposals.

Given the many structural impediments, the most feasible study designs may only be quasi-experimental or even one-group designs. Proponents must not be daunted. To enhance public and professional appreciation of the validity of non-experimental epidemiologic research designs, the field has recently embarked on a major new policy initiative, the Project on Scientific Knowledge and Public Policy (SKAPP; see www.defendingscience.org[§]) (Michaels, 2005). Although there can be little doubt that RCTs are best at controlling threats to internal validity (Cochrane Library, 2004), in situations where RCTs are not feasible, it is essential to evaluate the merits of proposals using appropriate scientific criteria. Specifically, we recommend "weight-of-evidence" standards, like Hill's criteria, based on items such as biological plausibility, consistency in association, dose–response relationships (Hill, 1965), and triangulation of multiple methods to strengthen confidence in the research results. The critical point is that review criteria must be reasonable, in the sense of providing adequate assurances that the research will produce the most robust results possible in a given context.

Conclusion

In conclusion, we want to reaffirm that calls for community participation should not be confused with sanctioning unwitting concessions or excuses for lowering scientific standards. A rapidly growing literature in bioethics has laid the foundations for establishing a new ethical requirement for community collaboration in health research (Emanuel, Wendler, Killen and Grady, 2004; Dickert and Sugarman, 2005; Brody, McCullough and Sharp, 2005). Yet, properly understood, community collaboration is an ethical mandate, and hence, must be evaluated in terms of meeting moral standards, such as those outlined here, which are independent of questions of scientific standards and rigor in research.

That said, it is equally important to note that it will frequently be difficult and require a depth of judgment and discussion—in community partnerships and in study review panels—to determine whether a more

[§] The Project on Scientific Knowledge and Public Policy (see www.defendingscience.org) examines the nature of science and how it is used and misused in government decision-making and legal proceedings. Through empirical research, conversations among scholars, and publications, SKAPP aims to enhance understanding of how knowledge is generated and interpreted. SKAPP promotes transparent decision-making, based on the best available science, to protect public health.

rigorous research design, such as an RCT, in a given context is feasible or not. To work through these issues, trust is critical, and therefore, as CBPR advocates have long argued, it is critically important for funding agencies to allocate support for a startup "pilot" period of 2 or 3 years to allow the partners to develop confidence and respect for their mutual integrity. Although it will often not be possible to conduct an RCT, the collaborators have an obligation to seek the most generalizable knowledge possible to maximize the social value of the research.

References

American Indian Law Center. 1999. *Model tribal research code: With materials for tribal regulation for research and checklist for Indian health boards. 3rd ed.* Albuquerque, NM: American Indian Law Center, Inc.

Beauchamp, Tom, and James Childress. 2001. *Principles of Biomedical Ethics*, 5th edition. New York: Oxford University Press.

Belsky, Leah and Henry Richardson. 2004. "Medical researchers' ancillary clinical care responsibilities." *British Medical Journal* 328(7454): 1494-1496.

Brody, Baruch, Laurence McCullough and Richard Sharp. 2005. "Consensus and controversy in clinical research ethics." *JAMA* 294 (11):1411-14.

Buchanan, David, and Franklin G. Miller. 2007. "Justice in research on human subjects." In *The Blackwell Guide to Medical Ethics*, edited by Rosamond Rhodes, Leslie Francis, and Anita Silvers, 373-392, New York: Blackwell.

Buchanan, David, Susan Shaw, Amy Ford and Merrill Singer. 2003. "Empirical science meets moral panic: an analysis of the politics of needle exchange." *Journal of Public Health Policy* 24:427-44.

Chen, Donna, Loretta Jones and Lillian Gelberg. 2006. "Ethics of clinical research within a community-academic partnered participatory framework." *Ethnicity and Disease* 16 Supplement 1: S118-35.

Cochrane Library, editor. 2004. *Cochrane collaboration*. 2nd ed. Oxford: Oxford University Press.

Community Intervention Trial for Smoking Cessation (COMMIT). 1995a. "I. Cohort results from a four-year community intervention." *American Journal of Public Health* 85(2): 183-192.

Community Intervention Trial for Smoking Cessation (COMMIT). 1995b. "II. Changes in adult cigarette smoking prevalence." *American Journal of Public Health* 85(2): 193-200.

Daniels, Norman, and James Sabin. 1997. "Limits to health care: Fair procedures, democratic deliberation, and the legitimacy problem for insurers." *Philosophy and Public Affairs* 26: 303-350.

Dickert, Neal and Jeremy Sugarman. 2005. "Ethical goals of community consultation in research." *American Journal of Public Health* 95(7):1123-7.

Dresser, Ruth. 2001. *When science offers salvation: Patient advocacy and research ethics*. New York: Oxford University Press.

Emanuel, Ezekiel, David Wendler, and Christine Grady. 2000. "What Makes Clinical Research Ethical?" *JAMA* 283: 2701- 2711.

Emanuel. Ezekiel, David Wendler, Jack Killen, and Christine Grady. 2004. "What makes clinical research in developing countries ethical? The benchmarks of ethical research." *Journal of Infectious Diseases* 189:930-7.

Evidence-Based Working Group. 1992. "Evidenced-based medicine: A new approach to teaching the practice of medicine." *Journal of the American Medical Association* 268(17): 2420-2425.

Flay, Brian. 1986. "Efficacy and effectiveness trials (and other phases of research) in the development of health promotion programs." *Preventive Medicine* 15:451-74.

Glasgow, Russell, Lawrence W. Green, Lisa M. Klesges, David B. Abrams, Edwin B. Fisher, *et al*. 2006. "External validity: We need to do more." *Annals of Behavioral Medicine* 31: 105-8.

Green, Lawrence. 2003. "Tracing federal support for participatory research." In *Community based participatory research for health*, edited Meredith Minkler and Nina Wallerstein, 410–418. San Francisco: Jossey-Bass.

Green, Lawrence, M. Anne George, M. Daniel, Charles Frankish, Carol Herbert, W.R. Bowie, *et al*. 1995. *Study of participatory research in health promotion: Review and recommendations for the development of participatory research in health promotion in Canada*. Vancouver, B.C.: The Institute of Health Promotion Research, University of British Columbia and the B.C. Consortium for Health Promotion Research, Royal Society of Canada.

Green, Lawrence and Russell Glasgow. 2006. "Evaluating the relevance, generalization, and applicability of research." *Evaluation and the Health Professions* 29(1): 126-53.

Hill, Austin B. 1965. "The environment and disease: Association or causation?" *Proceedings of the Royal Society of Medicine* 58: 295-300.

Holder, Hal. 2000. "Community prevention of alcohol problems." *Addictive Behaviors* 25: 843-859.

Holder, Hal. 2002. "Prevention of alcohol and drug 'abuse' problems at the community level: What research tells us." *Substance Use and Misuse* 37(8–10): 901-921.

Institute of Medicine. 1998. *Scientific opportunities and public needs: Improving priority setting and public input at the National Institutes of Health*. Washington, DC: National Academy Press.

Israel, Barbara, Eugenia Eng, Amy Schulz and Edith Parker (Eds.). 2005. *Methods in Community-Based Participatory Research for Health*. San Francisco: Jossey-Bass.

Israel, Barbara, Amy Schulz, Edith Parker, Adam Becker, Alex Allen, J. Ricardo Guzman and Richard Lichtenstein. 2003. "Critical issues in developing and following community based participatory research principles." In *Community based participatory research for health*, edited by Meredith Minkler and Nina Wallerstein, 31-44. San Francisco: Jossey-Bass.

Kass, Nancy. 2001. "An ethics framework for public health." *American Journal of Public Health* 91(1):1776-82.

Malone, Ruth, Valerie B. Yerger, Carol McGruder, and Erika Froelicher. 2006. " 'It's like Tuskegee in reverse': a case study of ethical tensions in institutional review board review of community-based participatory research." *American Journal of Public Health* 96(1):1914-9.

Michaels, David. 2005 "Scientific evidence and public policy." *American Journal of Public Health* 95(S1): S5-7.

Minkler, Meredith. 2004. "Ethical challenges for the 'outside' researcher in community-based participatory research." *Health Education and Behavior* 31:684-97.

Minkler, Meredith and Nina Wallerstein (Eds.). 2003. *Community-based participatory research for health*. San Francisco: Jossey-Bass.

Murray, David. 2001. "Efficacy and effectiveness trials in health promotion and disease prevention: Design and analysis of group-randomized trials." In *Integrating behavioral and social sciences with public health*, edited by Neil Schneiderman, Marjorie Speers, Julia Silva, Henry Tomes, and Jacquelyn Gentry, 305-320. Washington, DC: American Psychological Association.

Rosen, Laura, Orly Manor, Dan Engelhard and David Zucker. 2006. "In defense of the randomized controlled trial for health promotion research." *American Journal of Public Health* 96(7): 1181-6.

Viswanathan, Meera, Alice Ammerman, Erling Eng, Gerald Gartlehner, Kathleen Lohr, *et al. Community-based Participatory Research: Assessing the evidence.* 2004. Rockville, MD: Agency for Healthcare

Research and Quality; August 2004. Summary, Evidence Report/ Technology Assessment No. 99, AHRQ Publication 04-E022-1.

Wallerstein, Nina, Bonnie Duran, Meredith Minkler, and Kevin Foley. 2005. "Developing and Maintaining Partnerships with Communities." In *Methods for Community Based Participatory Research*, edited by Barbara A. Israel, Eugenia Eng, Amy J. Schulz, Edith A. Parker, 43-68. San Francisco, CA: Jossey Bass.

13. THE CEPA PROJECT: A NEW MODEL FOR COMMUNITY-BASED PROGRAM PLANNING

DAVID BUCHANAN, JOANI MARINOFF, EDNA APOSTOL, NANCY O'HARE, DALILA BALFOUR, MARIA RODRIGUEZ, CARMEN CLAUDIO, CARLOS SANTIAGO

Over the past two decades, there has been a growing interest in "community-based" approaches to health promotion and disease prevention. A number of authors (Chavis and Florina, 1990; Fawcett, Paine, Francisco and Vliet, 1993; Grace, 1990; McKnight, 1987) have made a distinction between community-based strategies and what could be termed "social planning" approaches, borrowing from the classic typology by Rothman (1979). In the social planning model, the goals, objectives and implementation activities are identified by public health professionals who design the programs based on their own training and expertise. The pioneering heart disease prevention programs, such as the Stanford three- and five-community studies, the North Karella project, the Minnesota Heart Health plan and the Pawtucket (RI) project, are well-known examples of the social planning approach to community interventions. But, for a variety of reasons, many people have become disenchanted with expert-driven interventions and have called for new approaches in which lay citizens play a central decision-making role.

There are many reasons supporting a shift from expert-led to citizen-led interventions. First, there is a growing recognition that expert models have been, at best, only modestly successful and not with all populations. Also, there is a sense that, if many public health problems are rooted in community disintegration and anomie (e.g., alcohol and drug abuse, suicide, violence, unsafe sexual behaviors, etc.), then a rekindling of community *civitas* (Bell, 1976) may be necessary to alleviate these problems. This kind of communal rejuvenation is not something that can be imposed by outsiders. Similarly, if a sense of powerlessness contributes to health problems, then a reliance on outside experts may foster or exacerbate feelings of dependency and incompetence.

In the larger picture, many people think government-run programs benefit middle class program managers more than the populations in need. Some authors have gone even further to suggest that bureaucratic programs do more harm than good (McKnight, 1987; Murray, 1984). Furthermore, there is a growing disillusionment with the ability of positivist social science methods to determine truths about the human condition, and hence, there have been renewed calls for moving away from the idea of a "scientifically-guided" society and toward a "self-guiding" society (Lindblom, 1990). Within the field of health education, there have long been injunctions to "start where the people are" (Nyswander, 1967). Finally, a powerful democratic impulse provides a moral imperative to open up any processes that might allow people to control the conditions that affect their lives.

Based on the foregoing, the call for community-based health promotion programs is well justified. In this chapter, we present a case study of a program that was developed as an innovative approach to community-based public health programming. The *Centro de Educación, Prevención y Acción* (CEPA) project is designed to break down the barriers between program developers and program recipients to the greatest degree possible. The program described here illustrates both the possibilities and the limitations of intensive citizen involvement. The case study presents some of the lessons learned in the process in hopes that they may be of value to others trying to engage in community-based approaches to health promotion.

Background

The *Centro de Educación, Prevención y Acción* (CEPA) project is a collaborative endeavor between the Holyoke Latino Community Coalition and the University of Massachusetts School of Public Health. The CEPA program is one part of a larger project funded under the "Community-Based Public Health" initiative of the W. K. Kellogg Foundation. To set the context for the discussion, a brief description of the overall initiative is in order.

The Community-Based Public Health initiative grew out of the recommendations contained in the Institute of Medicine's *Future of Public Health* (1988) report, the "Faculty-Agency Forum" meetings and original thinking from within the W. K. Kellogg Foundation. The Community-Based Public Health initiative was unique in at least two respects. Where both the IOM report and the Faculty-Agency Forum focused on building stronger ties between academic programs and public health agencies (health departments), the Kellogg Foundation thought it essential to include community groups as well in any new efforts to revitalize the field of public health (for many of the reasons cited here). Hence, they required a tripartite relationship: academics, professional practitioners, and community-based organizations.

Second, realizing that the creation of viable linkages among these three major partners was going to be an unprecedented and undoubtedly difficult process, the Foundation established a two-stage proposal process. The Request for Proposals (RFP) called for the submission of brief concept papers. From over 100 submissions, the Foundation selected fifteen semi-finalist consortia from across the country to participate in a year-long "Leadership and Model Development" phase. The LMD phase was unfunded (except for travel expenses) and, over the course of five national meetings, culminated in the development of full proposals.

The Massachusetts Community-Based Public Health Consortium is composed of five major member organizations: the University of Massachusetts School of Public Health; the Massachusetts Area Health Education Centers (AHEC); the Massachusetts Association of Health Boards; the University of Massachusetts (Worcester) Medical School; and, four communities located in central and western Massachusetts. The project is located in semi-rural New England, with two distinct population groups participating: rural, white, working class communities and rural Latinos (predominantly Puerto Ricans) now living in urban centers.

The initial contact that led to the creation of the Consortium was between the School of Public Health and the Massachusetts AHEC. At that time, the MAHEC had initiated and was staffing three community coalitions. In addition, the Executive Director of one of the local AHEC offices was also the co-chair of the Holyoke Latino Community Coalition. Thus, collaboration with the MAHEC was instrumental in initiating contacts between the university and the community coalitions.

The CEPA program is based in the city of Holyoke, a small city (pop. 42,463) in the throes of industrial decline. Holyoke has experienced large demographic shifts over the last two decades, with a major influx of Puerto Rican migrants who now compose over one-third of the population. Holyoke has among the highest rates in the state for infant mortality, pregnancy, children living in poverty, Latinos living in poverty, substance abuse problems and people with HIV and AIDS. In a recent report, the Massachusetts Civil Rights Commission cited Holyoke as one of five cities in the Commonwealth likely to experience widespread civil disturbances in the next five years. By any measure, the health status indicators for Holyoke are grim. This report describes the two phases of the CEPA program, the planning and initial implementation phases, which occurred during the first two years of the project.

The CEPA Program: Planning Stage

During the Leadership and Model Development stage of the Community-Based Public Health initiative, a collaborative needs assessment process was undertaken in each of the participating communities. One of the major advantages of this initiative is that there were no pre-conceived notions about the types of public health problems to be addressed. This opportunity enabled the Consortium to conduct a true community needs assessment, with free rein to pursue whichever community priorities emerged, rather than–as is more commonly the case–responding to funding agency's mandates.

In Holyoke, a faculty member began working with the Health Promotion group of the Holyoke Latino Community Coalition (HLCC). The HLCC is one of the longest standing independent community organizations serving the health needs of the Holyoke Latino community. The Health Promotion group is one of four action subgroups of the HLCC; the group ranges in size from six to ten members. The Health Promotion group is made up of Latinos who are Holyoke residents or health and human service providers working in Holyoke.

In the planning stage, the Health Promotion group used three methods to gather needs assessment information: focus groups with residents, personal and telephone interviews with providers, and a community forum. The basic protocol for the focus groups, interviews and community forum is shown in Table 13.1. Information was collected in Spanish or English, whichever was more comfortable for the participants.

Table 13.1: Focus Group and Individual Interview Protocol
1. ¿Qué cosas necesitan las personas/comunidades para ser saludables? [What things do communities/persons need to be healthy?]
2. ¿ Qué problemas de salud existen en Holyoke? [What are the health problems in Holyoke?]
3. ¿Cuales de estos problemas son los tres mas importantes? [Which of these health problems are the three most important?]
4. ¿ Qué tipo de programas tu puedes sugerir para ayudar a resolver algunos de estos problemas? [How can these problems be addressed?]
5. ¿ Qué tipo de ayuda puede proveer la Escuela de Salud Publica en Holyoke? [How can the UMass School of Public Health help with some of these problems?]

A total of six focus groups were conducted by members of the Health Promotion group. Focus groups were held with: teenagers (two groups), residents in a public housing project, elders, and residents recruited on street corners (two groups). The responses gathered in the focus group interviews are notable for their insight into the health needs of the community. They also serve to illustrate the differences between a community-based approach and standardized needs assessment protocols (such as the CDC's Behavioral Risk Factor Survey).

For example, focus group participants were asked "¿Qué cosas necesitan las personas/comunidades para ser saludables?" (What do people/communities need to be healthy?). Among the residents' responses were: "a person you can trust," "leaders who care," and "role models." While these answers may not fit into the response categories of standardized instruments (e.g., seat belt use, low-fat diets, and the like), they do offer insight into the limits of current epidemiological thinking.

In addition to the focus groups, the Health Promotion group conducted personal and telephone interviews (n=25) with representatives from virtually all health agencies located in Holyoke. The use of a community-driven interview protocol, developed and implemented by members of the Holyoke community, again elicited remarkably perceptive responses. For example, in reply to questions about what people need to be healthy, providers answered: "purpose in life," "a sense of moral coherence," "good relationships," "a good basis for spiritual growth," as well as more conventional answers such as non-smoking and exercise.

Finally, the Holyoke Latino Community Coalition organized a community forum to allow other community members the opportunity to provide input into determining priority health needs. The forum was advertised through coalition mailings, the community newspaper, phone calls and flyers distributed in the community. The community forum resulted in a lively discussion about current social conditions in Holyoke. Many pointed questions were directed at the academics regarding their motives for pursuing the project in the Holyoke community. The community forum was tape-recorded, transcribed and analyzed by a consultant to the coalition.

The focus groups, telephone interviews and the community forum resulted in the identification of four priority issues: 1) HIV/AIDS, 2) substance abuse, 3) domestic violence, and 4) medical interpreting services. Since the first three problems are closely related, the Health Promotion group decided to focus on HIV/AIDS prevention, with the expectation that any program that could have an impact on reducing the risk of HIV infection would also necessarily have to have an impact on issues like substance abuse and domestic violence. The needs assessment results were bolstered by Department of Public Health data that show that Holyoke suffers a vastly disproportionate share of the AIDS epidemic.

In summary, in using a community-engaged approach, the CEPA project called on community members to identify their own questions and to collect information from other community members on their own terms. The academic partners played a minor, secondary role. The results of this process were not only robust but in many respects more thought-provoking than standardized needs assessment protocols.

Initial Implementation Stage

From the community needs assessment, the HLCC Health Promotion group proposed to initiate an innovative, community-based HIV/AIDS prevention program. The HP group (now joined by a faculty member and a graduate student) re-constituted itself as an Advisory Board for the CEPA project. Because of the history of Puerto Rico's colonial status, gross inequalities in economic status, and extensive personal experiences with discrimination, the HP group decided that the CEPA program should be based on a participatory, critical thinking and empowerment model.

The basic philosophy of the CEPA program is that people in high risk environments know better than anyone else what will be effective in preventing HIV infection given their circumstances. Therefore, the fundamental strategy of CEPA is to reduce the gap between program developers and program recipients to the greatest extent possible. This strategy ensures that program activities will be the most relevant, culturally appropriate and well-suited to meet the needs of those at risk

To put this strategy into practice, the CEPA program has developed a three-stage process: 1) *Concienciización*/Education, 2) Planning, and 3) Action (C-E-P-A). The stages are dynamic, not sequential; they overlap and inform one another.

Concienciización/Education

In stage one, the CEPA staff (a project coordinator and an outreach worker) participated in an intensive self-led educational process with the Advisory Board. The *concienciización*/ educational process (Freire, 1970, 1973) focused on community development, community organizing, community empowerment, critical consciousness and participatory education. The Advisory Board thought these topics were essential because of their experiences with discrimination and social and economic disenfranchisement in Holyoke. Particular readings were also identified by the Advisory Board. Sessions were conducted as a process of mutual self-education and consciousness-raising, with weekly meetings extending over a three-month period.

Growing out of the *praxis* of *concienciación*, the Advisory Board and CEPA staff developed an eleven-session training program to carry out with community residents. Even though the Advisory Board is composed of community residents and community providers, they felt they needed to get even closer to the population at risk, and hence, work directly with local neighborhood residents.

Like the staff development experience, the resident training program is based on models of empowerment and participatory education. Based on the work of Paulo Freire, the empowerment process has been described by Wallerstein (1991); it consists of listening, dialoguing, problem-posing and action. As the Advisory Board discovered, the respective models (empowerment and participatory) are not entirely compatible, with an inherent bias toward examining the "root causes" of health problems in the empowerment model and a more open, self-directed approach in the participatory education model (CUSO, 1985; Hall and Kidd, 1978; Knowles, 1978; Mezirow, 1985). The challenges in balancing these approaches will be examined in greater detail in the discussion section.

Planning

In stage two, planning, the CEPA staff went door-to-door in a neighborhood selected because of its high level of risk factors (i.e., poor, rundown housing stock, high unemployment rates, high numbers of school drop-outs, presence of sex industry workers, and presence of drug dealers and shooting galleries). The staff also met with community agencies, social organizations, church representatives, tenants' groups, and so on. They introduced themselves and the program and invited community residents to participate in planning the program.

The objective at this stage was to recruit a small group of eight to twelve neighborhood residents to form a Residents Planning Board. After lengthy discussions, the Advisory Board decided to enlist a planning group as diverse as possible, rather than seek out specific subgroups (e.g., sex workers, adolescents, etc.). Board members were opposed to the idea of recruiting community members according to pre-selected categories (a la "market segmentation" as propounded in Social Marketing). In contrast to expert planning models, they thought that such a process would further fragment the community by stressing differences over more significant, shared commonalities.

Based on a successful outreach effort, a highly diverse group was recruited in the initial round. The ten participants ranged in age from thirteen to fifty-five. There were two men and eight women, two people with AIDS, and one family unit (father, mother, and daughter). They work in a variety of occupations, from insurance, to homemaker, teacher, counselor, unemployed, and student. All are Puerto Rican.

All sessions were planned originally to be conducted in Spanish. As the group evolved, however, they decided to encourage people to speak in whichever language they felt most comfortable, as virtually everyone was bilingual. The residents received stipends for their participation. The stipends are not motivational incentives, but due compensation for the time, knowledge, and labor supplied by the residents.

The community residents then met once a week for two hours in the evening to participate in a series of structured discussions designed by the Advisory Board. At the heart of the community-engaged approach, these sessions are designed to have people living in high risk environments identify the needs, barriers, and resources they personally experience in trying to respond effectively to the threat of AIDS. The purpose of these discussions is to have those at highest risk decide for themselves the types of services, support, and actions that will best address the causes of their susceptibility.

(To recall the overlapping nature of the three identified stages, these sessions are also clearly a part of the community *conciencización* and education process and a part of the Action of the CEPA project.)

An outline of the objectives for the eleven sessions is shown in Table 13.2. The planning process took three months to complete. Each session was tape-recorded and each concluded with time for immediate feedback, so the process could be replicated and modified as needed. The end result of these sessions was the identification of the types of services needed for effective community-based HIV prevention. The desired program characteristics were framed in terms of a simple, user-friendly "request for proposals."

Growing out of the planning process, the Residents Planning Board decided that community programs should focus on work with the teenage population. They identified four major goals for community programming. To prevent HIV infection, they said programs should: 1) promote self-esteem, both individually and collectively; 2) promote life-enhancing family values; 3) create a public space for the Puerto Rican community; and 4) promote effective communication skills.

The goals identified deserve a couple of comments. First, it is important to note that the community residents did not think that clinical information about modes of HIV transmission was essential. In contrast to many conventional programs, they understood well that the problem of AIDS was due to more than a simple lack of information. As one member put it, "You have to feel pretty good about yourself to want to protect yourself from HIV."

Second, the goal of promoting life enhancing family values is a distinct reflection of Puerto Rican cultural values. In contrast to the high value placed on individualism in the United States, Puerto Rican community members situated the issue in the social context of inherent familial relationships. Echoing this priority, participants noted that the name of the project, "*cepa*," can be translated as "core" or "root," as in family roots of genealogical trees.

Table 13.2: List of Resident Training Sessions

Session	Objectives
1	To get to know group members To understand project expectations To understand individual/collective commitment and responsibilities To develop a schedule of next five meetings
2	To continue developing group cohesiveness To review project expectations To review schedule of meetings To introduce the topic of HIV
3	To share personal migration stories To share personal understanding of Holyoke To compare/contrast stories to connect collective experiences
4	To increase knowledge of HIV/AIDS To explore and begin to understand root causes of HIV infection To become more aware about why Latinos, specifically Puerto Ricans, are vulnerable to HIV To understand the social, psychological, and medical impact of HIV
5	To discuss further the root causes of HIV infection among Latinos To establish linkages among causes

	To illustrate with case studies how these linkages are interrelated
6	To continue discussing the root causes of HIV infection among Latinos To identify and discuss factors contributing to low self-esteem
7	To identify ways by which individuals can take individual and/or collective action to impact systems To identify individual/collective strengths that protect communities from low self-esteem and lack of well-being
8	To facilitate a process by which participants identify effective HIV prevention strategies To emphasize the individual's role as an impetus for change To connect the ideas that will be identified by this process with the resources that are available through the mini-grants
9	To continue the process of identifying the criteria for programs To prioritize the program proposals and ideas
10	To identify a process for announcing, selecting, reviewing and evaluating the program proposals To identify participants who would like to continue as voluntary members of the advisory board To evaluate the residents' training program
11	To establish a timetable for the RFP and projects To recognize the efforts of the participants To celebrate the planning process

The Residents Planning Board identified seven additional characteristics or criteria that would make programs more effective: 1) peer (teen) involvement in programming and outreach activities; 2) Persons With AIDS (PWA) involvement in all levels of programming; 3) the appropriation of leadership and guidance roles by program participants; 4) a focus on the strengths within the community; 5) well trained staff; 6) an on-going evaluation process; and, 7) guarantees of confidentiality for participants. They advised that programs should focus on self-esteem, self-determination, community development and the promotion of peer interaction. Typical activities included after-school activities, summer programs, sports and other team activities, peer support groups and drop-in neighborhood centers.

Action

In stage three, a call for community action was issued through requests for proposals, providing funding for grants up to $5,000. The proposal was widely circulated in the community through flyers, radio programs and announcements (PSAs), newspaper articles, outreach, handbills, mailings, community parties, presentations in agencies, a press conference, an open house, and word of mouth through informal interpersonal networks.

Members of the Residents Planning Board, Advisory Board, and CEPA staff jointly participated in reviewing the proposals and determining which groups received funding. In line with the project's philosophy, the reviewers decided from the outset to give preference in funding to non-traditional groups or agencies. Residents involved in the planning stage eagerly volunteered for a monitoring role in reviewing the progress of the community grants too.

In the first round, the reviewers decided to fund three proposals. One proposal was to lend partial support to a Latino teen theater troupe focusing on adolescent themes, one proposal was to set up a summer teen drop-in center (submitted and run by teenagers), and a third was to fund a mother's group to start dance, music, and basketball lessons for neighborhood teens. As a condition of funding, the CEPA project requested that each group participate in a shortened version of the residents critical thinking process.

The CEPA project successfully engaged community members in a substantive role in a community-based program planning process. In collaboration with community members, the Advisory Board made plans to monitor the progress of the community grants over the next three years. CEPA is also in the process of replicating the program in two other neighborhoods. Based on the CEPA experience, there are several points for discussion about the prospects for community-based program planning.

Discussion

Based on these experiences, the Advisory Board members are deeply impressed both with the difficulties in creating a fully participatory model (and not slipping into a "banking" mode of education that presumes people need to be filled with the experts' information) and with the benefits of such an approach. The dilemma of reconciling a commitment to a participatory, community-based approach with the aspirations and expectations of the program initiators has become a central theme in on-going discussions of the CEPA project. Several examples will serve to illustrate this point.

From the outset. the Advisory Board has wrestled with questions about how to define the project. Members were committed to a *process* of involving community members in designing the project. But we also recognized that funding agencies usually require quite specific delineation of the proposed program activities before extending their support. How, then, could CEPA specify the program activities before it had engaged the very people who were to decide which activities were most appropriate?

In the original grant proposal, the Health Promotion group compromised by describing the planned process and listing a number of *potential* activities. The W. K. Kellogg Foundation accepted the idea. But, when CEPA has sought additional funding, other foundations have responded as expected in demanding to know exactly what they were going to be getting for their money. The idea that program activities would emerge from the process and could take many unforeseeable forms has been difficult to sell (even to some of the other partners in the larger Kellogg CBPH project).

Then, the Advisory Board had to decide how to structure the residents training program. Again, we wrestled with the trade-offs. If the Advisory Board designed the training, then we would be assuming control, telling the participants what we expect them to do, and inevitably reproducing our own assumptions, interests, and biases. But if we did not provide any structure to the discussions, we feared people would think we were unprepared and did not know what we were doing. Again, a delicate, carefully considered balance emerged as the process proceeded.

In the event. we decided to plan all of the sessions in advance (see Table 13.2). But during the training, we tried–largely unsuccessfully–to encourage the residents to take over and lead the sessions. We struggled too over revealing the full plan of the sessions. Some of us thought that presenting a completed plan would discourage the residents from realizing they could re-direct the sessions; others thought that failing to tell them what was planned was even more manipulative.

As the process was underway, we decided to share plans for the next immediate session and ask the residents for their suggestions and approval. Few changes were made. The feedback from the residents was that they were generally comfortable with the direction of the sessions. But they also expressed concerns–on more than one occasion–that they did not fully understand why we were doing a few particular activities and that they wanted to move more quickly into designing the HIV prevention program.

Two further examples: In planning the sessions, the Advisory Board decided to dedicate one session to a discussion of the historical relationship between Puerto Rico and the United States. Here, the tensions between a critical empowerment model and a participatory model became most apparent. On the one hand, Advisory Board members thought it was important to make clear the connection between the history of US imperialist domination and the present disproportionate share of health burdens borne by the Puerto Rican peoples. On the other hand, Board members wanted just to hear and share personal migration stories and believed that collectively these stories would make the same point. So, the CEPA project was again faced with questions about how to proceed.

In the session at hand, the Advisory Board tried to prepare a concise history of Puerto Rico's colonial status. It was of course impossible to cover a complete history in such a short period of time. So, a member of the Advisory Board ended up presenting a long lecture that took up almost the entire time that evening. The community voices were left out, the residents reduced to a passive role of being fed information. More to the point, the session jarred us into thinking about the seductiveness of power and control and about how we too had internalized the banking system of education.

Similarly, we felt obligated to present the clinical perspective about HIV transmission in another session. We invited a guest speaker, but we knew we needed to prepare her for the CEPA mutual teacher-learner educational process. We also thought the standard medical model needed to be balanced with a broader socio-political perspective that we could present. But despite the best laid plans, the guest speaker wound up dominating the session and the residents were again treated as empty vessels waiting to be filled.

As was the case after each session, the Advisory Board and staff took time immediately afterwards to process these sessions and reflect self-critically on the experience. Like at many other points in the project, we came face-to-face with the possibilities and limits of community-based program planning. The experience brought home how difficult it is to set up a process that enables people to take control of the conditions that affect their lives and how difficult it is not to assume a powerful, controlling role in telling people what we think they need to know.

We shared our concerns with the residents at the next meeting. Collectively, we decided to repeat the AIDS 101 session, this time, however, listening to the knowledge each of us already had. The candor of the Advisory Board, admitting our mistakes, dropping any pretensions as experts with answers about how people should live their lives, changed the tone and dynamic of the. meetings. The distance between program developers and program recipients was narrowed. Community members and board members came a little closer in understanding that answers to questions about how to live in the face of the threat of AIDS could not be dictated, but must be generated through a process of mutual discussion, reflection and dialogue about the kind of community we want to live in together.

The Advisory Board was struck by the possibilities and benefits of this project as well. The most moving experience for everyone involved was a rekindling of pride in our Puerto Rican identity. The sense of confusion and ambivalence around having "dual identities"–and its relationship to a sense of low self-esteem was openly discussed for the first time for many of us. Discussions about the influence of cultural roles and how they shape perceptions, both positively and negatively, of possible choices and subsequent decisions were frank, deeply personal and collectively liberating. The experience reconnected each of us with the bonds of community.

In conclusion, the CEPA experience shows how program initiators inevitably make decisions that shape the direction of any resulting community programs. The idea that program developers can totally bracket their assumptions is difficult to maintain. The extent to which a program might be called "community-based" will always be a matter of degree. Hence, rather than presuming they have the best interests of the people at heart, public health professionals might better approach community development work by self-critically examining their own interests and biases first.

But these constraints are not insurmountable. As long as feedback is openly and continuously solicited and incorporated, the gap between program developers and recipients can continue to be narrowed. The CEPA project thus provides a powerful model for maximizing community involvement in issues vital to the health and well-being of community residents.

References

Bell, Daniel. 1976. *The Cultural Contradictions of Capitalism*. New York: Basic Books.

Chavis, David and Paul Florin. 1990. *Community Development, Community Participation, and Substance Abuse Prevention.* Santa Clara County, CA: Bureau of Drug Abuse Services, Department of Health.

CUSO. 1985. *Basic and Tools: A Collection of Popular Education Resources and Activities,* CUSO Education Department, Ottawa.

Fawcett, Stephen, Adrienne Paine, Vincente Francisco and Marni Vliet. 1993. "Promoting health through community development. In *Promoting Health and Mental Health in Children, Youth and Families,* edited by David Glenwick and Leonard Jason, 233-255. New York, NY: Springer Publishing Company.

Freire, Paolo. 1970. *Pedagogy of the Oppressed.* New York: The Seabury Press.

Freire, Paolo. 1973. *Education for Critical Consciousness.* New York: The Seabury Press.

Grace, Helen. 1990. "Building Community: A Conceptual Perspective." *International Journal of the W. K. Kellogg Foundation.* W. K. Kellogg Foundation, Battle Creek, Michigan, Spring/Summer: 1.

Hall, Budd and J. Roby Kidd (Eds.). 1978. *Adult Learning: A Design for Action*. Toronto, Canada: Pergammon Press.

Knowles, Malcom. 1978. *The Adult Learner: A Neglected Species*. Houston, TX: Gulf Publishing.

Lindblom, Charles. 1990. *Inquiry and Change: The Troubled Attempt to Understand and Shape Society.* New Haven, CT: Yale University Press.

Mezirow, Jack. 1985. "A Critical Theory of Self-Directed Learning." *New Directions for Continuing Education* 25:17-30.

McKnight, Jon. 1987. "Regenerating Community." *Social Policy* 17(3): 54-58.

Murray, Charles. 1984. *Losing Ground.* New York: Basic Books.

Nyswander, Dorothy. 1967. "The Open Society: Its Implications for Health Educators." *Health Education Monographs* 1: 3-13.

Rothman, Jack. 1979. "Three Models of Community Organization Practice, Their Mixing and Phasing." In *Strategies of Community Organization: A Book of Readings* (3rd Edition), edited by Fred Cox, John Erlich, Jack Rothman and John Tropman, 25-44. Itasca, IL: F. E. Peacock.

Wallerstein, Nina. 1991. "Powerlessness, Empowerment and Health: Implications for Health Promotion Programs." *American Journal of Health Promotion,* 6(3):197-205.

14. PROMOTING DIGNITY: THE ETHICAL DIMENSION OF HEALTH

These are tough times for public health, in general, and health promotion, in particular. Globally, the lack of viable alternatives to a competitive neoliberal capitalist economic order has put increasing pressure on state governments to cut taxes, cut social services, and demand greater accountability, typically based on cost-benefit analyses. As no government has unlimited resources to allocate to the health-care sector, the fair distribution of scarce resources must be justified by appeals to some standard of justice. These days, there is tremendous pressure to meet utilitarian standards of efficiency and effectiveness, where investments in health promotion must be shown to lead directly to measurable reductions in morbidity and mortality.

In the face of such pressures, a recent meta-analysis of interventions to promote physical activity and nutritious food consumption unfortunately found that the best programs to date have produced a conspicuously small effect (.21) (Kamath, Vickers, Ehrlich, *et al.*, 2008). According to standard statistical textbooks, an effect size of .20 accounts for approximately 1% of the explained variance (Fritz, Morris and Richler, 2012). Since efforts to establish the social sciences were initiated at the same time as the development of the modern natural sciences–writing in the 1650s, Hobbes sought to establish an empirical science of politics modeled on Galileo's laws of planetary motion (Bhattacharya 1987)–one has to wonder why the social sciences have not been nearly as successful in discovering the causal relationships that govern human behavior (e.g., the factors that lead to overeating) as the medical sciences have been in identifying the causes of malaria, which has, thereby, enabled the development of effective interventions to treat malaria. This chapter explains why the current goals and methods of health education may be fundamentally misdirected and why a new direction for the field, centered on promoting dignity, is essential both for improving individual health and for creating a good, just, and healthy society.

The essay addresses three points. First, for reasons having to do with the undeniable success of the natural sciences in controlling events in the natural world, researchers in health promotion have largely elected to try to duplicate that success by seeking to identify the most efficient means to engineer an optimal state of biophysiological functioning (in contrast to any more comprehensive definition of human well-being, as explained below); as a result, this approach denies the intrinsic role of autonomy in defining human identity and well-being. This approach is deeply flawed, both empirically, in the striking lack of success in developing effective interventions to change health-related behaviors, and ethically, in subverting the essential role that autonomy must play in any reasonably satisfactory account of human well-being. Second, I present one well-known definition of autonomy and one major research challenge related to that definition. Third, the analysis concludes with the call to promote human dignity, for which autonomy is an absolute precondition. A new direction will require careful reconsideration of one central assumption guiding current work in the field, and consequently, a major shift in attention toward articulating values that matter and assuring the fair distribution of people's capabilities to pursue socially valued life plans.

Science and the Denial of Autonomy

I want to come at the issue of the most problematic assumption underlying the field today indirectly. It is important to see how the usual everyday practices of conducting research in the health sciences have resulted in the unfortunate conflation of standards for ascertaining truth, with the power to control outcomes. This disturbing turn of events has led to the denial of the most distinguishing features of the human condition.

As we saw in Chapters 1 and 3, the archetype for conducting scientific research has been around for a long time, well-illustrated in the work of Sir Robert Boyle. Over time, people have come to believe that the criteria of prediction and control are the best, if not the only, way to know whether a statement is true or not. These procedures define the basic scientific framework used in health science research today.

Experimental research on biophysiological processes works remarkably well, the results of which benefit virtually everyone every day. For example, we have learned that, if raw milk is heated to a certain temperature, then it kills the *Brucella* bacterium, which has effectively eradicated brucellosis. If water is treated with fluoride, then it reduces dental caries. If hypercholesterolemia is treated with statins, then cholesterol levels drop, and consequently, heart attacks decline. If people with HIV/AIDS are treated with antiretroviral (ARV) therapies, then the reproduction of the virus is slowed and people live longer. The list goes on. Conversely, based on observational data, epidemiologists thought that beta-carotene reduced lung cancer risk, but this hypothesis was later disproven in a randomized controlled trial (RCT), which, in fact, found that it caused higher lung cancer mortality rates (Omenn, Goodman, Thornquist, *et al.*, 1996). Based on an impressive track record of results, behavioral health scientists now seek to apply the same research methods in order to develop comparably effective interventions to prevent smoking, overeating, and so on.

With the rise of evidence-based medicine (Evidence-Based Medicine Working Group,1992), it is now widely accepted that RCTs provide the gold standard for assessing the validity of claims about matters of health. As just illustrated, in applying the experimental method, an inherent by-product of establishing the validity of any hypothesized relationship is the power to control outcomes, the power to effect changes in the dependent variable by modifying levels of the independent variables. In standard practice, the more accurate the prediction, the more confidence one has about having identified a true statement about the way things are in actual fact, where the accuracy of the prediction is usually reported in terms of statistical power, confidence intervals, or the percentage of the variance explained. Moreover, great store is put in the idea that research in the health sciences will be incrementally progressive, where the goal is to explain a greater proportion of variance in each subsequent generation of experiments, as seen with each new generation of ARVs, which enable people with HIV/AIDS to live longer.

Given the success of this model, because so-called risky behaviors now account for the greatest proportion of the burden of disease (Mokdad, Marks, Stroup, *et al.*, 2004), tremendous resources are now allocated to research in the behavioral health sciences, where success in verifying hypotheses is likewise linked to developing the power to predict and control behaviors associated with these adverse health outcomes. Currently, of the roughly $30 billion annual budget of the NIH, $1.2 billion is specifically allocated to behavioral science research each year, while the total amount is actually much higher, as research with behavioral components in other areas such as alcoholism, anorexia, cancer, drug abuse, and so on, does not get parceled out in official government reports. The current mission of the Office of Behavioral and Social Science Research (2000) is stated as follows:

> The core areas of behavioral and social science research are those that have a major and explicit focus on the use of behavioral or social processes to *predict* or *influence* health outcomes or health risk factors. Basic research in the behavioral and social sciences is designed to further our understanding of fundamental *mechanisms* and patterns of behavioral and social functioning relevant to the Nation's health and well-being. It is

> designed to elucidate knowledge about underlying *mechanisms* and processes, knowledge that is fundamental to improving the observation, *explanation, prediction, prevention*, and management of illnesses, as well as the promotion of optimal health. [emphasis added]

As codified in evidence-based medicine's hierarchy of knowledge (see Table 7.1, and likewise evidence-based public health; Brownson, Fielding and Maylahn, 2009), it is important to reiterate that this state of affairs has come to pass because researchers accept that the criteria of prediction and control provide the highest degree of confidence about having identified valid and reliable knowledge. Just as Depo Provera has proven to be highly effective in preventing pregnancy, the goal of behavioral health research is to discover comparably effective methods to prevent behaviors associated with unhealthy outcomes.

The first point of this chapter is that virtually all funded research in health education accepts and has adopted the fundamental tenets of the natural sciences model, i.e., that the criteria of prediction and control provide the most compelling basis for confirming the validity of propositions and that human behavior is no different than the occurrence of any other event in the natural world. Just as the moon circles the earth due to the laws of gravity, so too the assumption is that human behavior can and will ultimately be explained as the product of similar yet-to-be-discovered causal laws that govern all physical events. If everything that happens in the world can be explained in terms of causal relationships and human beings are part of this same natural physical universe, then human behavior must likewise be the inevitable result of a particular constellation of antecedent causes that produce the particular outcome of interest. If that outcome is considered undesirable (e.g., smoking causes cancer), then the logic of this model dictates that the *causes* of smoking be identified, so that the causal chain of events can be disrupted and the initiation of smoking prevented. In standard practice, the causes of smoking are identified by experimentally manipulating hypothesized independent variables and observing the effects of these changes on the dependent variable (smoking initiation).

The success of the scientific method in developing effective treatments for HIV/AIDS, vaccines for Ebola, and so on, continues to capture the imagination of most researchers, government officials, and the general public in light of its truly remarkable and unquestionable success. Given the tremendous toll that certain well-known behaviors take on human health, the goal of most health education research today is to identify the causes of unhealthy behaviors (e.g., lack of self-efficacy, the social determinants, etc.), whereby the very methods used to verify the causes in the course of conducting the research can subsequently be replicated in implementing applied programs by conscientiously duplicating the same procedures to produce the targeted result: people will lose weight, stop smoking, wear condoms, and so on. In this framework, any hints of autonomy register simply as unwelcome noise, unexplained variance, where the goal and perceived value of the research are to account for and reduce such seemingly random variations as much as possible. In the modern scientific framework, autonomy does not exist anyway, as all phenomena are subject to the same cause-and-effect laws that govern all events in the universe. Regrettably, the scientific model of health promotion leaves out everything that makes human beings uniquely human, in particular, agency, free will, autonomy, values, volition, and dignity.

The Questionable Assumption Underlying the Natural Sciences Model

Contrary to the presuppositions of this huge research enterprise, however, the assumptions of scientific naturalism and the denial of human autonomy and free will have not gone unchallenged. Indeed, the eminent philosopher John Searle (2004, p. 4-5) sees the issue of free will as the most important question facing philosophy today. As he puts it,

> There is exactly one overriding question in contemporary philosophy . . . the question is, How can we square this self-conception of ourselves as mindful, meaning-creating, free, rational, etc., agents with a universe that consists entirely of mindless, meaningless, unfree, nonrational, brute physical particles?

In this light, it seems apparent that most behavioral health scientists operate on the mindless, meaningless, unfree, non-rational side of this basic operating assumption. In contrast, I find the most compelling evidence for questioning this assumption in the conspicuous lack of success that the legions of competent behavioral health scientists have had in developing interventions that are even roughly equal to the success found in the medical sciences. If one accepts that the health science model described here is the most appropriate framework for defining the goals and methods of health education, then the field is in deep trouble, because we have not been–nor, I think, will we ever be–able to deliver effective interventions that reliably reduce behaviors that we deem undesirable, precisely because this approach fails to take into account the essential role of autonomy in characterizing the human condition.

The Definition and Role of Autonomy in Human Conduct

If one allows that a central assumption underlying current practice in health promotion might be problematic, then it is important to consider the possibility of adopting the principal alternative assumption in formulating appropriate goals and methods for the field. In a humanistic perspective, health promotion would be guided by the assumption that the common everyday experience of making choices is not an illusion and that human beings have the capacity for free will. Following Dworkin (1988), the exercise of autonomy involves the unique human ability to step back and consider the implications of an action for the kind of person one wants to be, to ask ourselves whether we want to act on felt first-order desires or not, by assessing them in light of higher order values and the kind of person we would like to become.

Dworkin's definition introduces a distinction between *desires* and *values*, where the use of the two terms is intended to mark a categorical difference. The difference between values and desires is not a matter of degree of intensity, where values might be reduced to desires for things that people really, *really* want (Watson, 1975; Scheffler, 2010). The critical difference lies in the perceived independence of values, where their validity is not determined by individual feelings. To paraphrase Wolf (2015), values articulate the grounds for assessing the worth of felt desires from the point of view of someone other than one's own self: to claim that something is valuable is to claim that others have good reason to value it too. To simplify somewhat, desires are generally tied to feelings of pleasure and pain, whereas values generally relate to concerns for morality and meaning. Values can be discussed and defended in terms of reasons; desires are *de facto* wants, akin to hunger or thirst, where one is experiencing the sensation or not, without need for further explanation or justification. Or, to paraphrase Dworkin (1988), reasonable choices must be governed by standards that are not merely a reflection of our own preferences. It is at this point that questions about the nature of values raise critical issues for future research.

Research on Values

The crux of the research challenge here is that values (e.g., justice) do not have empirical properties; they are not constituted by anything that registers on sense perceptions (or their technological analogs); they do not have physical structures or give off emissions that can be seen, touched, heard, and so on. In essence, they are grasped only in human consciousness and become manifest only in language, wherein lie the limits of an empirical science (Antonaccio, 2012). Because their ontology is quite unlike the material found in the natural, physical domain, their validity cannot be tested and confirmed by the methods of empirical science. In an egregious error in early 20th century thought, however, because values are not amenable to sorts of empirical analyses that result in *objective* (note: in the strictly delimited sense of *tangible, sensory-dependent*) evidence, a particular strand of epistemological thought–positivism–insisted on asserting a categorical distinction between facts and values and then assigned values to the category of metaphysical nonsense, where value claims were alleged to be irredeemably irrational, because of their lack of accommodation to empirical verification.

In his analysis of this historical turn of events, Taylor (1995) shows how the move to equate values with subjective desires stems from a colossal categorical mistake—drawing conclusions about what things *are* (ontology) on the basis of *how they are known* (epistemology). If their existence cannot be empirically detected, measured, and confirmed, then many people in the modern world have been led to believe that values cannot be objectively real and cannot be anything more than mere personal feelings, subjective likes, and dislikes. In the positivist worldview, moral convictions about principles of justice thus fall into the same category as beliefs in Santa Claus, where the prospect of gaining valid knowledge on questions about the nature of the just society is considered impossible, a foolish waste of time.

In contrast, as noted in Chapter One, scholarship in the humanities has long focused on investigating the human experience of values, based on their undeniable impact on how people lead their lives. Historically, humanistic research has viewed values as real and independent of any particular individual's desires, and hence, appropriate topics for objective discussion and analysis. As the twin complementary pillar of human intellectual achievement (next to science), humanistic inquiry rejects the tenet that truth can be determined only by following certain correct methods (i.e., hypothesis-testing), by manipulating independent variables and observing the effect(s). Instead, research in the humanities proceeds on the basis that there are certain types of questions that command human attention, such as questions about the good life for human beings, that can be answered only in terms of substantive content, the depiction and elucidation of the experience (Altieri, 2015). In humanistic studies, researchers reflect on the experience of self-consciousness: encounters with the demands of justice, the joy of beauty, the love of another, and other values. Importantly, it appears that, as human consciousness grapples to find the words to articulate ideals of perfection (perfect justice, perfect beauty, etc.), these images of the good have not yet yielded to any final absolute characterization. Still, confidence in the truth of statements about the meaning and appeal of values grows through successive approximations that enable human beings to see more clearly lives worth living. Evidence of moral progress abounds, as seen in the significant reductions in human suffering and the tremendous expansion of the sphere of people considered entitled to live with dignity. For behavioral health researchers, the challenge outlined here is simply a reiteration of the call to expand programs of interdisciplinary research sounded on university campuses today.

Promoting Dignity

My third point concerns the relationship between autonomy and dignity. Perceptions of the meaning and scope of dignity have fluctuated over time, from an initial association with the nobility and dignitaries, to the Christian doctrine ascribed to all of God's creatures (including animals), to its modern meaning originally put forward by Immanuel Kant (Rosen, 2012). For Kant, dignity refers to a state of being, the manner of carrying oneself associated with living righteously, with an integrity found in upholding moral values. It is possible for human beings, and only human beings, to live with dignity because we are rational agents with the capacity for moral autonomy; it is only human beings who can make choices based on principled ideals, above and beyond the limited pursuit of satisfying carnal appetites, which is common to all living creatures (Kolnai, 1995). All kinds of creatures have desires, but it is only human beings who can evaluate a felt desire, specifically in terms of whether its satisfaction is worthwhile, in the sense of creating value. People know that they can sometimes be victims of their own desires, acting on an impulse that they only come to regret the next day, and beyond. Dignity is manifested by reflecting on the quality of one's desires and choosing the path that will yield the greater good, not just maximizing pleasure, but heeding the aspiration to be a better person (decent, honorable, and trustworthy) and to do something meaningful and fulfilling with one's life (Waldron, 2009). It is only human beings who can identify and choose to pursue projects that make the world a better place, enrich human experience, and offer a sense of fulfillment in living a life worth living.

I want to conclude the chapter with recommendations for promoting dignity. To live well, people need to decide or to discover what they care about and what they regard as important to them (Frankfurt, 1998). Caring about something provides purpose and gives meaning to action. It affects the kind of life one lives by imparting goals, ordering priorities, and giving direction in trying to accomplish something that may lead to happiness. Caring about something enables people to choose between the things that they really want to do, to become the person they really want to be, and simply acting on whatever whim pops into mind. The language of caring signals projects that people believe are worthwhile. For example, it is hard to think of parenting as being fun–often it is a struggle–but it can also bring great joy. Important projects usually involve a lot of work, but people are willing to make the effort for the pride of accomplishment, of being able to point to something that they think worthwhile, for what it tells them about themselves. Caring about something thus appears to be essential for exercising autonomy.

Conversely, not caring about anything leaves people without direction. People who do not care about anything have no aims or ambitions. Nothing stands out as being important and inviting, nothing really matters. Not caring about anything is characteristic of the state of anomie, a sense of meaninglessness, nihilism (Frankfurt, 1998). Acting on random urges is what people do when they do not have projects that they care about. If there is nothing that is more important, then it does not really matter what one does in the moment; there is nothing that might give one pause to reconsider whether there might be anything better to do than just getting high and sitting on the couch all day. People need to have projects that they care about in order to put the urge for immediate gratification into some larger context, a rational framework that provides reasons for choosing one option over another. To make a truly autonomous choice takes having something better to do. People are willing to forego easy indulgences if and when they see they have something more worthwhile to do.

Fingarette (1967) writes: "Responsibility emerges where the individual accepts as a matter of personal concern something which society offers to his concern." In this view, the choice or discovery of pursuits that one finds worthwhile is not something that can be instrumentally induced. Society cannot compel people to care about anything; it can only hold up examples of things that others have found valuable for them to see. The individual has to feel the pull of the options available to them. For individuals to find pursuits that they care about, the avenues open to them have to be attractive, they have to see and accept that the pursuits that society has to offer them are personally attainable and valuable. In this view, people develop a sense of caring to the extent that they see that there are real possibilities that can lead to accomplishing things that they consider meaningful, worth doing. The corollary is that, if someone comes to believe that there is nothing to do or be that matters, then she is left to do whatever she wants.

. . .

As we saw earlier, Sen (1992, 2009) defines capabilities in terms of a person's ability to do valuable things and attain valued states of being. He goes on to make a distinction between "capabilities" and "functionings," where functionings are capabilities realized, actually put into practice. Here is the rub. Extant social conditions can and often do impede people's motivation to act–to translate capabilities into functionings–by undermining their belief that they can achieve a life worth living. In such circumstances, many people are left to drift aimlessly, without feeling the pull of projects that are worth their time and attention, where the lure of immediate sensual gratifications looms larger, because the amount of pleasures appears to be the only good that life has to offer. To live well, people need to have something valuable to do with their lives (Griffin, 1986; Doyal and Gough, 1991). There is an irreducible ethical dimension to health signified by the longing to live with dignity.

It bears repeating that people who exercise the greatest degree of autonomy also experience the best health, and conversely, people with the least amount of autonomy have the poorest health (Marmot, 2003; Marmot, 2004; Syme, 1998). In the analysis presented here, the explanation for this observed relationship is that having activities, pursuits, and relationships that one recognizes as worth one's time and effort enables people to make meaningful choices from the barrage of desires that human beings constantly feel. Thus, the problem is not that people have too much autonomy; the most important challenge for health promotion today is that the capacity for exercising autonomy, in the ethically relevant meaning of the term, is unjustly distributed. People need to see that there are worthwhile things to do with their lives and that such social valued pursuits are attainable and not foreclosed due to social circumstances. It is the social conditions that nurture or stunt the development of human capabilities that has the most decisive impact on people's health.

References

Altieri, Charles. 2015. *Reckoning with the imagination: Wittgenstein and the aesthetics of literary experience*. Ithaca, NY: Cornell University Press.

Antonaccio, Maria. 2012. *A philosophy to live by: engaging Iris Murdoch*. Oxford, UK: Oxford University Press.

Bhattacharya, Nikhil. 1987. "Hobbes's theory of natural and social sciences." *International Archives of the History of Ideas* 111: 33–55.

Brownson, Ross C., Jonathan Fielding, and Christopher Maylahn. 2009. "Evidence-Based Public Health: A Fundamental Concept for Public Health Practice." *Annual Review of Public Health* 30:175-201.

Doyal, Len and Ian Gough. 1991. *A theory of human needs*. London, UK: MacMillan Press.

Dworkin, Gerald. 1988. *The Theory and Practice of Autonomy*. Cambridge, UK: Cambridge University Press.

Evidence-Based Medicine Working Group. 1992. Evidence-based medicine: a new approach to teaching the practice of medicine. *JAMA* 1992; 268: 2420–2425.

Fingarette, Herbert. 1967. *On Responsibility*. New York: Basic Books.

Frankfurt, Harry. 1998. *Necessity, volition and love*. Cambridge, UK: Cambridge University Press.

Fritz, Catherine, Peter Morris and Jennifer Richler. 2012. Effect size estimates: current use, calculations, and interpretation. *Journal of Experimental Psychology: General* 141: 2–18.

Griffin, James. 1986. *Well-being: its meaning, measurement and moral importance*. Oxford, UK: Clarendon.

Kamath, Celia, Kristin Vickers, Angela Ehrlich, *et al.* 2008. Behavioral interventions to prevent childhood obesity: a systematic review and meta-analyses of randomized trials. *Journal of Clinical Endocrinology and Metabolism* 93: 4606–4615.

Kolnai, Aurel. 1995. "Dignity." InRobin Dillon (ed.), *Dignity, character and self-respect*, 53-75. New York, NY: Routledge.

Marmot, Michael. 2003. "Self-esteem and health: autonomy, self-esteem, and health are linked together." *BMJ* 327: 574–575.

Marmot, Michael. 2004. *The status syndrome: how social standing affects our health and longevity*. New York, NY: Henry Holy and Company.

Mokdad, Ali, James Marks, Donna Stroup, *et al.* 2004. "Actual causes of death in the United States, 2000." *JAMA* 291: 1238–1245.

Office of Behavioral and Social Science Research, Mission. 2000. Appendix A in *Translating Behavioral Science into Action: Report of the National Advisory Mental Health Council's Behavioral Science Workgroup*. Bethesda, MD: Department of Health and Human Services, Public Health Service, National Institutes of Health, National Institute of Mental Health.

Omenn, Gilbert, Gary Goodman, Mark Thornquist, *et al.* 1996. Risk factors for lung cancer and for intervention effects in CARET, the Beta-Carotene and Retinol Efficacy Trial. *Journal of the National Cancer Institute* 88: 1550–1559.

Rosen, Michael. 2012. *Dignity: its History and Meaning*. Cambridge, MA: Harvard University Press.

Scheffler, Samuel. 2010. "Valuing." In Samuel Scheffler, *Equality and tradition: questions of value in moral and political theory*, 15-40. Oxford, UK: Oxford University Press.

Searle, John. 2004. *Freedom and Neurobiology: Reflections on Free Will, Language and Political Power*. New York, NY: Columbia University Press. Sen, Amartya. 2009. *The idea of justice*. Cambridge, UK: Belknap Press.

Sen, Amartya. 1992. *Inequality reexamined*. Cambridge, MA: Harvard University Press.

Syme, Len. 1998. "Social and economic disparities in health: thoughts about intervention." *Milbank Quarterly* 76: 493–505.

Taylor, Charles. 1995. "Explanation and practical reason." In: Charles Taylor, *Philosophical arguments*. Cambridge, UK: Harvard University Press.

Waldron, Jeremy. 2009. *Dignity, rank and rights. Tanner lectures on human values*. Berkeley, CA: University of California.

Watson, Gary. 1975. "Free will." *Journal of Philosophy* 72: 205–220.

Wolf, Susan. 1981. "The importance of free will." *Mind* 90: 386–405.

Wolf, Susan. 2015. *The variety of values: essays on morality, meaning and love*. Oxford, UK: Oxford University Press.

15. LOOKING FORWARD

The central thesis of this book is that, to advance research and practice in promoting the health and well-being of individuals and populations, we need to develop and utilize a more comprehensive body of knowledge about human motivation and action. The field needs to take into account an expanded view of the human condition, one that recognizes the role of values in inspiring human agency and the human capacity for ethical deliberation in exercising autonomy. Health promoters need to reject the scientistic assumptions of behaviorism and its disregard for human agency. In light of the shortcomings of a strictly empirical natural science framework, there is an unequivocal need for incorporating a humanistic approach that recognizes the key role of normative values in envisioning a better life that people strive to realize. While keeping the challenges of conducting humanistic research well in mind, it is time for the field to head a new direction.

In a humanistic approach to health promotion, the goal is to increase autonomy, as it is widely recognized in the scholarly literature as the defining characteristic of human wellbeing. The instrumental scientific approach is inherently set up to restrict autonomy as much as possible, even while the question of free will remains unresolved. Health promoters can and should choose which set of assumptions they think most closely matches their experience in working with fellow citizens and community residents. A humanistic approach acknowledges that human beings have the capacity to form conceptions of the good and to imagine, think and reflect critically about their life plans, towards realizing an authentic identity, fulfilling their role in the community, and upholding their responsibility for contributing to the Common Good (Taylor, 1992). Human beings can and will resist being scientifically manipulated to achieve externally-set health objectives, or to being cast in an inferior social status position by systemic structural forces (Nussbaum, 2011). To increase autonomy, we need to strengthen societal institutions to assure that all citizens gain the skills and capabilities that they need to find decent work, support their families, and experience the satisfaction of a life well lived, reforms that are essential to reduce the stress associated with social structural barriers.

The pre-requisite skills and capabilities for exercising autonomy are both characterological and pragmatic. The exercise of autonomy (from the Greek, "self-rule") is positive freedom; it involves practicing and becoming habituated in self-regulation, impulse control, conscientiousness, diligence, and self-determination, and not being carried away by momentary urges against one's better judgment. These character traits are essential for reflective self-awareness and can be instilled with attentive nurturance and strengthened by consistent regular practice in supportive institutional contexts (Heckman, 2006: Heckman, 2013; Jacobs, 2001, Mischel, Ebbesen and Zeiss, 1972; Mischel, Shoda and Rodriguez, 1989; Tangney, Baumeister and Boone, 2004; Kochanska, Murray, Jacques, *et al*, 1996). To develop these capabilities, children from an early age need to be protected from the stress of inadequate housing, insufficient food, ragged clothing and limited educational support to succeed in school (Duncan and LeMenestral, 2019; Shonkoff, *et al*, 2012). They need to be raised in households where parent(s) and guardian(s) have sufficient means not to be overwhelmed by inordinate exhausting stress. In terms of practical skills, all citizens need to gain skills in literacy, numeracy, history, science, and other stores of knowledge, which are essential to participate in the modern market economy.

In a humanistic approach to health promotion, the most significant challenge is to inspire a democratic majority to see the value of creating a society in which everyone can develop their potential skills and capabilities to the fullest extent possible. Are there grounds for thinking that strengthening autonomy will lead people to make better choices not only with respect to various health behaviors, but also attend to realizing a common vision of a good and just society? On the one hand, the challenge of defining a just society epitomizes people's frustrations with the humanities: we do not have a sharply discriminating, operational definition of justice ready at hand and achieving consensus on a definition of justice has thus far proven elusive. On the other hand, I do not see any viable alternative: creating a just society in which all citizens can realize a decent life is a moral and political problem, not a scientific problem to be solved.

Pulling the pieces together

The impetus for the issues raised in this book grew out of work that I was doing as a health promotion practitioner. Early in my career, I was working in adolescent substance abuse prevention and I was struck by how poorly programs fared. Not only did most programs not reduce or prevent drug use, but many actually resulted in increases in drug use after completion (even after adjusting for potential maturation effects). I found this fascinating and decided to pursue my doctoral degree so that I could better understand why they were not working as intended. Doctoral studies enabled me to locate my particular concerns in a broader intellectual landscape, from epidemiology and the social sciences, to epistemology and ethics. My interest in increasing program effectiveness soon opened onto ethical concerns about contributing to the development of powerful programs intended to effectively alter people's behavior. The lodestar guiding my thinking since that time has been the two sides of this same issue: (1) why aren't health promotion programs more effective, and what would it mean if the field developed programs that truly worked as intended, that were just as effective in preventing drug use as physicians are in treating syphilis? And (2) what are other potentially valuable approaches to designing health promotion programs, in terms of both goals and methods; and what approaches would be ethically compatible with an appreciation of the human capacity for moral deliberation and choice?

Over the course of my academic career, I have sought to understand the challenges facing health promotion today and here trace them to two key points. First, the epidemiological transition marks a major break in the etiology of the leading causes of morbidity and mortality. As a convenient marker, I date the watershed tipping point to the US Surgeon General's 1964 Report on *Smoking and Health*. From this time on, the focus of scientific attention shifted to discovering the means to alter behavior as effectively as streptomycin arrests the Mycobacterium tuberculosis (Medical Research Council, 1948). Second, there is general consensus in the philosophical literature that the question of free will remains unresolved. In light of this unknown, I have stressed the absolute *sine-qua-non* of human autonomy, arguing that it is the most distinguishing characteristic of the human condition and that which enables the whole of human morality.

Starting in epidemiology, it is important to appreciate the far-reaching repercussions of the germ theory of disease. It came into prominence at roughly the same time that the major health professional associations (i.e., the AMA and APHA) were being established and recommendations for (re)formulating academic programs in medicine and public health were being enacted to put them on firm scientific foundations. This outlook had such a profound impact that decades were spent searching in vain for the germ that caused heart attacks, to the point that the eventual shift in attention to behavioral risk factors has come to be referred to as the "second revolution" in public health (Neubrauer and Pratt, 1981).

Not only did the focus of attention shift, but also, our understanding of causality needed to be radically transformed. The etiology of infectious diseases is categorically distinct from the etiology of (most) chronic diseases. Where there is a direct one-to-one causal relationship between exposure to the agent and the onset of infectious disease, human behaviors are "merely" risk factors for chronic diseases, neither necessary nor sufficient to determine chronic disease onset. Not only does this shift mean that expectations for reducing chronic disease prevalence need to be tempered significantly–there is not going to be any behavioral equivalent to DPT vaccines–but it also prompts the thought that human behavior may likewise not be absolutely determined but rather made only more or less likely to occur in the face of psychological, social and structural risk factors. Put another way, there appear to be consistently small effect sizes and large degrees of unexplained variance when analyzing the effects of interventions on behavioral outcomes, which led me to turn to the epistemological literature for potential explanations.

One further point from epidemiological studies, there is now convincing evidence of a strong correlation between the social determinants of health (SDOH) and a wide range of health outcomes. Although I have pointed out how the term, "determinant," may overstate the case, the SDOH framework is helpful in conceptualizing what the sociologist Anthony Giddens terms the "agency-structure" problem, which recognizes the capacity of human beings for agency while acknowledging that one's agency is limited by social structural constraints to greater or lesser degrees related to social position.

I delved into the epistemological literature seeking to understand why the social sciences have not demonstrated the same level of success in producing desired outcomes as the natural sciences. In a curious coincidence of timing, while the "culture wars" between positivist and interpretive social scientists were erupting in social science departments across the US and Europe, researchers in the health sciences were producing and disseminating recommendations advocating "evidence-based" medicine and public health. These documents codified a lexical hierarchy of knowledge, where randomized controlled trials were dubbed the "gold standard" of health research and all other research designs flagged as less robust, less trustworthy. With greater numbers of threats to their validity, anything less than a RCT provides less confidence in drawing conclusions and making recommendations based on such study results.

Academic researchers who operate within the positivist/natural science paradigm are well aware of the poor track record of studies designed to modify health behaviors, but they have largely insisted on staying the course. When pressed for an explanation of the low rate of success in producing effective behavioral interventions, health scientists have responded in two main ways: by insisting that the social sciences are at a young immature stage in their development (Glanz, Lewis and Rimer,

1997); and/or that there are a multitude of factors that operate in non-linear, circular feedback loops, which thus requires the application of "complexity science" for analysis (Miles, 2009; Paley and Eva, 2011). In general, there has been little truck with the idea in the public health circles that the fundamental assumptions underlying the natural science paradigm need to be re-examined. Their reluctance to challenge the scientific method or propose a more comprehensive approach to knowledge-generation is particularly evident in applications for financial support from the National Institutes of Health, which places a premium on scientific rigor.

In tracing how we have come to find ourselves in this epistemological predicament, several prominent contemporary scholars, notably, Robert Bellah, Jürgen Habermas and Charles Taylor, hark back to the seminal distinction between *theoria* and *praxis* made by Aristotle. Aristotle recognized that knowledge about events in the natural world (*episteme*) was categorically distinct from knowledge about human affairs (*phronesis*) precisely because the constellation of factors and range of motives bearing on any particular human interaction are unique. In the realm of *praxis*, each individual in a given particular cast of agents brings her own personal history and distinct goals shaped by the specific context where the encounter occurs. As such, according to a long line of epistemological thought, human actions do not conform to the law-like generalizations and predictable outcomes found to govern events in the natural world.

From there, Taylor and Habermas show how Aristotle's original distinction has come down to us today in the difference between instrumental and practical reason. Instrumental reason focuses on identifying the most efficient means to a given end; practical reason focuses on identifying the most worthwhile goals to be achieved and recognizes that ends and means are not independent of one another: the methods chosen to get there inevitably influence the outcome. The great sociologist, Max Weber, was the first to foresee and explain how the growing resort to instrumental reason was one of the most disturbing developments in modern thought. In Weber's analysis, the growing recourse to instrumental reason has trapped humankind in what he termed "the Institutional of modernity." Weber saw this development as the most significant contributor to the rise of modern moral malaise and the perplexing loss of sense of purpose (*anomie*) plaguing modernity. As he put it, we are moving in the direction of knowing more and more about identifying the most efficient means, but less and less about why certain goals or ends are worthwhile, or some more worthwhile than others.

Taylor reveals another important insight to extend our understanding of the ramifications of scientism. He explains how questions of ontology–

what things are in their essence–have been erroneously conflated with questions of epistemology–how things are known. Positivists aver that any assertion that cannot be empirically tested is meaningless metaphysical nonsense. But just because something cannot be empirically detected does not mean that it cannot exist or influence behavior. Dismissing questions about the subjective experience of transcendent values as quaint hangovers from a benighted pre-scientific time in history has had a baleful influence on studies of the human condition.

At the heart of the matter, the philosopher John Searle considers the issue of free will the most important question facing philosophy today. From this perspective, it is one's choice of assumptions that drives debates about (potentially) different forms of knowledge, reasoning and research, whether *theoria/praxis*, instrumental/practical reason, or scientific/hermeneutic research. The unquestioned assumptions and errors in logic reviewed here have had many untoward effects on the behavioral health research enterprise: from questions about the distinction between facts and values, to the possibility of research into non-empirical subjective reality, the (perceived) relative value of qualitative (hermeneutic or interpretive) versus quantitative (positivist) research, and the acceptability of different forms of theory and theorizing; from the warrants for making knowledge claims, to the status of the social sciences, to different conceptions of justice.

Positivists do not know what to make of values. Because they do not have empirical properties that can be operationally defined and measured, empirical scientists have tended to treat them as cultural artefacts, epiphenomena that have evolved slowly over time as human beings sought to work out rules for living together in social groups on a trial-and-error basis, in order to reduce strife and increase bounty. In this framework, values are seen to be contingent and provisional, not part of an objective universe. Since subjective experience cannot be observed empirically, their perception has been dismissed as a product of a fantastical human imagination, like unicorns and Santa Claus, outside the domain of scientific research and impervious to claims about their truth or validity.

Following from this same line of thinking, the value of qualitative research has been systematically discounted, mainly because interpretive claims are necessarily *post-hoc* and so cannot be empirically tested and verified. Researchers operating within the positivist paradigm are charged with responsibility for developing theories that must take the form of statements from which hypotheses can be derived and tested. Under the assumption of determinism, the goal of research is limited to answering questions about the direction and magnitude of cause-and-effect relationships. Theories aimed at elaborating an abstract concept to dispel confusion, offer clarity, reveal new aspects or previously unrecognized dimensions, address (apparent) contradictions, and provide additional reasons for adopting a particular position or pursuing a certain course of action are considered to hold little value, except as a preliminary first step towards developing hypothesis-generating theoretical statements.

In response to these same pressures, although the status of the social sciences is still debated in academic departments, the role and status of health promotion research–as the "social science wing" of public health–has been thoroughly assimilated into the natural science paradigm that informs all research in public health. The mutually reinforcing nature of the assumptions underlying the naturalist paradigm across these many dimensions make challenging any one specific aspect particularly difficult for those who would like to see the field move a new direction. Yet, in the words of C. P. Snow (see Chapter 8), the split between the sciences and the humanities into two antagonistic camps prone to mutual incomprehension and antipathy has been intellectually ruinous (see also, Berlin, 1980).

As proposed here, one reasonable way out of the impasse between empirical scientists and humanistic scholars lies in the concept of emergence. Emergence rejects reductionism and claims that new properties–such as life itself, motility, language and communication and free will–have emerged over time, nascent capacities that could not have been predicted nor explained by testing hypotheses about the outcomes of interactions between compounds in lower (less complex) states. While I am well aware that invoking the concept of emergence will not put questions of free will to rest, it seems to me the most plausible explanation of human beings' capacity for making choices that are not irredeemably pre-determined. Emergence provides intellectually defensible grounds for adopting the alternative assumption, where human beings can and do make choices that are expressions of the agent's will. This position does not deny that there are limits to human freedom–material existence and the social structure constrain and channel human behavior in significant ways–but it goes a long ways towards making sense of the felt experience of truly choosing between different courses of action.

One's position on issues in epistemology influences how one sees and frames issues in ethics. Most immediately, if one accepts the natural science assumption of determinism, then ethical questions are rendered moot: if human beings do not have the capacity for making choices, then human morality is impossible. The consequences of choosing one set of assumptions over another reverberates across several other important ethical concerns facing the field today, from the selection of goals, to research funding priorities, charges of paternalism, the plausibility of different theories of justice, and reinforcement of the perceived priority of the right over the good. Starting with the latter point, although I have not been able to spend as much time on it as the subject deserves, the rise of scientism has played a major role in the perceived priority of the right over the good in modern thought (Rawls, 1988). To oversimplify, this state of affairs has arisen in large part because conceptions of the "good" are inextricably linked to values, which empirical scientists have relegated to the realm of idle speculation. As a result of this and other pressures, moderns tend to uphold the right of people to choose to do whatever they want (except harm others), no matter how much one might think it is not good for the person nor something they should do.

The commitment to an empirical science has pressed the field into adopting goals and objectives that can be readily measured, such that measures of physical fitness have squeezed out consideration of other potential goals, herein subsumed under the rubric of human autonomy and wellbeing. It is practically impossible to measure the exercise of autonomy empirically or the expansion of the sphere of justice in the world. Consequently, the field has adopted problematic markers, such as BMI and blood pressure, to evaluate progress. In counterpoint, I have argued that we would not consider work in health promotion successful if some combination of therapies, technologies and medications produced people with BMIs of 25 but also with the inability to choose for themselves what they would like to eat or whether they might choose to do other things with their time besides getting at least 45 minutes of vigorous aerobic exercise at least three times a week, believing they have more important things to do with their time.

Epistemological assumptions have also had a significant influence on ethical questions involving funding priorities. Because effect sizes in behavioral health research are always smaller, with higher levels of variance, they always look less promising than clinical studies in NIH grant reviews. At an even broader level, due to economic, political and practical constraints, it is rare these days to have large, population-level group randomized trials of health promotion interventions approved, especially when competing against small, well-controlled biomedical treatments. When based strictly on the criterion of which studies are more likely to produce more reliable results that demonstrate a significant effect, clinical RCTs win out in the scoring assessments conducted by grant review panels. But as a result, the effects of policy changes designed to have an impact on population groups are rarely conducted and evidence that might support the value of implementing systemic ecological policy interventions is sorely lacking. (As explained in Chapter Six, I would remind the reader that such policy prescriptions require the support of a democratic majority, in the exercise of community autonomy.)

I have also explained how it is the unwarranted adoption of certain assumptions that has left the field liable to charges of paternalism. Under the assumptions of naturalism, behavior is determined by antecedent causes (like any other empirical event), free will is an illusion, and thus, questions about respecting the principle of autonomy moot. Critics decry the disregard for individual liberties advocated by health promotion professionals intent on reducing the prevalence of obesity and other common behavioral health issues.

As reviewed in Chapter Six, the philosopher Sam Scheffler explains how the commitment to certain unquestioned assumptions has furthermore significantly shaped debates about theories of justice. He points out that a Rawlsian egalitarian conception of justice is grounded in a thorough-going naturalism (where everything that exists is composed of natural properties subject to deterministic cause-and-effect laws), which therefore rejects the possibility of human agency and free will, and consequently, any conception of justice based on merit or desert.

A positive alternative

Choosing to operate on the basis of the alternative assumption that human beings have free will has significant implications for conceptualizing the purpose of research, the position of the social sciences, and the differences between desires and values. It also raises legitimate concerns about grappling with the inherent uncertainty of justifying normative positions, including the priority of autonomy.

Instead of testing hypotheses, in a humanistic approach to research in health promotion, one of the principal aims is to clarify the basic human values at stake in addressing the health concern at hand. I have pointed out that this type of reasoning is not strange or unfamiliar to academic health scientists: it is inherent in writing up protocols for human subjects protections, and in the experience of teaching, where one strives to illuminate a concept through dialogue with students. As it applies to health promotion, the aims of humanistic research are best accomplished by conducting case studies and narrative analyses to understand how human beings find meaning and make sense of their lives. Narratives (re)construct how a person (or community) links their past to the present, and then, past and present to their aims and plans for the future. Like historical research, the investigator seeks to marshal diverse lines of evidence that lend credence to the major thesis/theses while acknowledging and seeking to explain discordant findings that do not fall neatly into place. As noted throughout, one's confidence in the validity of the analysis is not determined by *a priori* p-values but by exercising reasoned judgment about the coherence of the argument, just like researchers do in justifying studies of low-cost lead abatement investigations or setting early stopping rules (see Chapter 8).

In contrast to the wholesale assimilation of social scientific research into the natural sciences model, I have proposed that the social sciences might be more fruitfully seen to be positioned to address the interaction between objective and subjective realities. To appreciate the distinct status of the social sciences, they are more accurately located at the intersection of the natural sciences and the humanities, drawing on and synthesizing both realms of knowledge. Positioning the social sciences here is helpful for thinking carefully about the role of the social determinants of health in health promotion practice and research, especially with regard to the agency-structure relationship. It takes agents to change the social structure: this is a moral and political challenge that will take the will of the democratic majority to make substantive changes (see below for further discussion).

In locating the social sciences with one foot in the natural sciences and one foot in the humanities, research in health promotion will be better positioned to appreciate the significance of autonomy in human affairs and for examining and clarifying different aspects or dimensions of this moral principle. One important area of research here is deepening our understanding of the differences between desires and values, especially in elucidating the concept of autonomy and distinguishing it from raw unbridled freedom.

In an example of humanistic reasoning, I have cited three lines of evidence in support of the priority of autonomy as a higher, more important goal for the field. In his comprehensive review of theories of wellbeing, the philosopher James Griffin indicates that autonomy is best understood to fall under objective accounts of human wellbeing. Likewise, Doyal and Gough (1991) explain that the exercise of autonomy is best understood as an objective human need. Arriving at the same conclusion from another direction, I have pointed out how one of the more well-known definitions of autonomy makes an important distinction between desires and values. In large part, the distinction is critical because many philosophers caution that basing moral choices on personal preferences is an extremely unsatisfying and precarious position, variously referred to as hedonism or subjectivism. They reject the idea that morality is irretrievably tied to cultural relativism, or in the extreme, to sheer individual preferences, because the logic of this line of reasoning inexorably presses toward nihilism: if all choices have equal value, then none is any better than another, and hence, it does not matter which one an individual may choose (O'Sullivan, 2008; Pangle, 1983; Stauth and Turner, 1988).

To press the point, it is important to be clear that I am not advocating that people should be free to do whatever they desire. I am saying that people will experience a higher sense of purpose when they can make choices responsive to higher-order values, values that matter, values that enable human beings to put momentary desires or urges in perspective by providing grounds for reflecting on whether there are other considerations that they should take into account as they work out the kind of person they most long to become. Here, Taylor emphasizes the need for making qualitative distinctions of worth, differences expressed in terms of higher vs. lower, profound vs. superficial, principled vs. debauched. Susan Wolf explains the sense of objectivity involved here: values articulate the grounds for assessing the worth of felt desires from the point of view of someone other than one's own self. That is, to claim that something is valuable is to claim that others have good reason to value it too.

To conclude this book, I would like to draw out the implications of adopting a humanistic approach to health promotion in three areas: the focus of efforts to improve population health; the skills and training needed for a new generation of health promotion professionals; and reflections on the struggle for creating a just society.

Health promotion to change the social structure

The field of public health is keenly focused on the social determinants of health these days. As discussed in Chapter Ten, however, I see little difference between aiming to alter psychological (e.g., perceived susceptibility, self-efficacy, etc.), social (e.g., social support, perceived norms, etc.) or social structural variables (e.g., food insecurity, safe neighborhoods, etc.) in terms of the overall formal structure of thinking about the issues at hand. It is an instrumental line of thinking that aims to identify variables at each respective level of analysis (individual, interpersonal, institutional) typically organized into a schematic Logic Model to guide planning for targeting independent variables to effect the outcomes prescribed in official government documents (such as *Healthy People 2020*). An important corrective is to re-cast the social determinants framework as calling attention to the tensions between agency and structure.

The social structure has both direct and indirect effects on human decision-making. It can restrict the exercise of autonomy by eliminating choices or making them much more difficult for people to attain (especially for those with limited resources), and conversely, by making unhealthy choices cheap and readily accessible. It also generates acute and chronic stressors, directly as a result of unemployment, poverty and racism, which have both physical and mental health effects. Exposure to stress causes a physiological response; the body releases the stress hormone, cortisol (and other physiological markers of allostatic load), which has a number of physical effects, including elevated blood pressure, sleep loss, and weight gain. Difficulty in sleeping, agitation and irritability, in turn, interfere with thoughtful reflective decision-making. Furthermore, experiencing chronic stress distorts one's perceptions of the relative value of satisfying an immediate desire versus foregoing it in order to pursue longer range plans (Graham, 2017). It is more difficult to think carefully about making plans for some distant future when one is facing a slew of urgent demands right now and the future so uncertain. Given these differential social structural pressures, a major challenge for the field is to think about how we collectively can go about reforming our major institutions to distribute the burdens of stress fairly.

To the extent that stress interferes with our ability to exercise autonomous judgment, the most significant step that the field can take to prevent unnecessary suffering and reduce health disparities is to relieve the chronic stresses associated with unemployment, poverty and racism. To do so, we need to bring the will of the majority to bear on reforming current institutional practices. To gain the support of the majority of the population, politically, we must respect the fact that we live in a pluralistic society (Berlin, 1991). The field of public health tends to attract members with a liberal progressive outlook, where justice is generally defined in egalitarian terms. In contrast, one prominent conservative position (arguably now supported by a majority of the American electorate) defines justice in terms of desert or merit (Kekes, 2006; Sandel, 2010). As Anderson has argued (see Chapter One), the essence of reasoned argument is that we persist in trying to persuade our antagonists that there is some crucial element of the matter at hand that their case neglects, while at the same time, we remain open to the prospect that we may *learn* from the exchange and come to see that the case we have been trying to make is flawed, because we will see a more significant, a larger truth in the matter.

Discussions about the nature of the just society will necessitate frank discussions about our mutual rights and responsibilities, towards the goal of assuring that all citizens have the capabilities–the substantive freedom–to pursue their life plans and live lives worth living. Although not without its critics, I think most citizens think about fairness in terms of reciprocity and an implicit social contract (Becker, 1986; Schmidtz, 2006):

I will uphold my end of the bargain if you uphold yours. In this light, we need to ask: What are the responsibilities of community members to those who are disadvantaged, and reciprocally, what are the responsibilities of those who are less well-off to try to reduce dependency on taxpayer support? (Becker, 1986). Both liberals and conservatives need to acknowledge that it is not a simple, either/or dichotomous choice between social structural forces or personal responsibility (Young, 2011). As recommended here, one potentially fruitful way to open a space for dialogue is to think about the issues in probabilistic terms. Just as smoking is neither necessary nor sufficient to cause cancer, so too the social structure does not determine people's behavior, but it does make certain outcomes more or less likely. Conversely, just as people are not free to escape the effects of smoking by choosing to ignore or deny the effects of the many chemical compounds in cigarette smoke on one's lungs, so too they are not free to pursue their life plans when they are denied the necessary capabilities. To strengthen the capacity of all citizen to make autonomous decisions such that they can assume responsibility for them, we must address the corrigible social structural factors that contribute to stress, especially for poor and minority groups.

To protect citizens from excessive stress and nurture the capability for exercising meaningful autonomy, we need to assure that everyone has access to decent affordable housing. Collectively, we need to expand family support and early childhood education programs, so that all children can succeed when they enter school. We need to enable all families to raise their children in safe neighborhoods with access to open green space and other public amenities. We need to hash out a funding formula so that all schools can offer their students a decent education. We need to assure access to healthy foods, which will also require strengthening our public transportation system. To achieve such goals, it will require building consensus, a democratic majority. Health promotion must resist the lure of a scientific, technological fix, the instrumentalist impulse to tame human nature just as we have so successfully gained the power to predict and control events in the natural world. To do so, health promotion needs to embrace a humanistic approach that fosters informed discussion and debate about the kind of society we want to share and live in together.

Preparing a new generation of health promoters

In the US, the structure, organization and curriculum of the first Schools of Public Health were established with the publication of the Rose Report in 1913. Like the 1910 Flexner Report for medicine, the Rose Report sought to put public health on a firm scientific foundation at a time when the germ theory of disease was becoming ascendant. It is time now to reflect upon the changes that have occurred in the field over the last hundred years and the challenges facing the field today.

Concern about the quality of preparation of public health professionals to address modern public health challenges has become a consistent lament in reports on the state of education in the field over the last 30 years, especially with respect to a potential mismatch between skills taught academic programs and the skills needed in professional practice. Published in 1988, the landmark *Future of Public Health* report decried the state of "disarray" of public health in the US, noting that, among other concerns, academic researchers had become "somewhat isolated" from the practice of public health (Institute of Medicine, 1988). During the 1990s, there was major interest and investment in community-based participatory research, which largely grew out of frustration with the slow pace of progress in reducing health disparities (Green, 2003). Over the last 10-15 years, the Council on Education for Public Health (CEPH, the accrediting body for schools and programs of public health in the US) has steadily increased requirements for applied practical field work experience in academic training programs. Green has issued a call for "practice-based science," which he sees as necessary to make the research conducted by academic investigators more relevant to the practice of public health (Green, 2006). The recent "roadmap for translational research" at the NIH stems from this same underlying concern about the distance between the conduct of scientific research and the development of interventions that demonstrably reduce the prevalence of chronic diseases and improve population health (Zerhouni, 2007). I believe the common underlying basis of these concerns stems directly from the failure to appreciate the significance of the epidemiological transition and the distinct ethical concerns raised by the singular quest to identify more effective methods to alter human behaviors.

To address these shortcomings, a humanistic approach to health promotion appreciates that scientific knowledge has limited utility in the sphere of moral and political action (Flyvbjerg, 2001; Sayer, 2011). Public health training programs need to be revised to adapt to the shift in disease etiology. When the occurrence of disease can be wholly explained by processes in the natural world, those diseases are best investigated by the methods of the natural sciences. When the chain of events that leads to health problems is initiated by people adopting unhealthy behaviors, however, the most appropriate methods of investigation and analysis necessarily shift to the social sciences. Where infectious diseases provide relatively well-defined scientific problems to tackle, health problems associated with human behaviors raise complex questions inextricably bound up with moral and political matters. Based on the shift in etiology, the skills and competencies that health promoters need be successful–to operate proficiently while demonstrating respect for the principle of autonomy–are quite different than those needed by medical scientists to cure infectious diseases with antibiotics or manage chronic disease symptoms (e.g., hypertension). Proficiency in deciding the most appropriate course of action is gained by developing sensitivity in perception and maturity in judgment, which grow with experience. As Aristotle (1962) noted long ago, "Nor is intelligence about universals only. It must also come to know particulars, since it is concerned with action and action is about particulars. Hence . . . some people who lack knowledge but have experience are better in action than others who have knowledge."

Experiential Learning

In his seminal *Experience and Education* (1938), Dewey advocated "experiential learning" as an explicit alternative to "traditional" education's reliance on foundations, universal truths and the quest for certainty, arguing instead for the need for active learning that is thoroughly contextualized, action-oriented and attuned to the contingencies of a changing world (Dewey, 1938; Roberts, 2008). In Dewey's view, education has an irreducible ethical dimension linked to citizenship, authenticity and the commitment to discovering and framing common purposes among citizens. For Dewey, it is only when people confront the dilemmas and predicaments raised by the conflicting values, aims and responses of others (a common characteristic of life in a modern pluralistic democracy) that one can dislodge pre-existing, deeply-entrenched subconscious schemata and spark the sense of curiosity that leads to social and moral growth. As Dewey states, "Thinking begins in what may fairly enough be called a forked-road situation . . . Demand for resolution of a perplexity is the guiding factor in the entire process of reflection."

To provide a concrete example, consider the following event, an experience encountered by one of my former students. A local board of health held community hearings about a proposed ban of the sale of all tobacco products in the town (Seelye, 2014). At the meeting, a large majority of the residents spoke out against the regulations. Under these circumstances, what should the health promoter say or do in this situation? The contention of this book is that knowledge of the independent evidence-based variables to be modified to produce the desired result of community resident support for the proposed policy change seems irrelevant and misguided. What the health promoter needs is the astute discerning judgment that comes with greater experience and a broader education that recognizes that human beings are not only affected by material reality but also by their hopes and dreams for a better life, the aspiration to pursue and fulfill their own life plans.

The purpose of revising the current science-based academic training programs is to enable future professionals to engage fellow citizens in collectively figuring out how to make things better, where the operative words here are "things" and "better." Health promotion must focus on engaging fellow citizens in discussions about the value of changing behaviors associated with chronic diseases (as well as many injuries and infectious diseases). The field must also work to build consensus about the most appropriate way to proceed to create a just society, one that does not put certain readily identifiable population groups at higher risk due to social position. In this light, programs need to prepare the workforce to be less naive, less green and to become more sophisticated, more nuanced in their analysis of each particular situation. The capacity for conducting such analyses involves both the sensitizing and sense-making functions of theory (see Chapter Three). Familiarity with the scholarly works reviewed here is essential, at a minimum to assure that future professionals are knowledgeable about the problematic assumptions underlying a strictly scientific curriculum. Not only do future professionals need to get better at noticing a broader range of the often subtle dynamics at work in a given situation (which they may have previously missed or overlooked), but they also need to become more astute at assessing their significance and assigning an appropriate weight to their relative importance, giving lesser weight to some while recognizing the greater significance of others. Programs need to prepare people to become more perceptive and insightful in developing a more comprehensive picture of what is fully going on.

Fieldwork is not merely an opportunity to increase the number of times that nascent professionals can practice a particular technical skill (on the analogy of taking blood pressures, but in health promotion, say, the skill involved defining operational ["SMART"] objectives, etc.). More significantly, it is an essential part of improving one's ability to apply a distinct epistemology, one aimed at becoming more adept at recognizing, distinguishing and characterizing the different values and principles that people bring to bear on a particular situation. With more robust academic training programs, health promoters can then turn their full attention to the issues at the root of health disparities.

Structural injustice as shared responsibility

In a humanistic approach to health promotion, we need to engage community members in advocating for social structural change, not only to reduce stress and make healthier decisions easier for more people, but also for the purpose of engaging people in exercising autonomy. We need to open up spaces in civil society for dialogue among citizens about their respective visions for a good and just society.

Structural injustice is a shared responsibility. Our lives are characterized by mutual interdependencies and mutual responsibilities. We are deeply interdependent as our lives unfold in and through institutional relations. We owe each other care due to these interdependencies; we have positive responsibilities towards one another. Because we are all involved in social practices that produce and reproduce the causes of health and social inequities, citizens collectively have a responsibility for changing the social conditions that have led the most vulnerable to suffer significant health disparities.

In her *Responsibility for Justice* (2011), Iris Marion Young makes the provocative case that attributing social ills to an impersonal structural system may have the paradoxical effect of individuals absolving themselves of their responsibility for righting these wrongs. Because it is difficult to identify a particular person who has committed the wrong and should be held morally accountable, it is not clear who should be blamed or who should mete out justice. There is no particular agent who committed a specific wrong, yet people still suffer injustice. Adopting the social structural view tends to reinforce the view that the workings of society have evolved like developments in the natural world, such that levels of unemployment, for example, are widely viewed as an inevitable and inescapable byproduct of modern market economies. But to paraphrase Young (2011), to call a situation unjust implies that we recognize that it is at least in part caused by human beings. Because human beings created it, it is a corrigible state of affairs. As such, we must carefully scrutinize and acknowledge the extent to which each of us individually and as members of society collectively are causally embedded in social practices that produce and reproduce unjust vulnerabilities. (See also Chapter Ten for a similar analysis of public health's embrace of the social determinants framework.) As Young concludes, each of us individually must assume personal responsibility for redressing the social conditions that exacerbate vulnerabilities and elevate risk for suffering diminished quality of life, impairments, premature disability, disease and death and so deny people the opportunity to achieve their full potential (Daniels, 2001).

Conclusion

Public health has always spanned the scientific and political worlds, from John Snow marching down to remove the pump handle, to Mayor Bloomberg's call for banning large sugary drinks. But controlling the spread of cholera raises categorically distinct challenges from trying to change human behaviors. Nowadays public health professionals need to acknowledge the conflicting values embraced by modern pluralist societies and associated claims about the appropriate role of the state in promoting and brokering different visions of justice. Health promoters need to become familiar with the legitimate counter-arguments levelled by both sides and muster their best case for persuading others to adopt the values that characterize one's vision of the good society (see, for example, Bellah, *et al*, 1991). There is no simple scientific formula for producing the political ends that public health professionals hold dear. Health promoters need to listen to opposing points of view, sort out where they stand on such issues, and learn how they can most effectively engage with others in identifying means and ends acceptable to all parties with a stake in the decision. Ensuring that professionals become more adept in grappling with the complex moral and political dynamics involved in working with different stakeholders with different agendas and often conflicting values as one attempts to build public support for different public health policies and programs is the most important task facing health promotion today.

** - There is a school of thought called "compatibilism," which posits that free will and determinism are mutually compatible and that it is possible to believe in both without being logically inconsistent; alas, space constraints preclude an adequate discussion; see Dennett, 2003.

References

Aristotle. 1962. *Nichomachean Ethics*. Translated by Martin Ostwald. Indianapolis, IN: Bobbs-Merrill.

Becker, Lawrence C. 1986. *Reciprocity.* New York: Routledge and Kegan Paul.

Bellah, Robert, Richard Madsen, William Sullivan, Ann Swidler and Steven Tipton. 1991. *The Good Society*. New York: Alfred Knopf.

Berlin, Isaiah. 1980. "The divorce between the science and the humanities." In Isaiah Berlin, *Against the Current*, 101-139. New York: Viking Press.

Berlin, Isaiah. 1991. *The Crooked Timber of Humanity.* New York: Alfred Knopf.

Daniels, Norman. 2001. "Justice, Health and Healthcare." *American Journal of Bioethics* 1(2): 1-6.

Dennett, Daniel. 2003. *Freedom Evolves*. New York: Penguin Books.

Dewey, John. 1938. *Experience and Education*. New York: Collier Books.

Doyal, Len and Ian Gough. 1991. *A Theory of Human Need.* London, UK: MacMillan Press.

Duncan, Greg and Suzanna LeMenestral (Eds.). 2019. *A Roadmap to Reducing Child Poverty.* A Report of the National Academies of Science, Engineering and Medicine, Washington DC: National Academies Press.

Flyvbjerg, Bent. 2001. *Making Social Science Matter: Why Social Inquiry Fails and How it Can Succeed Again.* Cambridge: Cambridge University Press.

Glanz, Karen, Frances Lewis and Barbara Rimer (Eds.). 1997. *Health Behavior and Health Education: Theory, Research and Practice.* Second Edition. San Francisco, CA: Jossey-Bass Publishers.

Graham, Carol. 2017. *Happiness for all? unequal hopes and lives in pursuit of the American dream*. Princeton NJ: Princeton University Press.

Green, Lawrence. 2006. "Public Health Asks of Systems Science: To Advance Our Evidence-Based Practice, Can You Help Us Get More Practice-Based Evidence?" *American Journal of Public Health* 96(3):406-9.

Heckman, James. 2006. "Skill Formation and the Economics of Investing in Disadvantaged Children." *Science* 312 (5782): 1900–02.

Heckman, James. 2013. *Giving Kids a Fair Chance*. Boston: The MIT Press.

Institute of Medicine. 1988. *The Future of Public Health.* Washington, DC: National Academy of Sciences Press.

Jacobs, Jonathon. 2001. *Choosing Character: Responsibility for Virtue and Vice*. Ithaca, NY: Cornell University Press.

Kekes, John. 2006. "Justice: A Conservative View." *Social Philosophy and Policy*, 23: 88-108.

Kochanska, Grazyna, Kathleen Murray, Tanya Y. Jacques, Amy L. Koenig, and Kimberly Vandegeest. 1996. "Inhibitory Control in Young Children and Its Role in Emerging Internalization." *Child Development* 67: 490-507.

Medical Research Council. 1948. "Streptomycin treatment of tuberculous meningitis." *Lancet* 1: 582-96.

Miles, Andrew. 2009. "Complexity in medicine and healthcare: People and systems, theory and practice." *Journal of Evaluation in Clinical Practice* 15(3): 409-410.

Mischel, Walter, Ebbe B. Ebbesen, and Antonette Raskoff Zeiss. 1972. "Cognitive and Attentional Mechanisms in Delay of Gratification." *Journal of Personality and Social Psychology* 21(2): 204–18.

Mischel, Walter, Yuichi Shoda, and Monica L. Rodriguez. 1989. "Delay of Gratification in Children." *Science* 244: 933–38.

Neubauer, Deane, and Richard Pratt, R. 1981. "The Second Public Health Revolution: A critical appraisal." *Journal of Health Politics, Policy and Law* 6(2): 205–228.

Nussbaum, Martha. 2011. *Creating Capabilities: The Human Development Approach*. Cambridge: Belknap Press.

O'Sullivan, Noel. 2008. "Liberalism, Nihilism and Modernity in the Political Thought of John Gray." In *The Political Thought of John Gray*, edited by John Horton and Glen Newey, 173-192. New York: Routledge.

Paley, John and Gail Eva. 2011. "Complexity theory as an approach to explanation in healthcare: A critical discussion." *International Journal of Nursing Studies* 48(2): 269–279.

Pangle, Thomas. 1983. "The Roots of Contemporary Nihilism and its Political Consequences according to Nietzsche." *Review of Politics* 45(1): 45-70.

Rawls, John. 1988. "The Priority of Right and Ideas of the Good." *Philosophy and Public Affairs*, 17(4): 251-276,

Roberts, Jay. 2008. "From Experience to Neo-Experiential Education: Variations on a theme." *Journal of Experiential Education* 31(1):19-35.

Sandel, Michael. 2010. "Aristotle: Who Deserves What?" In Michael Sandel, *Justice: What's the Right Thing to Do,*184-207. New York: Farrar, Straus and Giroux.

Sayer, Andrew. 2011. *Why Things Matter to People: Social Science, Values and the Ethical Life*. Cambridge: Cambridge University Press.

Schmidtz, David. 2006. "Reciprocity." In David Schmidtz, *The Elements of Justice,* 73-74. New York: Cambridge University Press.

Seelye, Katharine. 2014. "Firestorm erupts in anti-smoking Massachusetts town." *New York Times*, November 14, 2014. Available at: http://www.nytimes.com/2014/11/18/us/disgusted-by-smoking-outraged-by-a-plan-to-ban-tobacco.html?_r=0.

Shonkoff, Jack, Andrew S. Garner, and The Committee on Psychosocial Aspects of Child and Family Health. 2012. "The Lifelong Effects of Early Childhood Adversity and Toxic Stress." *Pediatrics*, 129(1): e232–e246, 2012.

Stauth, Georg and Bryan Turner. 1988. *Nietzsche's Dance*. Oxford: Basil Blackwell.

Tangney, June, Roy Baumeister, and Angie Boone. 2004. "High Self-Control Predicts Good Adjustment, Less Pathology, Better Grades, and Interpersonal Success." *Journal of Personality* 72 (2): 271–324.

Taylor, Charles. 1992. *The Ethics of Authenticity.* Cambridge: Harvard University Press.

Young, Iris Marion. 2011. *Responsibility for Justice*. New York: Oxford University Press.

Zerhouni, Elias A. 2007. "Translational Research: Moving Discovery to Practice." *Clinical Pharmacology and Therapeutics*, 81(1): 126-8.

INDEX